CONGENITAL MENTAL RETARDATION

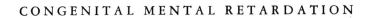

ADVANCES IN MENTAL SCIENCE I

# Congenital Mental Retardation

A SYMPOSIUM ARRANGED BY

*William M. McIsaac, M.D., Ph.D.*

*James Claghorn, M.D.*

*Gordon Farrell, M.D.*

PROCEEDINGS EDITED BY GORDON FARRELL, M.D.

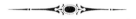

PUBLISHED FOR THE FACULTY FOR ADVANCED STUDIES OF

THE TEXAS RESEARCH INSTITUTE OF MENTAL SCIENCES

BY THE UNIVERSITY OF TEXAS PRESS, AUSTIN & LONDON

Standard Book Number 292-70008-3
Library of Congress Catalog Card Number 79–94051
Copyright © 1969 by the University of Texas Press
All Rights Reserved

Type set by G&S Typesetters, Austin
Printed by The Steck-Warlick Company, Austin
Bound by Universal Bookbindery, Inc., San Antonio

# PREFACE

THIS VOLUME is the first in a continuing series that will contain the proceedings of annual international symposia sponsored by the Texas Research Institute of Mental Sciences in Houston. This series will provide a forum for the presentation and discussion of the most recent discoveries, concepts, and theoretical considerations in the study of diseases of the mind.

The Texas Research Institute of Mental Sciences (TRI) is the principal facility for training and research of the Texas Department of Mental Health and Mental Retardation. This commission carries deep responsibilities; in the state are some 30,000 institutionalized patients with mental disease or mental retardation; thousands more need care but are not hospitalized.

TRI takes as its objective the upgrading of mental health care through research and training. The institute has ongoing service activities for psychoses, neuroses, alcoholism, drug abuse, gerontology, and mental retardation. Linked with these services are rapidly developing, potentially powerful research laboratories in neurochemistry, medicinal chemistry, behavioral pharmacology, biochemistry, neuroendocrinology, metabolism, and psychophysiology. Under the direction of its Faculty for Advanced Studies, TRI has a graduate and postgraduate training program that is designed to produce Mental Science Research Specialists. The emphasis transcends conventional educational methods to explore innovative approaches to research and treatment.

TRI organized the first International Symposium in Mental Science in November 1967 as part of its graduate training program. The subject was mental retardation with emphasis on the new discoveries about congenital diseases that damage the central nervous system. Important research in this area is going on in many parts of the world; it is critical to stay in the mainstream of this research at the very time it is being done, and to know about new developments in the leading research centers. This need was one of the most important reasons for holding the international symposium.

There were other reasons, too. Nothing is more inspiring to the students, the young people in science, than meeting the giants in the field. It motivates and stimulates them and sets the mood for their work. I well recall the delight I had in meeting and visiting Nobel Laureate Bernardo Houssay; an autographed picture hangs in my office and is still a source of pride. Men like Mason, Tait, Evans, Hench, St.-Gyorgy, immediately recognized by people in endocrinology, were only names in journals until I met them as a young postdoctoral fellow, when they became my heroes. We wanted our young students to have this experience.

Also important is the sense of a professional community engendered by an international symposium. Old friendships are renewed, new friendships made, scientific discussion is enkindled, and competitive research becomes more competitive—but in a spirit of fellowship.

One of the brightest chapters of medicine is unfolding: the age-old tragedies accompanying mental retardation are gradually yielding to the penetration of medical investigation. Many forms of mental retardation hitherto unexplained or improperly explained are now known to be the result of abnormalities transmitted from parent to offspring; sometimes the abnormality involves the mutation of a single biochemical reaction, often hidden for generations because of genetic characteristics; sometimes it is amenable to treatment.

The symposium in 1967 attempted to assemble a number of active workers in the field for discussion of these newer developments. From Ireland we brought Nina Carson, the discoverer of homocystinuria and the international authority. We found her to be a delightful young person. For phenylketonuria we invited the "doctor of phenylketonuria" herself, Helen Berry from Cincinnati. George Donnell, the top man in the country for galactosemia came from Los Angeles; for hyperhistidinemia, the discoverer of the syndrome, H. Ghadimi, came from New York. For Nyhan's disease we brought William Nyhan. In methodology we brought a rising young neurologist-pediatrician, Harvey Levy from Massachusetts. From Mexico came Dario Urdapelleta Bueno, leader in pediatric mental hygiene; from Guatemala, Roberto Rendón, international authority on malnutrition in mental retardation. From Ann Arbor came John Opitz, controversial, brilliant, witty. Patrick J. Doyle flew in from Washington to represent the President's Committee on Mental Retardation. The Texas Department of Health sent Ernest Cunningham to chair a meeting. Texas State Representatives Bill Archer and Glenn Vickery were here; Texas House Speaker Gus Mutscher took part, and lovely Ann Hughes graced a panel. We invited all the medical directors from the state institutions and members of their staffs. We blended people of influence, knowledge, and insight from our community and created a meeting that has been acknowledged as outstanding. The people who came to Houston for the symposium left with an impression of the city's cordial Southern hospitality and its unquestionably high level of medical competence.

What of the retarded subjects in the institutions whom the show was all about? The meeting helped to launch in Texas a statewide detection program for the newly discovered diseases which is backed up by sophisticated diagnostic facilities at TRI. This program is now in operation and is gaining momentum. Even more exciting, our own team, youthful as it is, is now making significant discoveries in mental retardation and epilepsy on its own.

We will have a symposium every year. The subjects will vary so that in time each of the major problem areas in mental health will be covered; then the sequence will repeat. Future symposia will be held on the topics of drug abuse, the major psychoses, alcoholism, and gerontology. The proceedings will be published and over the years a series of volumes will accumulate, reflecting the growth and advancement in our chosen field of endeavor.

So many of our staff and friends helped that to mention them all would make a list almost as long as the employee roster of the institute. A few contributed so much that justice demands their citation. My dear wife, Elizabeth Rauschkolb, M.D., put aside leisure and many of her professional pursuits to help with the arrangements. Gladys Smith transcribed miles of tape and unscrambled numerous manuscripts. Gail Cox has been of inestimable help in the final stages of this symposium and in the organization of the next. Our thanks go to the Pauline Sterne Wolff Memorial Home Foundation, The Lilly Research Laboratories, Wyeth Laboratories, Merck, Sharp & Dohme, Roche Laboratories, Sandoz Pharmaceuticals, and Schering Laboratories for financial help. We pay tribute to those powerful and good friends in education and in the community who lent their support to the cause; prominent among these are Frank C. Erwin, Jr., Charles A. LeMaistre, R. Lee Clark, Sumter S. Arnim, John L. Hill, David Peden, Leon Jaworski, John H. Freeman, John T. Jones, J. H. Creekmore, Henry J. N. Taub, and Miss Mildred Thornton. Finally if one dedicated a proceedings volume, this volume would be dedicated to V. John Kinross-Wright, a man of gentle ways but steadfast purpose, whose idea all of this was in the first place.

GORDON FARRELL, M.D.

# CONTENTS

xi

CONGENITAL MENTAL RETARDATION

# Phenylketonuria: Diagnosis, Treatment, and Long-Term Management

HELEN K. BERRY, M.A.

*Children's Hospital Research Foundation and the Department of Pediatrics, University of Cincinnati College of Medicine, Cincinnati, Ohio*

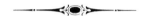

## Differential Diagnosis of Phenylketonuria

Screening tests among newborn infants for blood phenylalanine concentration are now common practice. Several procedures for screening specimens for the presence of increased amounts of phenylalanine are in common use. These procedures include the inhibition assay, fluorometry, and paper chromatography (Guthrie and Susi 1963; McCaman and Robins 1962; Berry *et al.* 1965). The level above which phenylalanine concentration is considered abnormal is 4 to 5 mg. per cent. At the time of discharge from the newborn nursery approximately one baby in five hundred has phenylalanine concentration of this magnitude. Since the incidence of phenylketonuria is probably not greater than one in ten thousand, the majority of babies with initially positive screening tests do not have phenylketonuria.

The procedure followed in our laboratory for examination of an infant with positive results in an initial blood screening test is as follows:

1. Request that the infant be given 100 mg. of ascorbic acid at least twenty-four hours prior to collection of a second blood specimen.

2. Obtain a blood specimen for quantitative measurement of phenylalanine and tyrosine concentration.

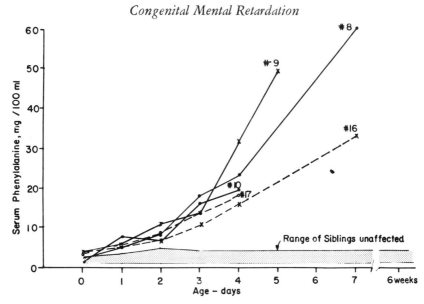

FIGURE 1. Serial serum phenylalanine levels of infants born into families with histories of phenylketonuria.

3. Obtain a urine specimen; test for increased amounts of phenylalanine and orthohydroxyphenylacetic acid; test for presence of tyrosine and tyrosine derivatives.

The biochemical characteristics of phenylketonuric infants include the following:

1. Serum phenylalanine over 15 mg. per cent—sometimes as high as 60 to 80 mg. per cent.

2. Urine phenylalanine over 100 $\mu$g. per ml.

3. Urine orthohydroxyphenylacetic acid over 10 $\mu$g. per ml.

4. Serum tyrosine below 5 mg. per cent.

Present evidence indicates that children with high serum phenylalanine concentrations accompanied by high excretion of phenylalanine and orthohydroxyphenylacetic acid have phenylketonuria. Phenylpyruvic acid may or may not be excreted, depending on the age of the child. While there is no direct evidence that high phenylalanine concentration in the blood leads to mental retardation, most children with high concentrations are mentally retarded if the disease progresses unrecognized to as late an age as one year. The chances that a child with phenylketonuria may have

4

normal development are greater if treatment with a low phenylalanine diet is used than if no treatment is given.

Infants born into families in which an older child is known to have phenylketonuria have a 25 per cent chance of also having the disease and constitute a high-risk group available for study. Arrangements were made to test newborn siblings of retarded phenylketonuric patients at birth and at one, two, three, and four days of age, and again at one, two, three, and six weeks of age, so long as the blood phenylalanine levels were normal (Berry, Umbarger, and Sutherland 1964). Results of testing fifteen newborn siblings in high-risk families are shown in Figure 1. Phenylalanine levels of cord blood were normal. By twenty-four hours of age phenylalanine levels between 6 and 8 mg. per cent were noted in infants 8, 9, and 10. The rising trend continued in specimens obtained at forty-eight hours of age. By three days serum phenylalanine levels were over 15 mg. per cent in infants 8 and 10; serum phenylalanine was over 15 mg. per cent on the fourth day in infant 9. Infants 16 and 17, tested by Dr. Richard Koch in Los Angeles Children's Hospital, showed similar increases in serum phenylalanine. This rapid rise in the phenylalanine content of the blood is characteristic of the phenylketonuric infant, up to 50 and 61 mg. per cent at ages five and seven days, the time treatment was begun. None of the other infants tested in these families have shown elevations of blood phenylalanine levels, although half of them may be assumed to be heterozygotes.

The most common factor contributing to increased frequency of elevated blood phenylalanine levels is prematurity or immaturity of the tyrosine oxidizing system. This immaturity accounts for approximately 90 per cent of positive initial screening tests. The reaction by which tyrosine is oxidized to dihydroxyphenylalanine (DOPA) and subsequent metabolites is inhibited by excess substrate (La Du and Zannoni 1955). Tyrosine accumulates to ten to twenty times the normal concentration. The inhibition of the enzyme, parahydroxyphenylpyruvic acid oxidase, is readily reversed by ascorbic acid. In a study of premature infants born at the Cincinnati General Hospital, 25 per cent of premature infants who were given ascorbic acid supplements of 25 mg. per day or less developed elevation of tyrosine and phenylalanine in the blood and excreted large amounts of tyrosine and tyrosine derivatives (Light, Berry, and Sutherland 1966). Figure 2 shows an example of an infant with tyrosine concentration elevated at one week. By the third week serum phenylalanine concentration was over 8 mg. per cent and tyrosine was 33 mg. per cent.

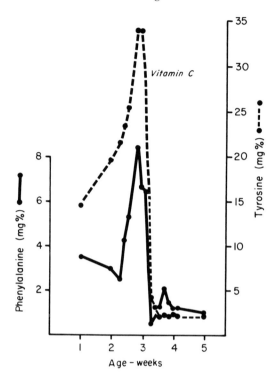

FIGURE 2. Phenylalanine and tyrosine concentrations in serum from a premature infant before and after administration of 100 mg. of ascorbic acid.

Both amino acids decreased to normal range within twenty-four hours after administration of 100 mg. of ascorbic acid and remained normal thereafter.

Phenylketonuria and conditions associated with abnormal tyrosine metabolism can also be distinguished on the basis of characteristic urinary metabolites. Figure 3 shows chromatograms of urine specimens from two children with phenylketonuria (demonstrating orthohydroxyphenylacetic acid, the most characteristic metabolite in phenylketonuria) and from one child with tyrosinemia (demonstrating tyrosine derivatives characteristic of abnormal tyrosine metabolism).

Phenylalanine-restricted diet for treatment of infants with phenylalanine elevation secondary to abnormal tyrosine metabolism is not recommended. The condition is best corrected by prompt administration of ascorbic acid.

Another group of infants, about 5 per cent of those with positive pre-

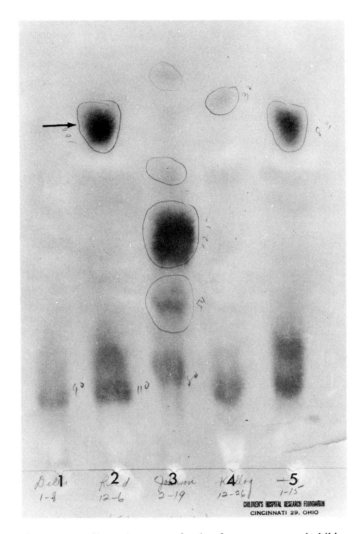

FIGURE 3. Chromatograms of urine from 1. a normal child, 2. an untreated phenylketonuric child, 3. a child with tyrosinemia, 4. a treated phenylketonuric child, 5. an untreated phenylketonuric child. The arrow points to orthohydroxyphenylacetic acid. (Solvent: butanol-ethanol-concentrated ammonium hydroxide [80–20–20]; Reagent: diazotized sulfanilic acid-sodium carbonate.)

liminary screening tests, show a slow rise of serum phenylalanine to 15 to 20 mg. per cent by three to six weeks of age. Tyrosine concentration is normal and the infants may have increased urinary excretion of phenylalanine. This group, commonly designated "hyperphenylalaninemic," presents the greatest problem both in terms of diagnosis and follow-up. Mild elevations of serum phenylalanine occur occasionally in an atypical heterozygote for phenylketonuria. In other instances, the syndrome may result from a partial deficiency of phenylalanine hydroxylase, or, as Woolf, Cranston, and Goodwin (1967) have suggested, it may be due to the presence of a different allele or an isozyme for phenylalanine hydroxylase, similar to the different alleles that produce the various types of hemoglobin abnormalities. Other possibilities are a deficiency of the cofactor pteridine or its reductase, or a deficiency of a related enzyme such as phenylalanine transaminase. The practical question arises as to whether or not phenylalanine-restricted diet should be used in such cases.

Because it is still not clear whether, or at what level, high blood phenylalanine concentrations are associated with defective mental development, treatment should be undertaken if phenylalanine levels are persistently elevated over 15 mg. per cent. Treatment can be given in such a way that infants are protected from further marked increases in serum phenylalanine if they have phenylketonuria, or from phenylalanine deficiency if they do not have phenylketonuria. Regular formula should be replaced by formula of low-phenylalanine content. Milk should be added to the formula in increments of 2 oz. per day for a week, increasing the amount of phenylalanine received daily from 100 mg. on the first day to 700 mg. on the last. Serum phenylalanine levels should be measured daily. In our experience, when a low-phenylalanine formula replaces the normal protein intake for the phenylketonuric infant, the serum phenylalanine level falls slowly over a period of two to five days; then as the phenylalanine intake is increased, the level rises again. If serum phenylalanine levels drop to 2 mg. per cent or less within twenty-four hours, a diagnosis of phenylketonuria is unlikely. Phenylalanine intake can be adjusted to maintain blood levels above 3 mg. per cent. This procedure represents a modified form of the phenylalanine tolerance test in which phenylalanine is given in the form of whole protein so that no unusual stress is imposed on a possibly deficient enzyme system. The results of loading young infants with phenylalanine alone have been misleading (Allen *et al.* 1964). At present the data on factors that affect phenylalanine hydroxylase activities in infants are so limited that it is not known if a routine liver biopsy

8

would offer a more clear-cut basis on which to make a decision for or against treatment.

## Treatment

The immediate objective of treatment for phenylketonuria is the reduction of the concentration of phenylalanine in an infant's blood by reducing the phenylalanine in his diet. Thereafter, the objective is to adjust phenylalanine intake to maintain blood phenylalanine levels in a range that assures sufficient phenylalanine for growth without permitting accumulation of excess phenylalanine and its by-products. The long-range purpose of treatment of a child with phenylketonuria is to allow him to grow and develop normally in spite of his metabolic defect.

The treatment diet is composed of a protein substitute, Lofenalac, which is combined with small measured amounts of natural foods to furnish the additional amounts of phenylalanine required for growth. Individual children vary in the amount of phenylalanine required for protein synthesis and growth and in the amount of phenylalanine that can be metabolized or excreted without danger of increasing serum phenylalanine levels beyond a safe range.

Once the decision has been reached to treat the child, the infant is taken off his regular formula and the low-phenylalanine formula is begun. Dietary prescriptions for the individual infant are calculated on the basis of his protein, caloric, and fluid requirements. An intake of approximately 3 gm. of protein per kg. per day, including approximately 5–6 gm. of protein from natural foods has permitted growth among children in the 25–90 percentiles while maintaining serum phenylalanine levels generally between 3 and 7 mg. per 100 ml. The phenylalanine content of the diet is adjusted according to individual needs as determined by the results of blood and urine testing.

Our treatment program is characterized by:

1. Frequent monitoring using microtechniques for serum phenylalanine and for urinary phenylalanine and its metabolic by-products.

2. Dietary alteration based on monitoring results and dietary information supplied routinely by the parents.

3. Establishment of individual dietary requirements based on monitoring results.

4. Creation of the most normal eating atmosphere possible under an unusually restrictive regimen.

Early in the treatment program parents are taught to collect blood from a finger or heel puncture. They are provided with microhematocrit tubes, sealing material, and a protective package in which to mail blood specimens to the laboratory. Blood is collected daily during the first week of treatment, weekly until the end of the second month, and, thereafter, at intervals of two weeks until one year of age. Specimens are obtained at monthly intervals after one year except during illness when they may be requested more frequently. Blood specimens are usually collected about two hours after a meal. Filter paper urine specimens are collected daily during the first month of treatment, twice weekly to the end of the first six months, and weekly or every two weeks afterward. Parents are supplied with a list giving a wide variety of foods for which the phenylalanine content is indicated for one tablespoon of each food, permitting ready substitution. The mother records daily intake: the amount of Lofenalac and the type and amount of other foods and liquids that are actually consumed. The records are mailed with the daily urine samples.

Administration of the diet requires continuous biochemical monitoring. Serum phenylalanine determinations are performed using the fluorometric procedure. Urinary phenylalanine and orthohydroxyphenylacetic acid determinations on the filter paper specimens are carried out using paper chromatography.

The following examples illustrate the relations between dietary phenylalanine intake, serum phenylalanine concentration, and urinary excretion of phenylalanine and orthohydroxyphenylacetic acid. We selected 3 mg. per cent as the minimum safe level for serum phenylalanine concentration in treated phenylketonuric infants because early in our experience attempts to maintain phenylalanine levels in the normal range of less than 2 mg. per cent resulted in growth failure. The upper limit of 7 mg. per cent was selected arbitrarily and further studies may show that higher blood phenylalanine levels up to 10 or 12 mg. per cent may be permitted without adversely affecting the outcome of the treatment. The periods are arbitrarily chosen to facilitate interpretation of the graph. Figure 4 represents an infant who had a positive blood screening test at three days of age. Repeat serum phenylalanine determination at eleven days showed a level of 25 mg. per cent. The baby was first seen in our clinic when three weeks old. The diagnosis of phenylketonuria was confirmed as shown in period 1: serum phenylalanine of 33 mg. per cent, urine phenylalanine of over 100 μg. per ml., orthohydroxyphenylacetic acid of 60 μg. per ml. The urine was also positive for phenylpyruvic acid. On the basis of the confirming tests a decision was made to treat the infant.

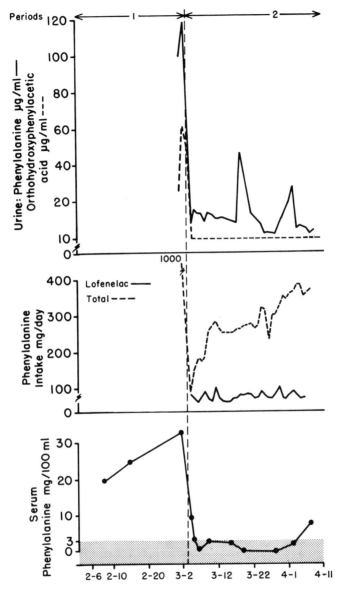

FIGURE 4. Monitoring of the initial stages of treatment of an infant with phenylketonuria. Note the decrease in serum phenylalanine and in urinary metabolites when phenylalanine intake was reduced and the increase in phenylalanine intake required to raise serum phenylalanine levels above 3 mg. per cent.

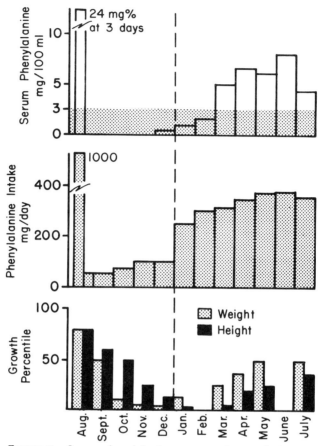

FIGURE 5. Serum phenylalanine concentrations and phenylalanine intake compared to growth percentiles for a child with phenylalanine deficiency.

Period 2 shows the first step in treatment. Lofenalac formula was substituted for the regular evaporated milk formula. By the second day serum phenylalanine had decreased to 3 mg. per cent. Urine phenylalanine decreased and orthohydroxyphenylacetic acid was no longer detected. Phenylalanine was added to the diet in the form of milk, 50 mg. of phenylalanine per ounce. Serum phenylalanine continued to drop and milk was added to raise the intake to nearly 400 mg. per day until the serum phenylalanine levels rose above 3 mg. per cent. Additional phenylalanine was added more cautiously until phenylalanine concentration in serum approached 7 mg. per cent. During the first few weeks of life phenylalanine intake is adjusted with milk. The milk additions are evenly distributed throughout the day and are given with the Lofenalac formula so the child does not receive an amino acid mixture severely deficient in phenylalanine at any time. The phenylketonuric baby is introduced to strained infant foods at the usual time. At six weeks he is offered Lofenalac as a semi-solid food, somewhat like a baby cereal.

If the phenylalanine intake is not increased to meet the needs of the rapidly growing infant during the first months of life the resulting deficiency causes growth failure; anemia, bone changes, and death may occur. Figure 5 shows data from a child with some of these symptoms. Treatment was begun at age two weeks. The diet consisted of Lofenalac alone for about three months. Lofenalac was designed to be deficient in phenylalanine, an amino acid essential for human growth. The essential amino acids in Lofenalac cannot be utilized for protein synthesis without additional phenylalanine derived from natural foods. When three months old the infant was severely anemic with hemoglobin of 8 gm. per cent. She was transfused and one ounce of milk was added to the daily diet. Weight dropped from the seventy-fifth percentile at the time treatment was started to the third percentile at four months. Height decreased more slowly. The patient was referred to our clinic at five months after spending the prior two months in the hospital. Hemoglobin was 9 gm. per cent; height and weight were below 10 per cent of normal. There were minimal bone changes suggestive of rickets. Hair was sparse; serum phenylalanine was below 0.5 mg. per cent. These are characteristic symptoms of phenylalanine deficiency. Phenylalanine intake was raised immediately to 250 mg. per day. Attempts to raise it still higher were not successful because the child had never had solid food. Three months were required to correct the phenylalanine deficiency and raise serum phenylalanine levels above 3 mg. per cent. The growth rate increased, with weight improving more rapidly than height.

Phenylalanine deficiency is one of the most common pitfalls in the treatment of phenylketonuria. There is no reason to believe that the phenylalanine requirements of phenylketonuric patients are different from those of normal infants who are given adequate amounts of tyrosine. Phenylalanine is required equally by both as an essential component of body protein. The range for phenylalanine requirements of normal infants

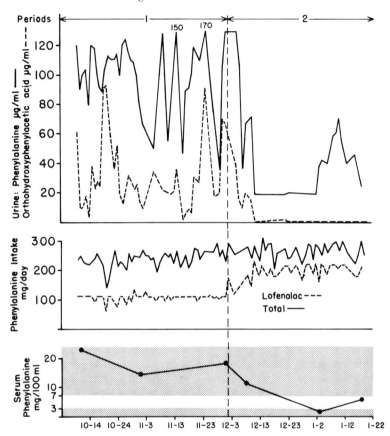

FIGURE 6.  Monitoring of a child with suboptimal protein intake, showing increased serum phenylalanine concentration and marked excretion
of urinary metabolites during a period when intake of Lofenalac was
low. Serum phenylalanine decreased to control range when additional
protein in the form of Lofenalac was added to the diet without a decrease in the total phenylalanine intake.

in the presence of tyrosine (determined by Snyderman, Pratt, *et al.* 1955)
was 47 to 94 mg. per kg. per day. Kennedy and others (1967) found
phenylalanine requirements for phenylketonuric infants in the same age
group to range from 38 to 110 mg. per kg. per day—requirements similar to those for normal infants. They noted that the traditional basis of
expressing requirements by weight needed modification. Increasing body

weight combined with a decreasing per kilogram need for phenylalanine produced an absolute requirement for all ages ranging from 200 to 400 mg. per day. Woolf (1962), in reviewing the phenylalanine requirement in phenylketonuria, noted a considerable variation in the amount of phenylalanine required by phenylketonuric infants during the first year of life, both from infant to infant and at different times in the same infant.

Contrary to generally held opinions, we find the first year of life the most difficult, and perhaps the most critical, period in treatment of phenyl-ketonuria. During this time phenylalanine requirements are changing most rapidly. This early period is critical to the establishment of feeding patterns. Careful attention must be paid to stages of eating development to ensure that the child acquires eating practices and habits that make management of the severely restrictive diet possible over a long period. The introduction of Lofenalac in a concentrated form is of great im-portance. This protein substitute must constitute the major portion of the child's diet and must be fed in sufficient amounts to provide for increasing protein requirements as the child grows. By one year of age it is difficult if not impossible to meet the protein requirement if Lofenalac is offered only as a liquid formula. The amount of Lofenalac must be in-creased at intervals. The child on a low-phenylalanine diet should be introduced to cup feedings, chopped foods, and self-feeding practices at the same ages as are other children. If the child is to grow up normally it is important that he be allowed to develop eating habits that are as normal as possible within the limits of the restricted diet. Satisfaction with the low-phenylalanine diet in later years depends on the taste pref-erences and eating attitudes the child acquires while very young.

If protein requirements are not met, growth suffers; the small amounts of phenylalanine allowed may not be utilized. An example of suboptimal protein intake is shown in Figure 6. The patient was three years old at the time. The earlier years of treatment had been uneventful and the mother had previously been quite successful in making necessary dietary ad-justments. Period 1 shows several weeks characterized by elevation of serum phenylalanine in the range from 15 to 25 mg. per cent, with increased excretion of phenylalanine and orthohydroxyphenylacetic acid, so that the pattern was not much different from an untreated phenyl-ketonuric patient. No marked alterations had been made in the total phenylalanine intake, and there was no reason to believe the child was obtaining food without the mother's knowledge. She had never become

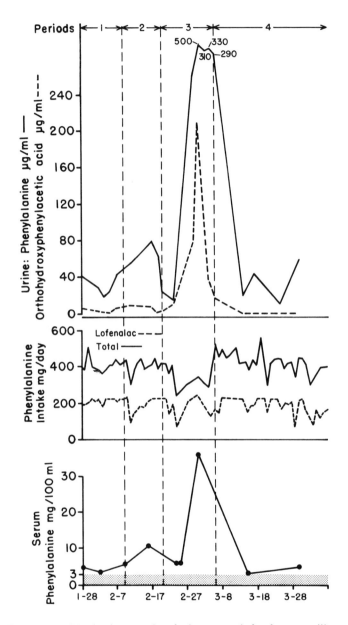

FIGURE 7. Monitoring results during a period of severe illness, showing increased serum phenylalanine and increased excretion of urinary metabolites in spite of a decreased intake of phenylalanine.

accustomed to taking Lofenalac in the more concentrated semisolid form. She consumed approximately 30 oz. of Lofenalac daily, supplying 21 gm. of protein, or about 1.45 gm. per kg. per day. Her protein intake should have been 44 gm., or the equivalent of 62 oz. of liquid Lofenalac. During the six-month period from July to December the weight percentile had dropped from 50 to 10 per cent. In period 2 the intake of Lofenalac was increased first by using a more concentrated liquid formula and then by gradually increasing the amount of Lofenalac in the semisolid form. No change was made in the total phenylalanine intake. Serum phenylalanine decreased to less than 7 mg. per cent and the urinary excretions decreased.

It is difficult to maintain biochemical control during illness. Figure 7 illustrates the effect of an acute episode of illness. During period 1 phenylalanine concentration in serum was between 3 and 7 mg. per cent; urinary phenylalanine was 20 to 40 $\mu$g. per ml.; and orthohydroxyphenylacetic acid was not detected. Phenylalanine intake was 400 mg. per day. In period 2 there was elevation of urinary phenylalanine to 80 $\mu$g. per ml. and traces of orthohydroxyphenylacetic acid were excreted. A brief period of refusal to eat was followed by an increase in serum phenylalanine to 11 mg. per cent in spite of the decrease in phenylalanine intake. Period 3 includes an episode of diarrhea, vomiting, and refusal to eat. For two days following the sharp drop in food intake serum phenylalanine remained at 6 mg. per cent. The total food intake remained low during the illness and serum phenylalanine rose to 37 mg. per cent, urine phenylalanine excretion was 250 to 500 $\mu$g. per ml., and orthohydroxyphenylacetic acid was 80 to 220 $\mu$g. per ml., all similar to the pattern of untreated phenylketonuria. We have no explanation for the magnitude of the increase in serum phenylalanine. During period 4 the phenylalanine intake was increased to 500 mg. per day for a week; urinary metabolites decreased and serum phenylalanine dropped to 3 mg. per cent. During periods of illness we have found it desirable to increase the phenylalanine intake by about 50 per cent until the acute phase is over. Loss of appetite and refusal to eat frequently accompany illness. Such situations are no cause for concern in a normal child, but in a phenylketonuric child a minor illness with temporary decrease in food intake can precipitate phenylalanine deficiency. To maintain the phenylalanine requirement, high-protein foods, soups, gelatin, eggnog, may be substituted for solid foods. When a patient must be hospitalized for elective surgery, for example, we have found it most convenient to permit the child to eat as another surgical patient might, returning to the low-phenylalanine diet after several days.

## Long-Term Management

Adequacy of nutrition in the phenylketonuric child is assessed by height and weight during growth phases. General physical growth and development should be comparable to that of the nonphenylketonuric child of similar age. Hematologic examinations at regular intervals aid in determination of nutritional adequacy. Roentgenologic evaluation should include X ray for determining adequate skeletal maturation and bone density or cortical thickness as indices of adequate nutrition. Presence of spicules in the epiphyses of the wrist represent advanced phenylalanine deficiency. Neurologic examination should be performed for establishment of normality. The electroencephalogram can be used as an adjunctive examination for deviation from normal during the therapeutic regimen. Speech and hearing evaluation may be helpful in establishing normal development. Mental development should be evaluated by psychologic testing at appropriate intervals. For children under three years of age the major tests are the Gesell Development Scales, the Cattell Infant Intelligence Scale, and the Bayley Mental and Motor Scales. For children between two and three years of age both the Stanford-Binet Intelligence Scale and the Wechsler Intelligence Scale for Children yield I.Q. scores. The Illinois Test for Psycholinguistic Ability may be used to describe deficits in psycholinguistic functions. The problems created in discipline, behavior, and language usage by the nature of treatment of phenylketonuria should be taken into account. It is important to differentiate between symptoms of the disease, signs of nutritional inadequacy, and problems created by the treatment program. Failure to recognize social and psychological factors may have long-range effects on the personality and social development of the child and of other members of his family.

In assessing the results of treatment, the previous record of untreated phenylketonuria may be reviewed. Over 90 per cent of patients with untreated phenylketonuria have I.Q.'s below 50 and eventually require institutionalization (Knox 1960). Some of our early patients fell in this category. Treatment of the older retarded patient was effective in improvement of behavior and manageability, but there was no marked alteration in mental ability. Thus the low phenylalanine diet may relieve a severely retarded child of the disturbed or autistic overlay and permit him to function more efficiently. With the younger child more improvement may be seen, but there may be no marked alteration in mental ability. It seems that for treatment to be effective, it must be started early in life, probably in the first three months of life (Bickel and Gruter 1963). Early detection and well-monitored treatment may allow an affected child to develop normally, both mentally and physically. We reported the results of treatment of twenty-seven patients recently, including eight in whom treatment was begun at less than three months of age (Sutherland, Umbarger, and Berry 1966). These eight children are all over two years of age at present and the group of treated infants has grown to twelve in number. With one exception children whose treatment was begun before three months of age attained height and weight ratings above 25 per cent of normal; several ranked in the ninetieth percentile. Suboptimal protein intake rather than phenylalanine deficiency was probably responsible for the poor growth pattern in one child. Anemia was not seen in the group of eight infants. We have recently had mild anemia develop in a premature phenylketonuric infant at six weeks of age, but the child responded to iron and increased phenylalanine intake. All bone densities were normal and bone ages were usually normal. We have recently encountered decreased cortical thickness of the metacarpus in some older children in whom serum phenylalanine levels had been maintained at low levels for long periods. Increasing the intake of both phenylalanine and protein has improved the condition. Speech and hearing evaluations showed that none of the patients had loss of hearing. Expressive language skills, sentence length, and vocabulary were related to I.Q., with variations in expressive abilities which appeared to be related to attention span and to personality characteristics. Neurological examinations showed that one of the eight patients whose treatment was begun at less than three months of age had positive neurological findings compared to five of nine whose treatment was begun later. All patients with treatment beginning later than three months of age had abnormal EEG's, while two of the children treated before three months had abnormalities. Mental development was evaluated by psychological testing at appropriate intervals. No effort was made to test infants under six months of age. Table 1 shows I.Q. scores of eight children whose treatment began when they were less than three months old. All have now been tested using the Stanford-Binet or the Wechsler Intelligence Scale, and all recorded I.Q. scores over 100. Also shown in Table 1 are I.Q. scores of ten unaffected siblings, ranging from 88 to 139. Five of the patients had older

TABLE 1

Comparison of I.Q. Scores of Early- and Late-Treated
Phenylketonuric Siblings with Unaffected Siblings and Parents

| Patient No. | I.Q. Scores | | | |
|---|---|---|---|---|
| | Early-Treated Patient | Unaffected Siblings | Affected Sibling (Late-Treated) | Parents |
| 5 | 118 | 110 ( 7–11)* | 70 (5–1)* | |
| | | 103 ( 3–2) | | |
| 3 | 114 | 139 ( 7–8) | 55 (5–2) | |
| 2 | 107 | 90 ( 6–0) | 63 (7–5) | |
| 4 | 102 | 94 ( 9–2) | 83 (4–9) | 126 (F) |
| | | 88 ( 7–5) | | 93 (M) |
| 7 | 112 | 100 (13–9) | 70 (8–0) | 112 (F) |
| | | 90 ( 4–9) | | 102 (M) |
| 8 | 102 | | | |
| 1 | 103 | | | 102 (F) |
| | | | | 96 (M) |
| 6 | 106 | 115 ( 3–10) | | 115 (F) |
| | | 126 ( 2–9) | | 123 (M) |
| Mean | 108 | 106 | 68 | |

* Age at test (yr–mo)
F=father; M=mother

phenylketonuric siblings who were treated at one year of age or later. Mean I.Q. of phenylketonuric siblings in the same family was 68, ranging from 55 to 83. Shown also are I.Q. scores from four sets of parents. I.Q. scores in the treated patients are consistent with those of the non-phenylketonuric family members.

Some of our older patients with mild to moderate mental retardation have been removed from treatment without any notable changes. We have not discontinued dietary treatment on any of the children whose treatment began before three months of life. They cannot be distinguished from normal children in any way. Two of them are progressing favorably in first grade.

Results by other investigators were summarized by Baumeister (1967). Data from his studies are tabulated in Table 2. Of early treated children, 45 per cent had I.Q. scores over 90; 14 per cent of those treated between sixteen and fifty-two weeks had I.Q. scores over 90; 6 per cent of those whose treatment was begun between one and three years of age had I.Q.

TABLE 2

Per Cent of Children with I.Q. Score of 90 or above
Compared with Age of Beginning of Treatment

| Age | Number of Children | I.Q. 90 or above |
|---|---|---|
| Under 15 weeks | 31 | 45% |
| 20 to 52 weeks | 29 | 14 |
| 1 to 3 years | 70 | 6 |

Recalculated from Baumeister (1967)

scores over 90. Mean I.Q. of eighty-seven children whose treatment was begun after six months of age was 51. Baumeister concluded that favorable results occurred most consistently in the group in which treatment began under fifteen weeks of age. Our data on children treated at nine months of age or later are consistent with those of other workers. The fact that over half the children reported in the literature whose treatment began early in life had subnormal intelligence is disappointing. However, we should ask why the children who were treated early achieve I.Q. scores around 70 to 90 reasonably consistently, rather than 50 to 55, as noted for the majority of children treated later in life. Results from additional reports in 1966 and 1967 are compared with three reports in 1965 and 1966 (Kennedy *et al.* 1967; Sutherland *et al.* 1966; Hsia 1966; Kang *et al.* 1965; Berman *et al.* 1966; Koch *et al.* 1967). In the first three reports, twenty-eight patients treated before three months of age were described. Of these, 36 to 50 per cent had I.Q. scores over 90—results similar to the data summarized by Baumeister. More recent reports, including our data, describe thirty-seven children treated before three months of age. All had I.Q. scores over 90. Distinguishing features in the latter children were normal growth, normal bones, and usually normal hematological indices. We cannot account for the discrepancies unless the severely restrictive diet has been handled too rigidly in the past. Certainly many people consider poor growth, abnormal bone changes, and hematologic abnormalities inevitable consequences of treatment of phenylketonuria. It is possible that the protein malnutrition that occurs is responsible for mild to moderate mental retardation in children maintained on diets severely deficient in phenylalanine and protein. The treatment diet need not be harmful. Normal growth should be a necessary criterion to assess adequacy of the diet. Phenylketonuric children treated early in life with diets that furnished adequate but not excessive amounts of phenylalanine have achieved normal I.Q. scores and normal growth fairly consistently. If significant improvements can be made in the quality of treatment of phenylketonuria, later studies may show more clearly whether dietary treatment can prevent mental retardation in phenylketonuric patients.

*Phenylketonuria*

# DISCUSSION

GLORIA COCHRAN: I first want to thank Dr. Farrell, in planning this program, for considering clinicians and other people who are directly involved in studying patients with inborn errors of metabolism as well as biochemists and nutritionists. These are the people who have the greatest experience, of course, and these are the people who have given us the answers today, as you can well tell from the paper that Mrs. Berry has presented. How far we have come from the question of whether we should screen infants, whether we should treat them, whom we should treat, how we should treat, what we should treat them with! All of these have been questions and areas of controversy in the past. I think they are gradually being answered by detailed studies such as those Mrs. Berry has shown us, which are possible in centers where a large enough group of children can be followed. This is one of the problems that Dr. Moore pointed out—you may be a specialist but not an expert because you cannot follow enough of these children as a clinician unless the program is set up so that a group of children can be followed in a given area by an interdisciplinary approach.

Some of the patients with whom I am familiar are here in our Child Development Clinic at Texas Children's Hospital (Houston). We have one patient who is a joint patient with Dr. Leighton Hill in the Metabolic Clinic (Texas Children's Hospital). This child, unfortunately, is not a well-controlled patient because we have not been able to control some factors in his management, mainly the psychosocial factors of parental understanding and follow-through. When I asked that the patient come back so I could give you recent weight and measurements, we were able to obtain his most recent laboratory studies, but the patient himself did not come in so I can only measure his chart and tell you that his chart weighs six pounds and is three inches thick.

We are more familiar with the patients whose progress was followed at St. Christopher's Hospital in Philadelphia, where there is a state program to provide Lofenalac free to the families where there is a need. There were also patients from New Jersey, who were seen at the Bancroft School and whose progress was followed by Dr. Warren Grover. We were able to see these patients in families where continuing supervision was provided. Many of the things that Mrs. Berry has discussed were found by these investigators who also noted similar problems of follow-up of the families. There is a real need to have other people involved in the team-approach work with the family, particularly social workers and psychologists. I wanted to make one additional remark about some studies that were done on the group at St. Christopher's by Dr. Wood, Dr. Freedman, and Dr. Steisel of the Department of Psychology. They attempted to study the psychosocial problems and interaction patterns in phenylketonuria.

They had set up an experimental program in which the child was placed in a simulated eating situation. They used questionnaires to evaluate the parents' basic understanding of the disease and interviewed the parents as to the problems of diet control. The categories of the parent's reactions were first, denial; second, perturbation, distress, and anxiety; third, an attempt to intellectualize, especially on the part of the fathers who would focus on a definition or statistics. Only a small number of the parents seemed to be realistic. When they asked the parents the difficulties that they had in following the program of diet control, they found that one of the underlying difficulties was the failure of the parents and particularly of other relatives to understand that things such as meat, eggs, and milk could actually be harmful to the child. They also encountered another problem: the child would beg a cookie or something else to eat from kindly neighbors. Clearly the people surrounding the child have to understand what the diet means. There were also conflicts when the family ate together because one child was on a special diet and others were not. Problems also developed when the child stole food or traded his possessions to other children for food. Other factors were the guilt the parents felt about denying the child something he wanted and the child's feeling that he was different.

There were indications that learning in the PKU child might be impaired by prohibitions against exploring and opportunities to try different things. These workers attempted to make some objective measurements by using an interaction scale to determine how the PKU children interact with people and with things in comparison to the retarded child, the normal child, or the psychotic child. They found that the PKU groups were significantly poorer than the normal children, but significantly better than psychotic children.

C. MOORE: Our program in the Health Department is primarily one of assisting in the screening for phenylketonuria and thank goodness my staff is here with me. Dr. Yerwood, Dr. Manning, and Mr. Tausch can answer some of the fine points that I will be unable to cover.

We have roughly 112,000 live births per year in Texas, and the average hospital stay across the state is 2.4 days for each newborn individual—and as I understand it (I am not a pediatrician) the children are not fed any protein for the first twenty-four hours—is that correct, Dr. Rouse? So, you can see that sometimes there is a great deal of doubt in our minds as to the validity of the Guthrie Tests or of any other screening techniques when a child has been on protein for such a very short time. The laboratory in Austin receives about 50 per cent of the screening tests for the state. We have no idea about the other 50 per cent of these children: whether screening is done; or, if it is done, what method is used and what the results are. We have approximately 8,000 deliveries by midwife in the state each year and we have no idea of the circumstances of the deliveries or of what happens to these children afterward. Do the midwives use the Guthrie technique or do they the use Phenistix? Just what does happen? It is rather difficult to find out. So, as you can see, since we receive only 50 per cent of the known live births during the year, it is quite difficult for us to provide any competent degree of follow-up services. We do send out information along with three papers by Mrs. Berry to the physicians. When we get a presumptive positive test we request that a serum specimen be sent in for re-evaluation or a more definitive chemical type of testing. But as far as being able to make a concerted effort toward securing the entire gamut of services needed by these children, we simply have not been able to do it.

Of course, we would like to see available in the state the type of staff that can go into the home, work with the children and the families, and provide follow-up with all the services that these children absolutely need. Time is short and I will not go any further, but you can see that there are many, many problems. If there are any questions, I will be happy to try to answer them. If I am unable to, I am sure that Dr. Yerwood, my co-worker, can help.

J. ALT: What happens to the parents of PKU children after the diagnosis is made? After the diagnosis, do we give them a simple explanation of what PKU means (simple to us may be anything but simple to parents), then give them the dietary instructions, send them home and tell them to come back at frequent intervals to have the child's phenylalanine levels checked? I am afraid people in the medical and paramedical fields too often lose sight of the family as a whole. If we do this, it is a tragic error on our part. If this is their first child with PKU, the parents probably are utterly confused—not only by the impact of the meaning of PKU but by concern about what is to follow in regard to the diet and worry about what the child will be like when it gets older.

First of all, let me talk about the infant who is diagnosed in the neonatal period. The dietary restrictions for infants are not as difficult for parents to handle as for the older child. Lofenalac is accepted more readily and the child is not actually aware that he is receiving something different —furthermore, he is not able to raid the refrigerator or get into the kitchen cupboards. It is another story with the child whose diagnosis of PKU is made at a later age. If the decision is made to place him on the Lofenalac diet, many problems may ensue. All of a sudden he is no longer allowed to eat many of the things the rest of the family eats, and, furthermore, he is required to consume some nasty-tasting liquid that certainly doesn't taste like his milk. I am trying to look at this in terms of the child, and I certainly would not want the parents to assume the negative attitude I have just given concerning the diet. Because the older child may also be retarded, there may be other feeding problems. A child has to learn how to eat and parents must help their children move through a continuous process toward adulthood. It is rewarding and gratifying to a mother to have her child readily accept the food she offers him. Many retarded children are difficult to feed and reject foods, especially during the transition to chunkier table food. Because of this, mothers may feel they are being rejected. In the case of children with PKU, where the diet is so drastically different, the problems are compounded. I feel, however, that in many instances this strict diet is more difficult for the parents than for the child. It is guilt-producing for the parents to deny their child food that the rest of the family enjoys. Parents may also feel guilty if the child's phenylalanine level is elevated even though they have adhered to the diet.

Since children with PKU spend relatively little time in the hospital, I would like to concentrate on the public health nurse in the community. She will have many opportunities to see these children in their homes and can be of great help in assisting the parents. First of all, the family is probably more relaxed in their own home environment. The nurse has an opportunity to observe the child in this environment and to detect factors that may help or hinder the child's development. What are the cultural values of this family? With proper knowledge about PKU and the diet, the public health nurse can help the parents adjust the child's diet to the family's eating pattern. For instance, if the family enjoys a snack in the evening, she can show the parents how to let the child with PKU save a food exchange so he may also snack. Or maybe there is a birthday party. The parents can learn to let the child with PKU trade his cake for the frosting. The diet for phenylketonuric children is necessarily a strict one, but parents must be helped to understand that these children will go on the same food jags as other children do. They will refuse certain foods and crave others, and their appetite will vary. We all have variations in our eating habits. I had never eaten Mexican food until I moved here two years ago; now I think I cannot survive without it. Public health nurses are and should be family oriented. They can help the parents see the needs of the other family members. If the parents become wrapped up in the child with PKU, certainly the siblings will suffer. If parents become involved in the dietary management alone, they may miss the signs of readiness in the child for new developmental tasks. Nurses can help the parents recognize when the child is ready to move into new tasks such as some of the self-help skills—eating, toilet training, and dressing. Whereas the normal child may attain these without too much effort on the parent's part, the child who is retarded may have to be taught how to learn. Nurses must have knowledge of normal growth and development in order to know at what level the child is functioning and where to begin in teaching him. Parents need to be made aware of the three R's in working with the retarded child: routine, repetition, and relaxation. And I might add that the three R's are not restricted only to the retarded child. They can work for normal children too. I feel that nurses need some knowledge of the genetic aspects of PKU. I do not expect them to be genetic counselors, but they should have enough knowledge to answer intelligently some of the questions that parents will ask.

I would like to tell you about some of my experiences with families of PKU children at the University of Iowa. One day a month was devoted to these children and their families. Depending on their age and dietary control, the children were seen from every one to four months. At different intervals they had physical examinations, psychological testing, social service case work, and speech and hearing evaluation. Guthrie Tests were given at each visit. The family was seen by the nutritionist at each visit, and the parents also met with the clinic staff. Dietary adjustments were recommended as necessary following the results of the Guthrie Tests. Public health nurses in the local communities visited these families to assist the parents in following the recommendations. I also participated in a study where the Guthrie inhibition assay test and the La Du quantitative serum phenylalanine test were performed simultaneously on the same blood samples in two different laboratories. Samples were obtained from children with PKU, from siblings and parents of these children, and from apparently normal children and adults. The results reveal that the Guthrie Test was reliable as the method for monitoring dietary control of PKU.

Another University of Iowa study which has also been published, concerned removing children with PKU from the diet. The sample was small, but the study was carefully controlled and the children had been given psychological testing just prior to discontinuing the diet. Testing was repeated at three-, six-, and twelve-month intervals. No significant change was found in intellectual performance on testing; however, some children improved in school performance and in behavior. This was reported by both the parents and the teachers. There was a more relaxed atmosphere in the home and family activities increased.

In another study, parental reactions to PKU were surveyed. Most parents were aware prior to seeking medical help that something was wrong with their child, and the fathers were the first ones to recognize a delay. The study revealed that these parents were completely unprepared to cope with the problems of mental retardation. Nurses as well as doctors need to be aware of the signs and symptoms of PKU and need to urge testing of children with developmental delay. Sad but true, one mother, after going to her physician numerous times saying that there was something wrong with her child, made the diagnosis of PKU herself after reading an article in a ladies magazine. We need to have empathy with these parents. Maybe it would be good for all of us to do what two nurses did several years ago in the state of Washington. They volunteered to babysit with two children with PKU and a normal sibling while the parents took a holiday weekend. The three older normal children in the family were kept by the grandparents. These two nurses certainly gained a better understanding of the day-to-day problems experienced by the parents.

Unfortunately, too often we forget that the parents have twenty-four–hour care of these children. As professional people interested in PKU, we must work together as a team to be effective in assisting parents who have phenylketonuric children.

E. CUNNINGHAM: I would like to direct this question to Mrs. Berry. At the meeting in Dubrovnik, Yugoslavia, this summer it was pointed out that it has been well established that excessive levels of phenylalanine interfere with initial myelinization. Is there evidence that in later years it can cause demyelinization?

H. BERRY: I cannot answer. There have been so few autopsies of phenylketonurics that it would be hard to make a firm statement. Perhaps, someone in the audience might have a more firm statement on this question. I do not think we know what causes the mental defect in phenylketonuria. It would be very convenient to say it is failure of myelinization, or later demyelinization, but I do not think we can be sure of that. Would anybody like to comment?

WINSTON COCHRAN: There has also been a suggestion, hasn't there, that serotonin levels are involved in some manner?

H. BERRY: There have been many proposals but each one of them falls down, particularly when you find that the phenylketonuric with normal intelligence—that rare individual who has gone through life with high blood phenylalanine levels but has escaped the mental defect—has the same biochemistry as the severely retarded one. If we could find out what happened in very early life, we might find a clue, but I would be loath to say what causes the damage. I wish I knew—it would be easier to handle the problem.

H. GHADIMI: In all fairness to opposing views, I would like to mention that the present dietary treatment of phenylketonuria is not based on properly controlled studies, is cumbersome, practically prohibits investigation of any other therapeutic approach, and probably should be discontinued indefinitely. It would be less difficult to put up with all the shortcomings of the present treatment if we knew (a) that all untreated phenylketonuric patients are going to be mentally retarded, and (b) that the present dietary treatment definitely prevents mental retardation. Unfortunately, this is not the case. Screening of affected families shows that 5–10 per cent of the biochemically affected children escape mental retardation. At present, in many centers, all newborn children with hyperphenylalaninemia are put on a cumbersome low phenylalanine diet. This is obviously superfluous, if not injurious, to at least 5–10 per cent of them. Thus, evaluation of the results of the treatment is difficult. At the time we learned that 5–10 per cent of phenylketonuric patients were

29

not mentally retarded, we believed that the occurrence of the disease was one in thirty or forty thousand. With the present widespread screening of newborns, the incidence has changed to one in ten thousand or even greater. Unfortunately, there is no way of determining what proportion of the patients will remain normal without any dietary treatment because all statistics now available are based on patients receiving the treatment. If all hyperphenylalaninemic infants are to be put on a low-phenylalanine diet, there should be attempts made to distinguish those who show minimum brain damage from those who may show no signs of brain anomaly. I realize this is a difficult proposition. Nevertheless, attempts should be made in this direction.

For instance, is anyone at present following these infants with periodic EEG's?

H. BERRY: This is what I was referring to in the troublesome "atypical phenylketonuria or hyperphenylalaninemia." If we could distinguish on any basis in early life the infant with the high blood phenylalanine level who is going to be retarded and the infant with the high blood level who is going to have normal intelligence, we would be able to plan the treatment more effectively. In practice, the best I can suggest is not to let treatment harm the child: do not cause mental retardation from protein malnutrition in case the child does not have phenylketonuria. This much could be done until we become more sophisticated in making the diagnoses. In studies of normal populations, there are several places where large groups of adult individuals are being tested for elevated blood phenylalanine concentrations and phenylketonurics with normal intelligence are not being found. On the other hand, all of us who deal with phenylketonuria know there are normal individuals going about their normal jobs, who have biochemical phenylketonuria and who somehow have escaped the damage from the disease. Such individuals occur in families where another phenylketonuric is severely retarded. Again, I simply say we do not have all the answers yet. I could not tell you how many of the eight infants we have treated who now have normal intelligence would have been retarded had they been left alone. Certainly, some of them had retarded siblings. On the other hand, one patient who was treated early had a phenylketonuric sibling with an I.Q. of 83. Who is going to argue with an I.Q. of 83? The same family had two normal siblings with I.Q.'s of 88 and 90. In that family we may not have done much. You must take care not to damage the child further by careless treatment.

R. HILL: What was the age of the infants referred to that were normal in which low phenylalanine diet was discontinued?

J. ALT: First of all, I will look at the age when the diet was started—anywhere from nine months of age to one who was seven years eight months when his diet was begun (his was begun mostly because his behavior was so bad). They were taken off at anywhere from five to nine years of age and their intelligence levels did not change significantly.

D. MARRACK: Does the negative nitrogen balance associated with fever and the associated raised serum phenylalanine have any measurable effect on the child especially in the first three to four months of life? Would nitrogen-retaining steroids be of value in such cases?

H. BERRY: Are you saying, "Do the blood levels go up?" We have some children who spent their whole first year with persistently elevated blood levels and persistent and recurring infections, possibly as the result of a suboptimal protein intake. The blood levels rarely go above 12 mg. per cent. These children seem to do just as well as those who have been kept at 3 to 4 mg. per cent.

D. MARRACK: I was thinking much more of an infant who has been reasonably controlled but who had an episode of fever.

H. BERRY: We have never been able to detect any relation between a high blood level and behavior. Sick children become fretful due to the illness. If the phenylalanine is low, they become very lethargic. Phenylalanine levels then may rise. We really cannot say that the high blood levels have damaged them.

H. GHADIMI: Our limited experience indicates that blood phenylalanine levels, as high as 12 mg. per 100 ml. can be tolerated without ill effects. Would you agree with this suggestion?

H. BERRY: There has been a study of use of anabolic steroids to reduce the blood phenylalanine levels in older patients. This seemed to work quite effectively. I know of no reason why it would not work. We have been equally successful in giving them small amounts of high-quality protein. It is better not to give more drugs than necessary in case we should disturb some balance about which we do not yet know enough. But that approach is certainly feasible.

D. MARRACK: No amount of dietary protein will keep a patient in nitrogen balance in the face of a sustained fever. The only way you can achieve this is by the administration of anabolic steroids. Then you can maintain the individual in nitrogen balance and normal plasma amino acid levels without any great effort during infection.

H. BERRY: Most of our children have been remarkably well. Our hospital charts are not large. As a matter of fact, we have never hospitalized any of these children for an illness. I cannot say what would be required. We recommend things that the mothers can carry out at home, keeping it as simple as possible, because the situation is difficult enough anyhow. If one wanted to use steroids under controlled conditions, they might work very well. But we have really not found them necessary. When the children are ill, we wait through the period and really do not worry about raised phenylalanine levels nearly as much as we used to.

C. MOORE: All my background and training is in obstetrics and I hate to be rather provincial and boorish, but our big problem is finding these youngsters. From the point of view of an obstetrician, is there any way a man in practice can anticipate the probability of a child being born with phenylketonuria?

H. BERRY: I do not think there is, if you are referring to testing the mothers during pregnancy. In our experience we have not found that the phenylalanine levels of mothers of phenylketonuric children have been elevated. Maternal plasma shows decreased levels of all the amino acids and the levels become lower as pregnancy advances. The finding of a high level might be significant, and I realize that this has been reported; but we simply have never observed phenylalanine elevated in blood during some twenty pregnancies of mothers who have had phenylketonuric children. They have all shown normal blood levels. The infants have all shown cord blood levels in the normal range. I do not know of any way you can know unless there is a family history. If there is already a phenylketonuric child in the home then the obstetrician should be very watchful!

H. GHADIMI: Recognition of the phenylketonuric infant of a heterozygote mother, prior to birth, does not seem to serve any practical purpose at this point. The enzyme capability of a heterozygote mother can well compensate for a homozygote fetus. I suppose that is why we assume that the central nervous system of the homozygote newborn is intact and prompt treatment is, therefore, advisable.

H. LEVY: Dr. Moore, you brought up a very interesting question today about which I could, perhaps, say a few words. I refer to your question regarding what the obstetrician can do. The answer does not directly concern phenylketonuria in the child but phenylketonuria in the mother. This is a problem that the people in Massachusetts, Dr. MacCready in particular, have been interested in for some time. There are reports from several places regarding the occurrences of brain damage in the offspring of mothers who had high phenylalanine levels and who in most cases were typical phenylketonurics. One of the questions asked is: "Does a high phenylalanine level in the mother cause brain damage to the fetus?" Of course, this has not yet been answered. But there are enough reports now to suggest that many of these fetuses have turned out to be mentally retarded children who do not have phenylketonuria. We have now in Massachusetts a mother who is slightly retarded with phenlyketonuria and who has three brain-damaged nonphenylketonuric infants in one of the state institutions, and another mother who has phenylketonuria and who has one nonphenylketonuric retarded child. One of the ways that obstetricians can be of help is by detecting phenylketonuria in the mother. This can be done by a very simple test and may be as simple as doing a Phenistix test on maternal urine. Dr. McCready is now consulting the Ames Company, who market both Phenistix and Clinistix, in an attempt to persuade them to incorporate the ferric chloride impregnated Phenistix principle into a multiple dip stick like Clinistix. This would enable the obstetrician when he is testing the urine of the mother who comes in for her first obstetric visit, to screen her for PKU. He now tests her urine for pH, which is ridiculous (he never uses this information anyway), so the Phenistix test could perhaps be substituted for the pH testing space. The question of whether or not one should treat the mothers who have phenylketonuria with a low phenylalanine diet during pregnancy in an attempt to prevent brain damage to the fetus is at this time a moot point. But the first step is to find out who these women are and learn more about them and their offspring.

E. AIRAKSINEN: How high do you allow the blood phenylalanine to rise in older age groups?

H. BERRY: We have liberalized our diet somewhat for older children. We previously kept them around 5 to 8 mg. per cent, but we find that as they approach six and seven years of age, there is a fall-off in growth rate and evidence of nutritional deficiency. Their protein intake seems difficult to maintain at a sufficiently high level. The only way we can increase the protein intake is to liberalize the diet with natural foods. There is a limit to how much Lofenalac a child can take even though he may have been trained from infancy to eat it. Some of the older children are now deliberately being raised to 10–12 mg. per cent phenylalanine in the blood. We have run into opposition from the mothers. They are extremely fearful and are reluctant to carry out this liberalization. This is somewhat different from other people's experiences when the diet is stopped. We try to assure them that nothing bad will happen, but parents find it difficult to allow the child to eat a little more liberally. So far we have increased serum phenylalanine levels to 12 mg. per cent in two children without much difference. How high we can go, I do not know. If we are to maintain nutrition during this second growth phase, we must do something; either stop the diet altogether or liberalize it to a marked degree.

## REFERENCES

Allen, R. J., Heffelfinger, J. S., Masotti, R. E., and Tsau, M. U. 1964. Phenylalanine hydroxylase activity in newborn infants. *Pediatrics* 33:512.

Baumeister, A. E. 1967. The effects of dietary control on intelligence in phenylketonuria. *Am. J. Ment. Def.* 71:840.

Berman, P. W., Waisman, H. W., and Graham, F. K. 1966. Intelligence in treated phenylketonuric children: A developmental study. *Child Development* 37:731.

Berry, H. K., Sutherland, B., and Umbarger, B. 1965. Procedures for monitoring the low-phenylalanine diet in treatment of phenylketonuria. *J. Pediat.* 67:609.

Berry, H. K., Umbarger, B., and Sutherland, B. 1964. Testing of newborn siblings in phenylketonuric families. *J.A.M.A.* 189:641.

Bickel, H., and Gruter, W. 1963. Management of phenylketonuria. In *Phenylketonuria*, ed. F. L. Lyman, p. 145. Springfield, Ill.: Charles C. Thomas Co.

Guthrie, R., and Susi, A. 1963. A simple phenylalanine method for detecting phenylketonuria in large populations of newborn infants. *Pediatrics* 32:338.

Hsia, D. Y.-Y. 1966. Phenylketonuria: A study of human biochemical genetics. *Pediatrics* 38:173.

Kang, E. S., Kennedy, J. L., Gates, L., Burwash, I., and McKinnon, A. 1965. Clinical observations in phenylketonuria. *Pediatrics* 35:932.

Kennedy, J. L., Jr., Wertelecki, W., Gates, L., Sperry, B. P., and Cass, V. M. 1967. The early treatment of phenylketonuria. *Am. J. Dis. Child.* 113:16.

Knox, W. E. 1960. An evaluation of treatment of phenylketonuria with diets low in phenylalanine. *Pediatrics* 26:1.

Koch, R., Acosta, P., Fishler, K., Shaeffler, G., and Wohlers, A. 1967. Clinical observations on phenylketonuria. *Am. J. Dis. Child.* 113:6.

# Phenylketonuria

La Du, B. N., and Zannoni, V. G. 1955. The tyrosine oxidation system of liver. II: Oxidation of p-hydroxyphenylpyruvic acid to homogentisic acid. *J. Biol. Chem.* 217:777.

Light, I. J., Berry, H. K., and Sutherland, J. M. 1966. Aminoacidemia of prematurity. *Am J. Dis. Child.* 112:229.

McCaman, M. W., and Robins, E. 1962. Fluorometric method for the determination of phenylalanine in serum. *J. Lab. Clin. Med.* 59:885.

Snyderman, S. E., Pratt, E. L., Cheung, M. W., Norton, P., and Holt, L. E., Jr. 1955. The phenylalanine requirement of the normal infant. *J. Nutr.* 56:253.

Sutherland, B. S., Umbarger, B., and Berry, H. K. 1966. Treatment of phenylketonuria: A decade of results. *Am. J. Dis. Child.* 111:505.

Woolf, L. I. 1962. Nutrition in relation to phenylketonuria. *Proc. Nutr. Soc.* 21:21.

Woolf, L. I., Cranston, W. I., and Goodwin, B. L. 1967. Third allele at phenylalanine hydroxylase locus in man. *Nature* 213:883.

# Homocystinuria in Northern Ireland[1]

NINA A. J. CARSON, M.D., I. J. CARRE, M.D., M.R.C.P.,
and D. W. NEILL, M.Sc., M.C. Path.

*Department of Child Health, The Queen's University of Belfast, Belfast, Ireland*

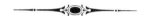

Homocystinuria was discovered in Northern Ireland when the urine specimens from two siblings with clinical histories of mental retardation and fits were examined as part of a screening study to detect inborn errors of amino acid metabolism in mentally retarded individuals. Urine specimens from these individuals were routinely subjected to two-way amino acid paper chromatography and to a battery of simple qualitative tests ( Carson and Neill 1962). One of the latter was the cyanide-nitroprusside test to detect sulfur-containing amino acids. A positive reaction to this test was obtained from the urine of these siblings. The oxidized chromatogram showed a normal amino acid pattern with an increase in what appeared to be cysteic acid. Because it is unusual to find an isolated increase in cystine excretion unaccompanied by either a generalized aminoaciduria or an increase in the dibasic amino acids—lysine, ornithine, or arginine—it was felt that further studies should be undertaken.

[1] This work was financed by a grant from the Medical Research Council.

We wish to acknowledge our debt to our medical colleagues, and in particular to Dr. C. M. B. Field, Dr. W. I. Forsythe, and Dr. T. W. Weir. The laboratory studies have been carried out by Misses P. Bradshaw, M. Harper, and Mr. J. A. Roche. Miss H. Wilson, B. Sc., Haematology Department of the Royal Bedfast Hospital for Sick Children, performed the investigation for platelet stickiness. We are also indebted to Mrs. Sadie Abernethy for her patient secretarial assistance, and to Mr. R. Wood for the photography.

Samples of the urine specimens were examined in University College Hospital, London, through the kindness of Professor C. E. Dent. Quantitative amino acid analysis using the Spackman, Moore, and Stein technique showed the abnormality to be an increase in homocystine and not in cystine. At the same time in Northern Ireland one of the patients had been given an oral cystine load. Paper chromatographic examination of the oxidized urine voided after the oral cystine showed that two spots were present side by side in the cysteic acid position, one of these being homocysteic acid.

## Clinical Findings

Since 1962 seventeen patients with this disorder have been discovered in Northern Ireland. After examination of the first few patients, it became clear that, apart from the excretion of homocystine in the urine, there was emerging a distinct clinical picture (Carson *et al.* 1965). The majority of the patients have fair hair, blue eyes, and a malar flush with poor peripheral circulation and *livedo reticularis*. With one exception, a nine-month-old infant (Mi. L., Table 3), all the patients have *ectopia lentis*, and all but two (Mi. L. and his five-year-old sibling, F. L.) are mentally retarded. Mi L., at one year of age, appears to be a perfectly normal child with no physical or mental stigmata of the disorder evident to date. It is of interest that in one group of American patients (Schimke *et al.* 1965), sixteen of thirty-eight patients were considered to have normal mentality.

The mental deterioration in our patients has been progressive, the early developmental history being normal. For example, A. McC. sat up at six months, starting talking at eleven months, and walked at eighteen months. By the age of two years, developmental quotient was recorded as 52, but at five years six months it was 15. In six patients fits occurred. Three of these patients (P. B., A.McC., and J. R.) had EEG recordings, and all showed a generalized abnormality. Patient P. B. had a normal record at the age of four years but progressed to generalized dysrhythmia by the age of seven years eight months. A. McC. at twenty-two months had a normal sleep record with some bursts of fast activity, of high voltage, and of sharp form, but by the age of seven years her record had deteriorated to a pattern showing general disorganization with epileptic features. At fifteen months J. R. showed no $\alpha$-rhythm, and a generalized abnormality was reported. Air pictures were performed on this child (who was

37

## TABLE 3

### Clinical Findings in Seventeen Patients with Homocystinuria

| Family | I | | | II | | III | | IV | | V | | VI | VII | VIII | IX | X | XI |
|---|---|---|---|---|---|---|---|---|---|---|---|---|---|---|---|---|---|
| Patient | Mi. L. | F. L. | Ma. L. | A. McC. | G. McC. | Pa. B. | Pl. B. | J. R. | S. R. | M. Rit. | J. Rit. | R. R. | A. S.* | G. M. | J. R. | M. McG.* | R. K.* |
| Sex | M | F | F | F | M | F | F | M | M | M | F | M | M | M | M | F | M |
| Age at diagnosis (in years) | 9/12 | 5 | 10 | 1 6/12 | 5 | 5 | 7 | 6 | 8 | 13 | 21 | 7 | 8 | 13 | 18 | 28 | 32 |
| Fair hair and malar flush | + | + | + | + | + | + | + | + | + | + | + | ± | + | + | ± | + | − |
| I.Q. | GQ 82 | 93 | 6-year level | 53 | 50 | 30 | 30 | 20 | 34 | 53 | ·70 | 70 | 50 | 50 | 30 | 25 | 50 |
| Ectopia lentis | − | + | + | + | + | + | + | + | + | + | + | + | + | + | + | + | + |
| Fits | − | − | + | +** | − | + | + | + | − | − | + | − | − | − | − | − | − |
| Peculiar gait | − | − | + | + | + | + | + | + | + | + | + | ± | + | + | + | + | + |
| Genu valgum/ Pes cavus | −/− | −/− | +/+ | +/− | +/+ | +/+ | +/+ | +/+ | +/+ | +/? | +/? | +/− | +/+ | +/+ | +/? | +/+ | ±/? |
| Long slender limbs | − | − | + | ± | ± | ± | ± | − | − | ++ | ++ | ++ | ++ | ++ | ++ | ++ | ++ |
| Cardiovascular disorder | − | ± | ± | + | + | + | + | + | − | − | + | ± | − | + | + | − | + |
| Thrombotic episodes | − | − | − | − | + | ++† | ++† | ++† | + | − | − | − | +† | − | − | ++† | − |

\* = Diagnosis of Homocystinuria made on urinary chromatographic evidence only. Patients died before full investigation could be undertaken.

\*\* = Developed fits at age of 7 years.

† Died as a result of thrombosis. A. S. and M. McG. not proven by post mortem.

+ + = Severe

+ = Slight

± = Probable

− = Value not obtained

TABLE 4

Differential Features between Homocystinuria and the Marfan Syndrome

| | Homocystinuria | Marfan Syndrome |
|---|---|---|
| Physical Features | Usually fair-haired. High malar flush. The majority are good-looking as children. | Usually pale, sad-faced individuals, older-looking than their actual age |
| Ocular Defects<br>*Ectopia lentis*<br>Spherophakia<br>Iridodonesis | Lens generally dislocated downward | Lens generally dislocated upward |
| Skeletal Changes | | |
| Arachnodactyly<br>Chest deformity<br>High arched palate | Frequently present in older patients | Present |
| *Pes cavus*<br>*Genu valgum* | Frequently present | May be present |
| Osteoporosis | Frequently present | Absent |
| Cardiovascular System | | |
| Transverse bands of intimal fibrosis | Described in all P.M. studies to date | Rarely described |
| Medial degeneration with fragmentation and disruption of elastic fibres | Present | Present |
| Thrombosis (Arteries and veins) | Frequent | Absent |
| Central Nervous System | | |
| Mental retardation | Present | Absent |
| Fits | Frequently found | Absent |
| Gait | Peculiar stiff-legged wide-based gait present | Normal |
| Fatty Change in Liver | Present | Absent |
| Inheritance | Autosomal recessive | Autosomal dominant |
| Homocystinuria | Present | Absent |

being investigated for what appeared to be a cerebrovascular accident) and reported diffuse cerebral atrophy, which, in the opinion of the neurologist, must have been present before the current episode.

Skeletal changes were present in fifteen of the seventeen patients. These vary from *genu valgum* and *pes cavus* in the younger patients to what appears to be typical Marfan-like features in the older patients, with arachnodactyly, chest deformities, and high-arched palate. These Marfan-like proportions appear in early adolescence and are not usually marked in the younger patients.

Because of this similarity to the Marfan syndrome in the older patients, urine was examined from fourteen individuals with the classical Marfan syndrome and forty-four first-degree relatives. No homocystinuria was found. It is, nevertheless, noteworthy that two of our patients with homocystinuria have been written up in the literature as classical examples of the Marfan syndrome (Lynas and Merrett 1958; Loughridge 1959).

Skeletal X rays performed on nine patients revealed that six of them (ranging from four to eighteen years) showed generalized osteoporosis, one (seven years) had retarded bone age, and two (nine months and five years) had normal bone density. The five-year-old child had a minor congenital anomaly of the dorso-cervical spine. Two of the older patients (fifteen and eighteen years) showed cupping of approximating surfaces of the vertebral bodies. S. W. Smith (1967) reported roentgen findings in three cases of homocystinuria and compared these with seventy-one other cases in the literature. He states that the only feature that differs from the Marfan syndrome is the presence of marked generalized osteoporosis. Table 4 lists the differential features between the Marfan syndrome and homocystinuria.

## Gait

A peculiar stiff-legged gait was present in fifteen of the seventeen patients. This gait has been variously described by other authors as "Chaplin-like," "ducklike," "shuffling," although our impression is that none of these phrases adequately describes the peculiarity.

The reasons for this peculiar gait, for the difficulty some patients experience when going up and down stairs, and for the pelvic girdle muscle weakness noted in three of the patients are not definitely known, but the following may be contributory factors:

1. These patients are inclined to misjudge distance in depth because of the dislocation of the lens and the associated myopia.

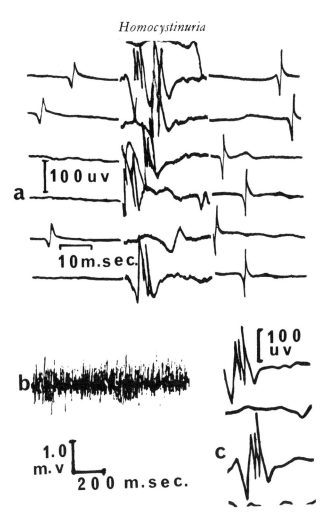

FIGURE 8.  Electromyographic tracing of the deltoid muscle for patient G. M. (a and b), and patient G. McC. (c).

2. *Pes cavus* was present in most of the patients and could cause difficulty in walking.

3. Poor intellectual development is often associated with peculiarities of gait which may stem from central nervous system involvement. Some of the patients in this study did have spasticity and increased lower limb reflexes.

TABLE 5

Muscle Function Studies in Homocystinuria

| Case | Patient | Family | Sex | Age | Muscle Weakness Clinically | Mean Duration Action Potential (Percentage Increase or Decrease) | Incidence Polyphasic Potentials (Percentage) | Amplitude of Interference Pattern (Millivolts) |
|------|---------|--------|-----|-----|----------------------------|------------------------------------------------------------------|----------------------------------------------|------------------------------------------------|
| 1 | G. McC. | II | M | 10 | ++ | −12 | 46 | — |
| 2 | A. McC. | II | F | 7 | + | −19 | 14 | 1.9 |
| 3 | G. M. | VIII | M | 18 | ± | −27 | 13 | 1.7 |
| 4 | R. R. | VI | M | 8 | 0 | + 3 (15) | 20 | 1.5 |
| 5 | Mi. L. | I | M | 1 | 0 | — | No apparent increase | — |
| 6 | F. L. | I | F | 5 | 0 | − 7 (8) | 14 | 1.0 |
| 7 | Ma. L. | I | F | 10 | 0 | −35 (11) | 27 | 2.5 |
| 8 | M. Rit. | V | M | 15 | 0 | −17 | 15 | 2.1 |
| 9 | J. Rit. | V | M | 20 | 0 | −26 | 16 | 2.1 |

Limb and/or pelvic girdle muscle weakness

++ = Severe

+ = Slight

± = Probable

0 = None

— = Value could not be obtained because of lack of cooperation

TABLE 6

Platelet Stickiness in Patients with Homocystinuria

| Patient | Platelet Stickiness (Percentage Remaining at 20 Minutes) |
|---------|:---:|
| Mi. L. | 80 |
| F. L. | 52 |
| Ma. L. | 61 |
| A. McC. | 62 |
| G. McC. | 59 |
| R. R. | 72 |
| M. Rit. | 61 |
| G. M. | 61 |
| J. R. | 65 |
| Normal Range | 65–80 |

4. Muscular weakness was also apparent in these patients.

In two patients (siblings) there was evidence of a rather marked pelvic girdle weakness. The patients were unable to rise from the floor without "climbing" up some support. A third patient rose from a lying position awkwardly and tended to use his hands in a "climbing the legs" attitude. An electromyographic study was undertaken (Hurwitz, Chopra, and Carson 1968) of nine patients (six males and three females) with homocystinuria aged nine months to eighteen years, of one unaffected twin, and of three sets of parents.

The deltoid muscle was examined by concentric needle electrodes 0.65 mm. in diameter using a three-channeled Disa machine. Figure 8 illustrates the electromyographic findings from patient G. M. (a and b) and from patient G. McC. (c).

The results in Table 5 show that electromyographic examination of seven of the nine patients with homocystinuria suggests a myopathy. The electromyographic examination was also abnormal and of myopathic type in two of the parents. As yet these findings have not been investigated fully using histochemical or histopathological techniques.

Thrombotic episodes have occurred in 43 per cent of patients. Three (and possibly five) patients have died as a result of thrombosis. Because the thrombi occurred in arteries and veins, attention was drawn to the possibility of a clotting diathesis. Investigations on platelet aggregation were carried out by L. McDonald and others (1964) on four of our patients, and the results showed increased platelet stickiness. At the same time Dr. McDonald found that homocystine added to blood from normal persons in concentrations similar to that found in the blood of homocystinuric patients caused increased stickiness to occur. Reports of studies from the United States have not confirmed this finding in all homocystinuric patients tested.

Platelet studies were performed on nine patients (including those in the McDonald study referred to above). A similar method was used. The results are seen in Table 6 and indicate that platelet stickiness of a minor degree was present in six of the nine patients. All the tests were performed by the same person under the same physical conditions. Studies of platelet aggregation are notoriously subjective, and rigorous standardization of technique is essential if the results are to have any significance. Many apparently unrelated factors are found to influence platelet stickiness, and it is not possible to attribute to this aspect of the study the degree of significance which applied to other features. For eight patients under treatment, platelet aggregation studies were performed at each visit with the most bewildering results. No correlation with improvement in biochemical status could be seen and no consistent trend was noted.

Centrilobular fatty degeneration of the liver was seen in four cases. Routine liver function tests gave normal results including alkaline phosphatase, serum glutamic oxaloacetic transaminase, and serum glutamic pyruvic transaminase. It is of interest, however, that isocitric dehydrogenase levels were moderately raised in seven of eleven patients studied.

There was clinical evidence of cardiovascular changes in the form of hypertension, sinus arrhythmia, and/or cardiac enlargement in eleven of the seventeen patients. In post mortem studies vascular changes have been noted in the form of fibrous intimal changes with fragmentation and disruption of elastic fibers in the media (Gibson, Carson, and Neill 1964). Probably all the patients will sooner or later develop cardiovascular involvement.

## Biochemical Defect in Homocystinuria

The finding of homocystine and the lack of cystine clearly calls for a study of methionine metabolism in these patients.

The three main functions of methionine in man are its role in protein synthesis; its role as methyl group donor in the synthesis of compounds such as choline, creatine, and adrenaline; and its role in the formation of cysteine with homocysteine as an intermediate metabolite (see Fig. 9).

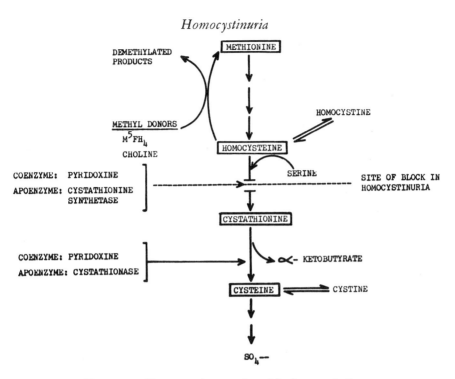

FIGURE 9. Known pathways of methionine metabolism.

Methionine is converted to S-adenosyl methionine, which is then de-methylated to form S-adenosyl homocysteine. This is hydrolyzed to homo-cysteine. The homocysteine is then condensed with serine aided by the enzyme cystathionine synthetase to form cystathionine. This thioether is then cleaved by the enzyme cystathionase to form cysteine. These last two reactions are $B_6$ dependent. Homocysteine may be remethylated to reform methionine with the aid of preformed methyl groups—that is, with be-taine and with a folic acid derivative (N-methyltetrahydrofolic acid). The equilibrium of this reaction, however, favors the formation of cys-tathionine.

Homocysteine may also undergo desulfuration to form hydrogen sul-fide and α-ketobutyrate. This is thought to be a minor pathway. Homo-cysteine is converted to homocystine both enzymatically and nonenzy-matically, the reaction being a reversible one. Most of the sulfur from cysteine is excreted as taurine and sulfate.

45

In homocystinuria this pattern of change is disrupted. There is now good evidence to show that the basic defect in this disorder is a deficiency or abnormality in hepatic cystathionine synthetase which prevents the formation of cystathionine from homocysteine (Mudd *et al*. 1964). The immediate result of this enzyme block is an accumulation of homocysteine in blood and tissues. This is a "nonthreshold" amino acid and is rapidly excreted in the urine in its oxidized form, homocystine. The back reaction to methionine is favored by the homocysteine accumulation and may result in high blood concentrations of methionine and in increased urinary excretion when its tubular reabsorptive capacity is exceeded.

Normally, cystathionine is present only in trace quantities in the blood and urine but in relatively high concentration in the brain. Autopsy studies reveal that cystathionine is low or absent in the brain of affected individuals (Brenton, Cusworth, and Gaull 1965). As cystine cannot be formed, it now becomes an essential amino acid and the patient depends on dietary intake for cystine requirements.

Nitrogen balance studies reported by Brenton and co-workers (1966) tend to confirm this fact. Brenton showed that in homocystinuric patients when methionine was the sole source of sulfur, negative nitrogen balance ensued. With the reintroduction of cystine, however, the patient returned to positive balance.

## Diagnosis

The biochemical diagnosis of homocystinuria is suggested by finding a positive nitroprusside-cyanide test in the urine. A positive reaction may be due to excess cystine or homocystine, and a chromatographic technique must be used to differentiate these two amino acids. Raised levels of homocystine are found in blood and urine. The syndrome may be accompanied by high blood methionine, although the levels of the latter vary greatly from patient to patient (for example, upper limits of normal to ten times normal). Two studies (Perry *et al*. 1966 and Komrower *et al*. 1966) report affected infants with methionine levels almost one hundred times the normal level. The mixed disulfide of homocystine and cystine is generally also raised in the blood. Cystine is either absent or only present in trace quantities.

It is important to note that in very young children there is little clinical evidence to suggest they are suffering from homocystinuria and, therefore, it seems to us particularly important that screening tests should be carried out on the urine of newborn children for the detection of this abnormality. It may be said that screening of this type is of little value without some hope of successful therapy, but it is surely valuable to parents to know at an early stage, should an abnormality of this type exist. Further, preliminary experiments suggest that it may be possible by treatment to modify the serum concentration of homocystine in affected children, and this modification might have an effect on the development of the clinical symptoms.

## Treatment

Treatment in the past has been directed toward giving these patients a diet low in methionine with added cystine and coenzymes $B_6$ and folic acid. This diet has been used in Northern Ireland in a severely retarded, hyperkinetic, five-year-old child without any clinical improvement being noted although with some biochemical success (Carson *et al.* 1965). Other workers (Komrower *et al.* 1966; Perry *et al.* 1966) have been more successful in treating cases discovered in the neonatal period. Their patients are still very young and attention has already been drawn to the fact that infants may have normal development for approximately the first to second year of life. Nevertheless, no mental deterioration or *ectopia lentis* has been reported thus far in their patients.

The logical step, the feeding of cystathionine, has not been attempted because of its expense, its high renal clearance, and lack of certainty that it would reach effective concentration in the brain.

M. C. Carey, J. J. Fennelly, and O. Fitzgerald (1967) have recently described low levels of fasting serum folic acid and have shown over-utilization of folic acid to occur. In 1961 A. R. Larrabee and his associates discovered that a folic acid derivative (N-methyltetrahydrofolic acid) was the direct methylating agent involved in the back reaction from homo-cysteine to methionine. Oral folic acid therapy when given to two siblings with homocystinuria resulted in increased transmethylation of homo-cysteine to methionine with a significant fall in urinary homocystine and an elevation in urinary methionine. This form of therapy may be of use in those patients who have methionine levels only slightly above normal.

In cystathioninuria, an inborn error also related to the metabolism of methionine, G. W. Frimpter, A. Haymovitz, and M. Horwith (1963) found that ingestion of high doses of $B_6$ caused a marked reduction in the excretion of cystathionine in the urine. Frimpter (1965) found that liver homogenates from two such patients cleaved radioactive cystathio-nine only slightly until excess of pyridoxine was added. The apoenzyme

47

TABLE 7

Change in Serum Levels of Homocystine and Cystine
after Two Weeks' Therapy with Oral Pyridoxine

| Patient | Age (in years) | Daily B$_6$ (in Mgs.) | Serum Homocystine* ($\mu$M/100 ml) | Serum Cystine** ($\mu$M/100 ml) |
|---|---|---|---|---|
| Mi. L. | 9/12 | 250 | 1.90–0.60 | 1.20–2.40 |
| F. L. | 5 | 300 | 3.05–1.50 | 0.80–2.04 |
| Ma. L. | 10 | 300 | 10.50–2.90 | 0–2.70 |
| A. McC. | 7 | 300 | 6.20–4.10 | 0–Trace |
| R. R. | 8 6/12 | 300 | 7.30–0.65 | 2.00–6.60 |
| M. Rit. | 15 | 400 | 7.30–8.60 | 0–0.40 |
| G. M. | 18 | 300 | 20.00–1.45 | 0–3.70 |
| J. R. | 20 | 450 | 16.00–30.00 | Trace–Trace |

\* No homocystine is normally present.
\*\* The normal range is 4.8 to 14.0 $\mu$M. per 100 ml. (ion exchange technique).

cystathionase failed to bind the coenzyme normally. C. R. Scriver (1960) in his article on Vitamin B$_6$ dependency and infantile convulsions suggested that the presence of an atypical apoenzyme may be the reason why children with this disorder require large doses of pyridoxine.

Preliminary communications on the treatment of homocystinuria with large doses of oral pyridoxine have been published by G. W. Barber and G. L. Spaeth (1967) and by C. Hooft, D. Carton, and W. Samyn (1967). These workers were able to reduce blood levels of methionine and blood and urine levels of homocystine. Barber and Spaeth had treated their patients for a six-month period with biochemical success.

We have attempted to treat nine homocystinuric patients with large doses of oral pyridoxine. The results are shown in Tables 7 and 8.

One patient J. Rit. has only been under treatment for two weeks at the time of writing but shows no biochemical response to date. M. Rit, her sibling, was also unresponsive to pyridoxine. The results to date in the remaining seven children are presented. We have achieved some success in modifying the biochemical picture in five of these children (Mi. L., F. L., Ma. L., R. R., and G. M.).

Levels of plasma methionine have been reduced to normal, although in most of the patients, traces of homocystine and mixed disulfide still remain. Serum cystine levels have increased. In two patients severely

TABLE 8

Results of Increased Dosage of Oral Pyridoxine Therapy

| Patient | Age | Initial Dose of $B_6$ (mgs/day) | Duration in Weeks | Serum Homocystine ($\mu$M/100 ml) | Present Dosage of $B_6$ (mgs/day) | Duration in Weeks | Serum Homocystine ($\mu$M/100 ml) |
|---|---|---|---|---|---|---|---|
| 1i. L. | $9/12$ | 200 | 3 | 0.95 | 250 | 5 | 0 |
| '. L. | 5 | 300 | 3 | 0.50 | 450 | 5 | 0 |
| 4a. L. | 10 | 300 | 3 | 1.0 | 450 | 5 | 0 |
| . McC. | $7\,6/12$ | 300 | 3 | 5.4 | 450 | 3 | 2.85 |
| . R. | 8 | 300 | 3 | 0 | 300 (unchanged) | 10 | 0 |
| i. M. | 18 | 300 | 4 | 1.9 | 450 | 14 | 1.2 |

affected clinically, one has shown no response and one has only now, after six weeks' therapy, shown a lowering of her homocystine levels.

These patients were all on a normal mixed diet, and no other vitamins or cystine supplements were given. They have been under treatment from six to thirteen weeks at the time of writing and no marked clinical improvement has been noted except that all have gained in weight over the period of treatment. One child, A. McC., has frequent petit mal fits and presents a particularly interesting case. Her fits became worse for the first two weeks after treatment commenced; then in the third and fourth week they moderated, and no fits were noted by the mother during the fifth and sixth weeks of therapy. This improvement may only be temporary, and we will have to wait for a longer period before claiming that pyridoxine treatment has been the cause of the improvement.

One other child, who was very nervous and excitable, has shown much improvement in his behavior at the hospital and during dental treatment (unsolicited report from the dentist, who did not know about attempted treatment). In contrast, the parents have not indicated any improvement in the home situation.

Complete understanding of the result achieved by high doses of pyridoxine must await further research, but experiments with homocystinuria liver homogenates to which have been added different quantities of $B_6$ would make an excellent study. It is difficult, from the printed work of S. H. Mudd (1964) on liver cystathionine synthetase and Frimpter

(1965) on cystathionase to compare the amounts of $B_6$ added to their liver homogenates.

## Complications

*Thrombosis.* Because of the tendency in these patients to form thrombi in arteries and veins, thrombotic episodes are to be expected and are treated with anticoagulants. Two of these patients have died as a result of a pulmonary embolus forming postoperatively after ophthalmic surgery. These deaths may be a coincidence. Nevertheless, the precaution of giving heparin to cover any surgical procedure and of continuing the medication until the patient is mobile again is now carried out in Belfast as a routine procedure. Under this regime, four patients have undergone ophthalmic surgery with no untoward results.

*Eye complications.* Three of our patients, aged eight, eighteen, and twenty-one years, first came to our attention through the Ophthalmic Department, where they were being treated for complete dislocation of a lens and secondary glaucoma. Clinically, they were mentally retarded, and all had Marfan-like physical features. Six other patients have also had eye complications requiring lens extractions in nine eyes. Ocular complications would appear to be more common in homocystinuria than in the Marfan syndrome. It is interesting that the dislocation of the lens in the latter syndrome is generally in an upward direction whereas in homocystinuria the dislocation is downward.

## Genetics

The familial nature of this disorder is evident from the fact that two or three affected siblings occurred in each of five families. The effective sibship data of the seventeen patients (eleven families) show that of forty-nine live individuals, seventeen were affected and thirty-two unaffected, with three early deaths and three miscarriages. The parents were all unaffected, and no history of consanguinity was elicited.

Family history indicated that three near relatives in three different families were possibly affected. These people were either dead or had left the country, and biochemical proof is, therefore, lacking. Of the seventeen affected relatives, ten were male and seven female. This data suggests an autosomal recessive type of inheritance in keeping with the type found in other inborn errors of amino acid metabolism.

The variability in the degree of mental retardation poses, as in other inborn conditions, questions that appear to strike at the fundamental concept of the genetically determined absence of an enzyme. If this concept be true, then it is necessary to postulate that in some affected individuals, ancillary pathways for the metabolism of methionine have been developed with the result that the brain is spared. One might suggest equally well that rather than the specific deficiency of cystathionine synthetase there is a deficiency of one isoenzyme, hepatic cystathionine synthetase. This deficiency would allow the individual reasonably normal mental development while at the same time he would show the other clinical stigmata of the disorder. There is abundant evidence for this concept of organ specificity of enzymes although we are unaware of any work relating the differential production of, say, myocardial and hepatic lactic dehydrogenase to different genes. Indeed, while it is known that certain properties of these two forms of lactic dehydrogenase are quite different, it is not clear whether these stem from differences in molecular formula or from differences in physical molecular association.

In the first family studied in Northern Ireland, a high incidence of schizophrenia was noted in the relatives. Similar findings have also been noted by other workers in England and America. Work on schizophrenia has suggested a disturbance in the process of transmethylation, and the significance of the findings in relatives of homocystinuric patients raises some interesting possibilities with regard to the etiology of schizophrenia (Osmond and Smythies 1952).

In this, as in other inborn errors of amino acid metabolism, the search must be for a definitive, yet practical, method to detect the heterozygotes. Theoretically, in homocystinuria, there should be a decreased level of cystathionine synthetase. Unfortunately, the enzyme has not been detected in skin, red blood cells, or white blood cells (Mudd 1964), the more readily available tissues for study.

J. D. Finkelstein and his associates (1964) have examined liver biopsies of the parents of affected children for cystathionine synthetase activity and have found the levels to be lower than the lowest values in a series of normal control subjects. This approach is, however, clearly not practical on a large scale. Methionine load tests have been performed, but the results on a few of the parents have been disappointing with regard to segregation of heterozygotes. One other possibility is electromyography, but again not enough parents have been studied to date.

Clearly, we are only now at the threshold of explaining this condition, but what has been done does at least point the way to specific fields for further investigation. Thus, there is obviously much further work to be carried out in tracing the association between the connective tissue and cardiovascular abnormalities and the primary biochemical lesion. The metabolism of cystathionine in the brain is fundamental to the mental retardation and requires elucidation. Of more practical importance is the elaboration of techniques capable of detecting the heterozygotes. Finally, our initial studies on the electromyography of muscle suggest that the biochemical abnormalities are also involved in the metabolism in these tissues.

# DISCUSSION

H. LEVY: Dr. Carson, we have had one experience in Massachusetts that was very interesting. We discovered a newborn in the Massachusetts screening program who had elevated levels of methionine in the blood and homocystine in the blood but did not have enough homocystine in the urine to yield a positive cyanide-nitroprusside test as late as three weeks of age even while on a normal diet. This finding is to some extent disturbing with regard to the process of screening newborns for homocystinuria by using the urinary cyanide-nitroprusside test. I might add that it contrasts with Dr. Perry's findings of a positive cyanide-nitroprusside test given within the first two weeks of life in a newborn homocystinuric. In view of this finding, we wonder if one can legitimately feel confident that one is screening effectively for homocystinuria in newborns by the use of the cyanide-nitroprusside test on the urine. It is our feeling at the present time (and again this is based on this single case) that one cannot effectively screen all newborns for homocystinuria by using only the cyanide-nitroprusside test, and, therefore, one must also look for an elevation of methionine in the blood. Dr. Carson, I would like to hear your comments about that. A second aspect of this business is that Dr. Perry's patient as well as Dr. Komrower's patient had marked elevations of methionine during the newborn period.

N. CARSON: How long have you followed this child?

H. LEVY: We have followed him now for about seven and one-half months. He is now eight months of age. This is the patient I wrote you about, as a matter of fact. His cousin is in an institution for the mentally retarded in Ireland. This patient's parents migrated from Dublin, I think, about three years ago. And because the cousin is mentally retarded, we felt certain she also had homocystinuria.

N. CARSON: Sorry to disappoint you.

H. LEVY: But, we have treated him now for seven and one-half months with a low methionine diet. The plasma methionine, which was initially about 13 or 14 mg. per cent on a normal neonatal diet, came down to the 4–6 mg. per cent range. The child has done extremely well in growth and development—including mental development. At the time of diagnosis, we discovered that his retarded sister, who is two and one-half years old, also had homocystinuria. We are guarded in our prognosis, however, since it is still far too early to tell how this infant will turn out. Interestingly enough, although we can get his methionine level down to 3 or 4 mg. per cent with a low-methionine diet, this is still about eight times normal by our standards. We have not been able to get his methionine down to lower levels than that; again, this experience is similar to Perry's findings. Recently, in the last month or month and a half, his methionine levels have bounced up to about 10 mg. per cent in the plasma on the same low-methionine diet. However, homocystine has remained absent from the plasma and quite low in the urine so we are encouraged by these findings. We have evidence that maybe methionine is not the compound causing brain damage. We have two patients now (two and one-half years of age and about nine or ten months of age) who have had elevations of methionine but no homocystine for the first four or five months of life. They have had no evidence of homocystinuria and they were not treated but were allowed to have high levels of methionine (as high as 25 mg. per cent) for these four or five months of life. Both children are now perfectly normal so we can say unequivocally that in these two children plasma methionine levels as high as 25 mg. per cent for perhaps as long as four to five months have caused no apparent brain damage. With this scanty evidence we would suspect that methionine does not do the damage. If an amino acid does cause the brain damage, perhaps it is homocystine.

N. CARSON: That is very interesting. The sister of the child with hypermethioninemia—did she have all the clinical features of the homocystinuric?

H. LEVY: She is now three years of age. When we saw her initially she was two and one-half years old. She has a very beautiful malar flush, a waddling gait that you have already described so beautifully, and she is developmentally retarded. The parents know she has been developmentally retarded from approximately the eighth to tenth month of life. At ten months she was just beginning to sit alone. She has no other neurologic findings. Dr. Mudd has now succeeded in demonstrating the presence of cystathionine synthetase activity in cultures of skin fibroblasts in normal individuals and has found that perhaps seven or eight homocystinurics have not had activity of this enzyme in their fibroblasts. It now appears that Dr. Mudd has provided a convenient method of looking at the enzyme. Perhaps in relation to what was mentioned about the vitamin $B_6$ business, we may now have an available method of checking its efficacy in vitro in these patients. We have, by the way, treated three or four patients with pyridoxine and have seen no effect whatsoever.

N. CARSON: We have had a mixed response among seven patients treated; five have responded and two were biochemically resistant to therapy.

H. LEVY: Our findings contrast, of course, not only with your findings but with other recently reported findings of biochemical amelioration by pyridoxine. We have wondered if there may not be different forms of homocystinuria—at least one form pyridoxine-sensitive and another pyridoxine-resistant.

N. CARSON: In fact, one form may be a genetic deficiency of the apoenzyme, and the other may be an abnormality in the apoenzyme itself or in the activation of apoenzyme with coenzyme. All our patients have had low methionine levels compared to some reports in the literature, and we wondered if by adding folic acid to the therapy, we could have a further decrease in the serum homocystine levels.

H. LEVY: We have not treated our two younger patients with folic acid. We have, however, determined serum folate activity in both and find that one is high normal while the other is low normal.

N. CARSON: Yes, ours are mostly right down to the lower limits of normal.

P. DOYLE: I wonder if I could ask a clinical question about the epidemic we had about twelve years ago with a deficiency of pyridoxine because Similac was autoclaved too vigorously. Many children developed convulsions. Many clinicians were giving high doses of pyridoxine for seizures with no result. In my trips to Latin America, I found that the German pharmaceutical companies were active. For example, every retarded child I saw in Ecuador had been given high doses of pyridoxine because the companies were pushing it as something that might yield the results that glutamic used to yield. They feel that the retarded patient can function better. Have you seen retarded patients improve with high doses of pyridoxine? Do you have comments on that?

N. CARSON: I have only had a few cases that I could honestly say were due to pyridoxine deficiency, and these patients have responded to pyridoxine therapy and are continuing on it. It certainly controls their fits.

55

# REFERENCES

Barber, G. W., and Spaeth, G. L. 1967. Pyridoxine therapy in homocystinuria. *Lancet* 1:337.

Brenton, D. P., Cusworth, D. C., and Gaull, G. E. 1965. Homocystinuria: Biochemical studies of tissues including a comparison with cystathioninuria. *Pediatrics* 35:50.

Brenton, D. P., Cusworth, D. C., Dent, C. E., and Jones, E. E. 1966. Homocystinuria. Clinical and dietary studies. *Quart. J. Med.* 35:325.

Carey, M. C., Fennelly, J. J., and Fitzgerald, O. 1966. Folate metabolism in homocystinuria. *Irish J. Med. Sci.* 6:488.

Carson, N. A. J., and Neill, D. W. 1962. Metabolic abnormalities detected in a survey of mentally backward individuals in Northern Ireland. *Arch. Dis. Child.* 37:505.

Carson, N. A. J., Dent, C. E., Field, C. M. B., and Gaull, G. E. 1965. Homocystinuria: Clinical and pathological review of ten cases. *J. Pediat.* 66:565.

Finkelstein, J. D., Mudd, H. S., Irreverre, F., and Laster, L. 1964. Homocystinuria due to cystathionine synthetase deficiency: The mode of inheritance. *Science* 146:785.

Frimpter, G. W. 1965. Cystathioninuria: Nature of the defect. *Science* 149:1095.

Frimpter, G. W., Haymovitz, A., and Horwith, M. 1963. Cystathioninuria. *New Eng. J. Med.* 268:333.

Gibson, J. B., Carson, N. A. J., and Neill, D. W. 1964. Pathological findings in homocystinuria. *J. Clin. Path.* 17:427.

Komrower, G. M., Lambert, A. M., Cusworth, D. C., and Westall, R. G. 1966. Dietary treatment of homocystinuria. *Arch. Dis. Child.* 41:666.

Hooft, C., Carton, D., and Samyn, W. 1967. Pyridoxine treatment in homocystinuria. *Lancet* 1:1384.

Hurwitz, L. J., Chopra, J. S., and Carson, N. A. J. 1968. Electromyographic evidence of a muscle lesion in homocystinuria. *Acta Paed. Scand.* 57:401.

Larrabee, A. R., Rosenthal, S., Cathon, R. E., and Buchanan, J. M. 1961. A methylated derivative of tetrahydrofolate as an intermediate of methionine biosynthesis. *J. Am. Chem. Soc.* 83:4094.

Lynas, M. A., and Merrett, J. D. 1958. Data on linkage in man: Marfan's syndrome in Northern Ireland. *Ann. Hum. Genet.* 22:310.

Loughridge, L. W. 1959. Renal abnormalities in the Marfan syndrome. *Quart. J. Med.* 28:531.

McDonald, L., Bray, C., Field, C., Love, F., and Davies, B. 1964. Homocystinuria, thrombosis and the bloodplatelets. *Lancet* 1:745.

## Homocystinuria

Mudd, S. H., Finkelstein, J. D., Irreverre, F., and Laster, L. 1964. Homocystinuria: An enzymatic defect. *Science* 143:1443.

Osmond, H., and Smythies, J. 1952. Schizophrenia: New approach. *J. Ment. Sci.* 98:309.

Perry, T. L., Dunn, H. G., Hansen, S., MacDougall, L., and Warrington, P. D. 1966. Early diagnosis and treatment of homocystinuria. *Pediatrics* 37:502.

Schimke, R. N., McKusick, V. A., Huang, T., and Pollock, A. D. 1965. Homocystinuria studies of 20 families with 38 affected members. *J.A.M.A.* 193:711.

Scriver, C. R. 1960. Vitamin $B_6$-dependency and infantile convulsions. *Pediatrics* 26:62.

Smith, S. W. 1967. Roentgen findings in homocystinuria. *Am. J. Roentgenology* 100:147.

57

# Histidinemia to Date

H. GHADIMI, M.D.

*Downstate Medical Center, State University of New York,
and Methodist Hospital of Brooklyn*

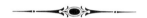

In 1960 at the Grand Rounds conducted at the Hospital for Sick Children in Toronto, a three-year-old girl, initials M. M., was introduced as "atypical phenylketonuria." The little girl with blue eyes and fair hair had no abnormal physical signs except for a speech defect and intention tremor of the hands. She used a certain amount of jargon so that her parent could understand more of what she said than an outsider could. She was somewhat emotionally unstable. She was not able to inhibit her anger or her pleasure in the normal way expected at her age. Her I.Q. was 93.

The laboratory work-up of the patient showed negative results except for persistent positive ferric chloride test of the urine. The patient was labeled as "atypical phenylketonuric" because, in spite of positive ferric chloride and Phenistix tests, the blood phenylalanine remained within normal range. The patient was being treated with a low phenylalanine diet.

Since blood phenylalanine remained within normal range, the diagnosis of phenylketonuria was challenged. This challenge resulted in intensive studies to establish the true nature of the disease. As a result of this research the "Inborn Error of Histidine Metabolism" was introduced to medical literature.

By recapitulating the story, I wish to emphasize the importance of avoiding the term "atypical." "Atypical something" most probably means an "atypical diagnosis," or an "atypical element in diagnosis," or an expedient, but not a realistic approach to the fine art of diagnosis.

## Histidinemia

Had we accepted the original diagnosis of "atypical phenylketonuria," the patient would have stayed on a cumbersome and superfluous diet of low phenylalanine.

Above all, the "Inborn Error of Histidine Metabolism" would still be pleading for recognition.

To date the number of reported "Inborn Error of Histidine Metabolism" cases exceeds twenty (see Table 9). I have heard of approximately twenty-five additional cases, which were recognized during the last four years but have not been reported. Two-thirds of the patients are female. Age range is one month to thirteen years. The oldest patient is the most retarded, but this finding does not mean that the degree of retardation necessarily increases with age. Excluding the three patients under one year of age, thirteen out of seventeen patients have speech defects. Except for high incidence of speech retardation, there is no special clinical characteristic for histidinemia. The speech defect per se has no pattern particular to histidinemia. With the high incidence of speech defect in histidinemia it is tempting to assume that a high concentration of histidine or one of its metabolites affects a particular area of the brain causing a specific defect. This explanation, of course, still remains in the hypothetical stage. It is possible that a speech defect is a forerunner or a mild manifestation of mental retardation.

The degree of mental retardation varies greatly. There are among those twenty cases, four normal-looking healthy children with a definite biochemical anomaly. On the other end of the scale there are six patients who are grossly retarded with an I.Q. of 50 or so. The I.Q. of the remaining seven range from 65 to 85. The limited data available at present suggest that the degree and incidence of retardation in histidinemia are much smaller than in phenylketonuria.

### Nomenclature

The name originally suggested was "Inborn Error of Histidine Metabolism." V. H. Auerbach and his associates (1962), when introducing the second report of the condition, suggested the name of "histidinemia," which was promptly accepted, perhaps because of its shortness and simplicity. The shortcoming of the new name is its lack of specificity, since transient histidinemia probably exists in early pregnancy. Moreover, it is possible that other conditions causing high blood histidine may yet be discovered. It is also unfortunate that the name describes a state in the blood, namely the presence of histidine, which is a normal and healthy state.

59

TABLE 9

Salient Features of Histidinemia Reported to Date

| Author | No. of Cases | Sex | Age | Speech Retardation | Intelligence | Other Symptoms | Plasma Histidine mg.% | Urine Histidine mg/24 hrs. | Histidase Activity in Skin |
|---|---|---|---|---|---|---|---|---|---|
| Ghadimi, H. et al. 1961 and 1962 | 2 | F | 3 Y | + | I.Q. 85 | Frequent infection, fair hair, blue eyes | 9.01 | 616 | Absent |
| | | F | 4 Y | – | Normal | | 7.13 | 819 | Absent |
| Auerbach, V. H. et al. 1962 | 1 | F | 4 Y 4 Mo. | + | I.Q. 83 | Small stature, fair hair, blue eyes | 15.8 | 506 | NS |
| La Du, B. N. et al. 1963 | 2 | F | 6 Y | + | Normal | Fair skin, blonde hair, blue eyes, mirror writing | 17.3 | 378 | Absent |
| | | M | 5 Y | + | Normal | | 13.4 | 850 | Absent |
| Andrews, B. F. et al. 1926 | 2 | F | 5 Y 6 Mo. | + | I.Q. 85 | Small stature, blue eyes | Higher than Normal | NR | NS |
| | | F | 7 Y | – | Normal | | | NR | NS |
| Hudson, F. P. et al. 1963 | 2 | M | 8 Y | + | Retarded | | Higher than Normal | NR | NS |
| | | NR | 1 Mo. | ? | ? | | | NR | NS |
| Davies, H. E., and Robinson, M. J. 1963 | 1 | M | 5 Y | – | Mildly retarded | Physical development below tenth percentile, brown hair, brown eyes | 9 | 312,578 | NS |
| Snyder, S. H. et al. 1963 | 1 | F | 8 Y | + | I.Q. 65 | Precocious puberty, hemivertebrae, dislocated patella | 15 | 26* | NS |

| Reference | N | Sex | Age | Mental status | | Clinical description | | | |
|---|---|---|---|---|---|---|---|---|---|
| Shaw, K. et al. 1963 | 1 | F | 13 Y | I.Q. 50 | + | Fair hair, blue eyes | 4.5-5.3 | 340-680† | NS |
| Gerritsen, T. 1964 | 3 | M<br>F<br>F | 3 Y<br>1 Y<br>10 Y 6 Mo. | Retarded<br>?<br>I.Q. 85 | +<br>?<br>- | ——<br>——<br>—— | 8<br>NR<br>NR | 600<br>NR<br>NR | NS<br>NS<br>NS |
| Holton, J. B. et al. 1964 | 1 | M | 6 Mo. | ? | ? | Frequent infection | 14 | 218 | Absent |
| Clarance, G., and Bowman, J. K. 1966 | 1 | F | 13 Y | I.Q. 54 | + | Height and weight below third percentile, short squat appearance, blue eyes, light hair | 11.2 | 599 | Absent |
| Woody, N. C. et al. 1965 | 3 | M<br>M<br>F | 11 Y<br>10 Y<br>6 Y | I.Q. 52<br>I.Q. 47<br>I.Q. 53 | +<br>+<br>+ | All have abnormal EEG's, fair hair, blue eyes. 10 Y has depigmented area of skin suggesting tuberous sclerosis | 1.8-4.3<br>1.5-6.4<br>1.4-3.4 | 500-2200†<br>500-2000†<br>250-800† | Present<br>Present<br>Present |
| Summary | 20 | 12 F<br>7 M<br>1 NR | 1 Mo.-13 Y | 6 I.Q. below 65<br>7 Mild retardation<br>4 Normal<br>3 Undecided | 13 +<br>4 -<br>3 ? | | Generally above 8 mg. % | 3-15 times normal | |

† = mg/gm creatinine
+ = Present
- = Absent

NS = Not studied
NR = Not reported
* = mg./kg body weight

Calling "Inborn Error of Histidine Metabolism," "histidinemia" is like choosing "glycemia" to name "diabetes mellitus." Altogether, the adoption of new terminology, namely adding the suffix "emia" to the name of the amino acid involved, leaves much to be desired. By no stretch of the imagination could it be used for all amino-acidopathies, since "Inborn Error of Amino Acid Metabolism" may exist without increased blood concentration of the incriminated amino acid—as, for example, in cystinuria and argininosuccinicaciduria. In conditions where the site of the enzymic block has been elucidated, the specificity of the nomenclature can best be retained by the use of the involved enzyme as the root of the new name. In this case, "histidinemia" would have been called "histidase deficiency."

## Biochemical Abnormality

A host of biochemical abnormalities results from deficiency or absence of histidase activity. Histidine (Fig. 10), as its chemical name (alpha-amino-beta-imidazolyl-propionic acid) implies, consists of an imidazole ring with an alanine side chain. We are not certain whether histidine is an essential amino acid, but the necessity for its presence in the diet in infancy has been established by S. E. Snyderman and his associates (1963).

Histidine forms carnosine by uniting with $\beta$-alanine. Carnosine is abundantly found in muscle. There was no indication of any gross muscular anomaly in the patient.

Histidine can be methylated on position 1 or 3 to make 1 or 3 methyl histidine. The presence of these methylated compounds in the biological fluids of the patient indicated that this pathway of histidine was open.

Enzymic decarboxylation of histidine results in histamine formation. Histamine eventually breaks down to imidazoleacetic acid. In animals, less than 1 per cent of ingested histidine forms histamine (Van Arsdel and Beall 1960). The skin of our patient reacted in a normal way after the injection of histamine liberator. The appearance of the wheel and flair, in the same size as in the control, indicated that histamine was present in the skin of the patient. These three pathways of histidine metabolism play a minor role in the economy of the substance, and therefore, a block in this direction could not have caused excessive accumulation of histidine in the blood.

Histidine, like other amino acids, participates in protein synthesis. The breakdown of protein in the body results in the release of histidine. We had no indication of any anomaly in protein synthesis. Hemoglobin is par-

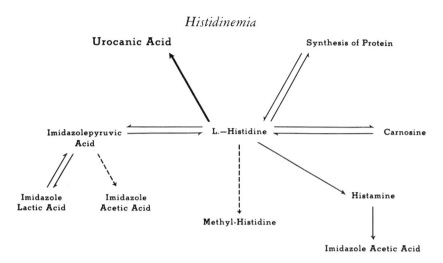

*Histidinemia*

FIGURE 10.  Metabolic pathways of histidine.

ticularly rich in histidine, yet there was no suggestion of any interference in hemoglobin formation. The patient did not have anemia. Starch block electrophoresis of the patient's hemoglobin revealed a normal mobility.

Histidine through deamination or transamination forms imidazole pyruvic acid. The latter then may be reduced to imidazolactic acid or converted to imidazoleacetic acid by undergoing decarboxylation. This route is similar to the subsidiary pathway of other amino acids and has the capacity to expand on demand. The high blood concentration of histidine may enhance the use of this pathway. However, even if this pathway operated at full capacity it still could not eliminate histidine as efficiently as the major catabolic pathway. Paper chromatography of the urine of the patients using specific staining techniques showed great excess of the aforementioned imidazole compounds, meaning that this pathway was fully exploited.

The major catabolic pathway of histidine starts with enzymic deamination of histidine to urocanic acid. The enzyme involved in this step is histidine deaminase, or histidase. Urocanic acid is then hydrolyzed to imidazolonepropionic acid by the action of the enzyme urokinase. Imidazolonepropionic acid is transformed to formiminoglutamic acid (FIGLU), and then to glutamic acid.

Considering the magnitude of the blood histidine concentration in histidinemia, we suspected from the beginning that the block was in the major catabolic pathway of histidine or in that pathway which leads to glutamic acid through urocanic acid. Further investigation proved that the block was indeed in the first step in this direction.

Abnormally low concentrations of glutamic acid in all biological fluids of our two original patients were noticed despite persistently high concentrations of histidine in the blood. This phenomenon was also observed in the samples obtained during the histidine loading test. Glutamic acid was not detectable on paper chromatograms of the fasting blood and urinary samples of the two controls. However, it appeared in substantial quantities after the administration of histidine accompanied by a temporary increase of glutamine. In sharp contrast, the corresponding paper chromatograms of the two patients' samples showed no glutamic acid, even after a histidine load (applying the conventional amount of sample on the filter paper).

Moreover, we found no trace of other metabolites of the major catabolic pathway in the biological fluids of the two patients, even under the stress of loading conditions. Urocanic acid, imidazolonepropionic acid, and FIGLU were not detected on the paper chromatograms of the samples showing the peak concentration of histidine.

This evidence indicated that the block in histidinemia was definitely in the conversion of histidine to glutamic acid, or, in the major catabolic pathway. To further delineate the site of the block in this direction, Auerbach and his associates (1962) studied the effect of the histidine load on excretion of FIGLU. They noticed that histidinemic patients failed to excrete FIGLU following oral administration of histidine, whereas controls did excrete FIGLU. This finding was also confirmed by B. N. La Du and his co-workers (1963).

Auerbach's group also observed that, after intravenous administration of urocanic acid (1 gm. sodium salt), to histidinemic patients, urocanic acid, imidazolonepropionic acid, and FIGLU appeared in the urine. Neither of these substances could be detected after administration of histidine.

Conclusive evidence of the absence of histidase activity in histidinemic patients came from La Du's laboratory. The ingenious observation that, in normal individuals, the *stratum corneum* contains histidase, made direct enzymic assay expedient. An enzymic assay based on the rate of urocanic acid formation was devised. In a procedure as simple as a manicure, the cuticles and dead skin around the nails can be removed and subjected to enzymic analysis. More tissues can be obtained from the sole of the foot. The tissues of La Du's two patients showed no urocanic acid formation and, therefore, no enzymic activity. The parents and a normal sibling showed about the lower limits of normal.

Recently, Dr. Vincent Zannoni, who worked with the original group of enzymic assays, has kindly analyzed the *stratum corneum* of our two patients and their parents. As expected, no enzymic activity was found in the tissue of the two patients. The rate of urocanic acid formation in the *stratum corneum* of the parents was about half the lower limit of normality.

## Abnormal Metabolites

With the block at the first step of the major catabolic route, accumulation of histidine in the blood and excessive excretion in the urine results. The exact level of blood histidine needed to trigger operation of the alternate or subsidiary pathway is not known. However, at a concentration of about 6 mg. of histidine per 100 ml., imidazolepyruvic acid, a product of the subsidiary pathway, is found in the urine. Such urine will react positively with ferric chloride and Phenistix.

The biochemical consequences of the histidase deficiency are:

1. Increased histidine concentration in the blood, urine, and CSF.

2. Excretion of large amounts of imidazolepyruvic acid, imidazolelactic acid, and imidazoleacetic acid in the urine of the patients.

3. Low blood concentration of glutamic acid.

4. High blood and urine concentrations of $\alpha$-alanine.

5. Perhaps, low blood serotonin due to interference with tryptophan metabolism.

The last two findings warrant some comment. The increased $\alpha$-alanine excretion was reported in our original paper (Ghadimi, Partington, and Hunter 1961). Later on, Auerbach and his co-workers (1962) reported similar findings. The most recent analysis of blood from our two patients by column chromatography revealed a concentration of approximately 9 mg. per 100 ml. An oral loading dose of 6 gm. of histidine monhydrochloride did not affect the $\alpha$-alanine levels. Therefore, $\alpha$-alanine could not result from breakdown of histidine to imidazole ring and $\alpha$-alanine chain. It is, however, of interest to note that in another condition associated with histidinuria, namely pregnancy, definite but not substantial increase of $\alpha$-alanine does occur. The chemical relation of $\alpha$-alaninemuria to histidinemia remains to be discovered.

A disturbance in tryptophan metabolism which results in low blood serotonin has been reported in phenylketonuria and may contribute to mental retardation. Low blood serotonin has also been reported in Auerbach's histidinemic patient. Holton (1964), reporting on a six-month-old boy with histidinemia, states that "the platelet 5-hydroxy tryptamine level, which was negligible on the uncontrolled diet, became normal on the reduced histidine intake." Our studies on our original patients have not supported this.

### Relation of Biochemical Abnormality to Clinical Manifestation

In histidinemia, as in phenylketonuria, the relation of the biochemical abnormality to the clinical manifestation is not clear. In histidinemia, however, there is a wider variation in clinical manifestations and more patients are spared mental retardation. Comparatively lower concentrations of histidine and, perhaps, the higher capacity of the subsidiary pathway of histidine than that of phenylalanine may account for the milder degree of mental retardation or for its absence.

The protein intake during early infancy may also play a role in the clinical manifestation of the disease. Our older patient has a definite metabolic anomaly but shows no sign of mental retardation or speech defect. This patient was on a regular diet during infancy. The younger patient, who has a speech defect, was put on a high protein diet during early infancy because of recurrent diarrhea. She consumed an average of 5 gm. of protein per kg. of body weight per day. We believe that this high-protein diet, administered during the crucial period of brain and speech development, resulted in a high concentration of histidine in the blood and has contributed to the manifestation of speech retardation.

### Diagnosis

Use of the ferric chloride test to screen patients in speech clinics may result in the detection of new cases, provided the patients are on a normal or high-protein diet. The urine of histidinemic patients with normal or high-protein intake will develop a green color with 10 per cent ferric chloride solution. However, the urine of histidinemics on a low-protein diet may not react positively with ferric chloride or Phenistix. Patients with mental retardation of unknown etiology should also be tested for histidinemia. For diagnosis of histidinemia in early infancy, a urinary ferric chloride test in the second week of life is recommended. The confirmation of the diagnosis should always include a quantitative determination of blood histidine. A histidine loading test, as well as determination of FIGLU in the twenty-four-hour urinary collection following administration of a histidine load, also aids the diagnosis. Finally, confirmation of the diagnosis by a direct enzymic assay is highly desirable.

## Genetics

The mode of inheritance is recessive. As in any recessive condition the first question asked is, "how can we recognize heterozygotes?" The answer is very simple. One day the sister of my patient asked, "Doctor, do you know how to catch a lion?" I answered "no." She told me that it is very easy, you catch two, and let one go. Here too, all you need to do is find a patient with histidinemia. The parents of such patients are heterozygotes. This, of course, is the most reliable way of diagnosis of heterozygotes.

The expression of the heterozygocity of the parents is well reflected in biochemical studies. Generally, parents have elevated concentrations of blood histidine and increased urinary output of the substance. However, some values may overlap the normal range. The response to an orally administered load of histidine may also point to heterozygocity. The percentage of the loading dose recovered in the urine is another way of detecting heterozygotes. The parents of our patients excreted 7.8 per cent and 13.2 per cent of the administered dose in contrast to 1.2, 2.1, and 5.7 per cent observed in three controls. Estimation of FIGLU in the twenty-four-hour urine collection after the administration of a histidine load offers another approach to identification of heterozygotes. Finally, La Du's test, the estimation of histidase activity in *stratum corneum*, would show values around the lower limit of normal.

## Treatment

The similarities between phenylketonuria and histidinemia make it tempting to institute a low-histidine diet in early infancy. The blood histidine should be kept within a permissible range, perhaps not higher than 6 mg. per 100 ml. This probably could be accomplished by administration of low-protein diet.

# DISCUSSION

W. McIsaac: Is it possible that any of the symptomatology could be due to urocanic acid deficiency? If so, since urocanic acid is readily available and inexpensive, might it not be used as a therapeutic agent?

H. Ghadimi: The use of urocanic acid as a therapeutic agent would have been indicated if we knew that the clinical manifestations of histidinemia were caused by a lack of that substance. In phenylketonuria it has been speculated that the comparatively low tyrosine level may play a role in the clinical manifestations of the disease. The analogy is permissible. Phenylalanine is converted to tyrosine, which is a very important amino acid because it is a precursor of very important substances such as adrenaline, noradrenal, and melanin.

In histidinemia, the block is in the major catabolic pathway. I am not aware of any particular significance of the metabolites of the catabolic pathways, except that a catabolic pathway is an outlet that does not permit the concentration of the substance to rise above a certain level. In other words, I assume that increased concentration of the metabolite, in this case histidine, plays a major role in the mechanism leading to the clinical manifestations. I may add that most of the metabolites of the catabolic pathways are nonthreshold substances. They are eliminated through the kidneys at a low blood concentration. That, too, may indicate that these susbtances are not important.

N. Carson: Dr. Ghadimi, is there any correlation between blood histidine levels and brain damage?

H. Ghadimi: Based on the limited data available, no correlation between the blood histidine levels and brain damage can be established. I believe that even in phenylketonuria, which has been studied so extensively, no such correlation has been established. Part of our problem, both in histidinemia and in phenylketonuria, arises from the fact that we do not know the levels of the incriminated amino acids at the crucial time of brain development. The oldest histidinemic patient reported so far happened to be the most retarded. Her blood histidine level was 4 to 5 mg.

per 100 ml.; this level is not very high. Obviously, we have no idea about her blood histidine level during early infancy. This patient was reported by Dr. Shaw and his co-workers from Los Angeles. Maybe Dr. Donnell will comment on their patient.

G. DONNELL: Dr. Ghadimi, the patient you allude to was one studied by Drs. Shaw and Elena Boder. She was a thirteen-year-old girl with normal physical development but severe mental retardation. Histidine concentration in blood ranged from 4 to 5 mg. per cent. Histidine concentration in urine was three to four times normal. By preference this girl selected a low-protein diet, a selection that may explain the relatively low blood histidine values in this girl.

H. LEVY: We have checked three cases of histidinemia as I mentioned in previous conversations. The first patient, discovered by Dr. Efron, was two and one-half years of age. The blood levels initially and on several subsequent occasions while the child was on a normal protein intake, were about 13 mg. per cent. He is perfectly normal although he had hypogammaglobulinemia during the first year of life. We have specimens on two other patients; one set of these specimens was sent to us by Dr. Maurice Kibel of Rhodesia. The Rhodesian child has had blood levels of 13 to 14 mg. per cent on two separate occasions. This child is severely retarded and has arachnodactyly. It was originally thought on clinical grounds that this child had homocystinuria, but much to everyone's surprise she turned out to have histidinemia. The third patient we have checked is five years of age, mentally retarded, and hyperactive. He has a histidine blood level of over 12 mg. per cent. I can say that out of three patients, two of them are severely retarded, and one is not retarded at all. There has been no essential difference in the histidine concentrations in the blood. May I say one other thing? Have you had any trouble in obtaining 25 mg. of *stratum corneum?*

H. GHADIMI: No, we did not encounter any difficulty.

H. LEVY: It is an ingenious test devised by an ingenious individual, and we think it is superb, but there is only one little problem—one needs at least 25 mg. of skin. This may not be much, but we cannot obtain by any means whatsoever short of major surgery 25 mg. of *stratum corneum* on anybody under four years of age. As a matter of fact, we cannot even get over 10 mg. of *stratum corneum* on anybody under four years of age. It is practically impossible because there is very little *stratum corneum* at this age and even less cooperation on the part of the patient.

H. GHADIMI: We had no difficulty in obtaining *stratum corneum* from our patients. They volunteered to supply it themselves. A sharp nail-clipper is all that is required. You can get an abundant specimen from the sole of the foot where *stratum corneum* is generally thick.

H. LEVY: Well, we think it is difficult, even using the feet. But in lieu of this type of test we have given a very simple test, which I think anyone could do with the basic chromatographic technique. We have now tested about sixty-four normals and three histidinemics and find it to be perfectly acceptable to substantiate the diagnosis of histidinemia. This is an indirect test for the enzyme, histidase. We take less than 2 mg. of *stratum corneum*, homogenize this skin in any way, apply the entire homogenate to Whatman 3MM chromatography paper, and chromatograph in butanol:acetic acid:water solvent overnight. We then stain with diazotized sulfanilic acid and look for urocanic acid. In the sixty or so normals this technique has revealed plenty of urocanic acid whereas in the three histidinemics no urocanic acid was found. This result, of course, is an indirect confirmation of Dr. La Du's findings, but, nevertheless, it is a step toward a simple indirect analysis for the enzyme which can be done in many clinical laboratories.

H. GHADIMI: Unless you wash your specimen thoroughly before homogenizing, I would suspect that the urocanic acid recovered on the paper chromatogram is from sweat, which is rich in this substance. Dr. Nyhan, I believe, has been using this approach for the diagnosis of histidinemia.

W. NYHAN: We have been testing for urocanic acid in sweat. The technique we have developed involved the separation of urocanic acid using a sephadex column. This method gives us an assay of very high specificity for the compound. On the other hand, the ultimate diagnosis of histidinemia involves the elegant assay for the enzyme developed by La Du and colleagues.

# REFERENCES

Andrews, B. F., Crosby, P. F., and Angel, C. R. 1926. Histidinemia: A new metabolic disorder. *Southern Med. J.* 55:1326.

Auerbach, V. H., DiGeorge, A. M., Baldridge, R. C., Tourtelotte, C. D., and Brigham, M. P. 1962. Histidinemia. *J. Pediat.* 60:487.

Clarance, G. A., and Bowman, J. K. 1966. Further case of histidinemia. *Brit. Med. J.* 1:1019.

Davies, H. E., and Robinson, M. J. 1963. A case of histidinemia. *J. Clin. Endocr.* 38:80.

Gerritsen, T. Histidinemia and mental retardation. 1964. In *Proceedings of the international Copenhagen congress on the scientific study of mental retardation.* 1:94. Geneva: Karger Publishing Company.

Ghadimi, H., Partington, M. W., and Hunter, A.

1961. A familial disturbance of histidine metabolism. *New Eng. J. Med.* 265:221.

1962. Inborn error of histidine metabolism. *Pediatrics* 29:714.

Holton, J. B. 1964. Histidinemia. In *Federation of European biochemical societies,* p. 117. Abstracts of Communications Presented at the First Meeting of the Federation. New York: Academic Press.

Holton, J. B., Lewis, F. J. W., and Moore, G. R. 1964. Biochemical investigation of histidinemia. *J. Clin. Path.* 17:671.

Hudson, F. P., Dickinson, R. A., and Ireland, J. T. 1963. Experience in the detection and treatment of phenylketonuria. *Pediatrics* 31 (pt. 1, no. 1): 47.

La Du, B. N., Howell, R. R., Jacoby, G. A., Seegmiller, J. E., Sober, E. K., Zannoni, V. G., Canby, J. P., and Ziegler, L. K. 1963. Clinical and biochemical studies on two cases of histidinemia. *Pediatrics* 32:216.

Shaw, K. N. F., Boder, E., Gutenstein, M., and Jacobs, E. E. 1963. Histidinemia. *J. Pediat.* 63:720.

Snyder, S. H., Myron, P., Kies, M. W., and Berlow, S. 1963. Metabolism of 2-C14-labeled L-histidine in histidinemia. *J. Clin. Endocr. & Metab.* 23:595.

Snyderman, S. E., Boyer, A., Roitman, E., Holt, L. E., Jr., and Prose, P. H. 1963. The histidine requirement of the infant. *Pediatrics* 31:786.

Van Arsdel, P. P., Jr., and Beall, G. N. 1960. The metabolism and functions of histamine. *Arch. Int. Med.* 106:714.

Woody, N. C., Snyder, C. H., and Harris, J. A. 1965. Histidinemia. *Am. J. Child.* 110:606.

# Recent Observations in Hyperglycinemia

WILLIAM L. NYHAN, M.D., Ph.D., and TOSHIYUKI ANDO, M.D.

*Departments of Pediatrics and Biochemistry, University
of Miami School of Medicine, Miami, Florida*

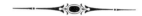

Hyperglycinemia is one of the new disorders of amino acid metabolism. It is characterized by the presence of abnormal concentrations of glycine in the blood, urine, and cerebrospinal fluid. Our initial description of this condition, the first case of hyperglycinemia, was reported in 1961 (Childs *et al.*). We have now had experience with five patients, and other cases have been reported from various parts of the world.

It is now apparent that there are at least two forms of glycinemia, and they appear to be distinct diseases. We have called the first type ketotic hyperglycinemia. It is characterized by recurrent episodes of ketosis leading to coma. The second type, which was first described by T. Gerritsen, E. Kaveggia, and H. A. Waisman (1965), lacked this and other clinical aspects of the syndrome but had convulsions and a decreased excretion of oxalic acid in the urine. Two siblings reported by C. C. Mabry and A. Karam (1963) may represent the same or an additional syndrome, and A. Prader (1967) has studied a patient with hyperglycinemia that was associated neither with ketosis nor with hypooxaluria. Tentatively, we have classified hyperglycinemia as ketotic and nonketotic. Glycine metabolism is complex, and I think it is likely that there will ultimately be a number of distinct disorders all of which are primary hyperglycinemia. We have felt that the patient described by J. M. Freeman and his colleagues (1964), in whom hyperammonemia and dimin-

TABLE 10

Clinical Manifestations of Hyperglycinemia

| Ketotic Type | Nonketotic Type |
| --- | --- |
| Developmental retardation | Developmental retardation |
| Neutropenia | Failure to thrive |
| Thrombocytopenia | Spastic paraplegia |
| Osteoporosis | Opisthotonos |
| EEG abnormalities or seizures | Seizures |
| Periodic ketosis with vomiting | Hypooxaluria |
| Dehydration, lethargy, and coma | |

ished carbamyl phosphate synthetase were associated with hyperglycinemia, represents an example of secondary hyperglycinemia.

The clinical manifestations of ketotic and nonketotic hyperglycinemia are indicated in Table 10. In the first type, the most striking feature is massive ketosis, which may begin as early as the first day of life. Hyperglycinemia is, then, one of the very few conditions, such as glycogen storage disease of the von Gierke type, in which ketones may be observed in the urine during the first day of life. Repeated episodes of metabolic acidosis and ketosis have persisted as the cardinal features of the disease. Vomiting has been of such severity that pyloromyotomy has been carried out in at least one patient. It seems very likely that this condition is considerably more common than our experience would indicate, but patients have probably died very early in life before the condition was recognized. Testing for ketonuria in very ill newborns may be an effective method of case-finding. Other clinical characteristics include thrombocytopenia and occasional episodes of *purpura.* These manifestations disappear spontaneously within the first six to nine months of life. Neutropenia has been observed regularly and has been persistent. Patients with this disease may have frequent infections. Infections in hyperglycinemia may lead to exacerbation of the metabolic defect, as they do in diabetes, in maple syrup urine disease, and in other metabolic disorders. Severe ketosis and coma have been observed in minor infections. The first patients reported were mentally retarded. Others reported have died too young to permit assessment of this feature. Data are, for this reason, inconclusive, but it appears that in surviving patients the untreated disease leads to severe degrees of mental retardation with I.Q.'s under 50.

Seizures and abnormalities of the electroencephalogram have been observed in about half of the patients, disappearing spontaneously, like the thombocytopenia, in patients surviving the first six months.

The nonketotic patient described by Gerritsen, Kaveggia, and Waisman (1965) was mentally retarded and had an extreme degree of spastic cerebral palsy. He had frequent seizures, failure to thrive, and a diminished excretion of oxalate in the urine. We have studied another patient of this type with Drs. Bray and Heiner of Salt Lake City. This patient was also mentally retarded. He had seizures and electroencephalographic abnormalities. He was hypotonic but also had increased deep tendon reflexes.

TABLE 11

Prognosis in Hyperglycinemia

| Case No. | Sex | Onset Symptoms | Age at Death | Reference |
|----------|-----|----------------|--------------|-----------|
| 1. E. G. | M | 18 hr. | 7 yrs. | Childs *et al.* 1961 |
| 2. M. S. | M | 4 mos. | 16 mos. | Freeman *et al.* 1964 |
| 3. | F | 3 days | 4 days | Tada *et al.* 1963 |
| 4. B. G. | M | 36 hr. | 4 days | Schreier and Muller 1964 |
| 5. A. S. | F | 2½ days | 9 days | Visser *et al.* 1964 |
| 6. | | 24 hr. | 11 days | Sass-Korsak *et al.* 1965 |
| 7. J. J. | F | 1–4 wks. | 6 wks. | Unpublished observations |
| 8. J. E. | F | 6 days | 3 wks. | Unpublished observations |
| 9. A. G. | F | 3 days | Living without CNS abnormality —3 yrs. | Unpublished observations |

Our first patient was obviously mentally retarded. He was also microcephalic. He had been repeatedly tested and found to have an I.Q. just under 50. He had increased deep tendon reflexes and ankle clonus. He became progressively osteoporotic through the years and developed two pathological fractures of his lower extremities. He survived for seven years but died in an acute episode of ketosis much like that seen in some of the newborns. He developed flaccidity and irreversible respiratory acidosis following a period of metabolic acidosis and ketonuria. Some of the very young patients with the disease have only respiratory acidosis and flaccidity, but it is our impression that these patients, too, probably went through an initial period of intractible metabolic acidosis with ketonuria which simply was not detected because of their very young age. The prognosis in hyperglycinemia is illustrated in Table 11. Evidence has been assembled from five of our own patients and from individual patients reported in Japan, Germany, the Netherlands, and Canada. Nearly all of the patients died in the neonatal period; only one of them is living. The patient A. G. is the sibling of the first patient. She has been studied with Drs. Brandt, Clement, and Childs and will be described in more detail later. We have recently heard of another surviving hyperglycinemic patient who has been managed by Dr. Donnell and his colleagues in Los Angeles. She also appears to be doing well at over three years of age, although she is somewhat retarded.

In most patients initial diagnosis of glycinuria was made by means of an intense glycine spot in a paper chromatogram of the urine. I would, however, like to emphasize that diagnosis can be made clinically, the better method. Documentation is not so easily carried out, and it is quite easy to miss a hyperglycinuria when using paper chromatographic methods for the screening of the urine. There is so much glycine in a normal urine that these patients are readily mistaken for normals or for patients with a generalized aminoaciduria. False positives are also commonly encountered.

Intense glycinuria may be documented by using the colorimetric method for glycine or by column chromatography. It is possible to be misled even by quantitative analysis of the urine for glycine. When the patient is most severely ill, he has been off protein intake for a number of days and treated with parenteral fluids. In these situations, urinary excretion of glycine falls and may reach the normal range. Furthermore, at least two forms of hyperglycinuria have been described in which there is no hyperglycinemia (DeVries *et al.* 1957; Kaser *et al.* 1962). In addition, the Fanconi syndrome, which results from reversible renal tubular damage, has been found in recovery to proceed through a phase of increased glycine excretion in the urine after all other aspects of the syndrome have disappeared (Cleveland *et al.* 1965).

Hyperglycinemia is readily documented by analysis of the blood. Again, quantitative determinations can be carried out either colorimetrically or by column chromatography. Perhaps cases will be detected during screening procedures that are now being carried out in some laboratories that use paper chromatography with spots of blood obtained in the course of screening for phenlyketonuria. The concentrations of glycine in the blood of patients in the untreated state may exceed by over ten times those of control populations. Even with extreme reduction in dietary protein and successful dietary management, the levels obtained in the blood are distinctly abnormal. Elevated concentrations of glycine are also found in the cerebral spinal fluid.

Further clinical experience with the ketotic type of hyperglycinemia is indicated in Table 12. This little girl represented an as yet unreported

TABLE 12

Case 7—J. J.

---

1 Week: Anorexia, vomiting, lethargy; breast-fed
2 Weeks: Symptoms worsened; bottle; convulsions
4 Weeks: Increased DTR, clonus; neutropenia; thrombocytopenia; hyperglycinemia; hyperglycinuria
Treatment: Parenteral fluids; most findings reversed
Fed Nutramigen: Died of intractible acidosis

---

patient with hyperglycinemia. She had anorexia, intermittent vomiting, and lethargy from the first week of life. She was a breast-fed infant, and she failed to thrive. She was seen at approximately two weeks of age by a nurse who recommended to the mother that, in view of the gastrointestinal symptoms, she be changed to a cows' milk mixture and fed by bottle. In response to this considerably increased protein load, her symptoms worsened. She developed convulsions. On admission she had increased deep tendon reflexes and ankle clonus. There was neutropenia and thrombocytopenia. She was promptly found to have markedly elevated levels of glycine in the blood and in the urine. On treatment with parenteral fluids, most of these findings reversed. The diagnosis was not universally accepted, and it was decided that she be fed a protein hydrolysate, which presents a high protein load in a readily absorbed state. Within a few days, she went into acidosis, which failed to respond to treatment, and died. This experience dramatically illustrates the tenuous hold on life which these patients have. We have reported experience with various provocative tests in a relatively old patient under carefully controlled conditions in a clinical research center. It is our conviction that provocative tests should never be performed in an infant with hyperglycinemia.

The metabolism of glycine is complex. A variety of metabolic pathways are open to this amino acid. Furthermore, glycine is a nonessential amino acid that is readily synthesized in the body. A number of the catabolic pathways have been assessed, and they function quite well in hyperglycinemia. For instance, hemoglobin synthesis is normal, and we have no information that there is anything wrong with purine synthesis. Glutathione, creatine, and oxalate are made quite efficiently in the ketotic form of hyperglycinemia.

On the other hand, there is clearly an abnormality in the utilization of glycine. If this abnormality was not clear from the simple documentation of elevated levels of glycine in the blood, it was clarified by the glycine tolerance test. Considerable loads have been employed amounting to 0.5 gm. per kg. of glycine (Childs *et al.* 1961). Nevertheless, in controls there was very rapid utilization. In contrast, astronomical levels were obtained in the patient. Interestingly, even this strikingly abnormal tolerance test was not associated with any change in clinical condition. The glycine tolerance test, unlike the other provocative tests, appears to be quite a safe method of challenge in this condition.

Glycine is not completely without toxicity. It has been possible to fractionate the syndrome to some extent and to isolate those features that are related to concentrations for glycine in the blood because certain methods, such as a low-protein diet or the administration of sodium benzoate, effectively reduce plasma concentrations of glycine. The neutropenia seen in the syndrome has, in this way, been found to be a manifestation of the toxicity of glycine itself. The percentage of polymorphonuclear leukocytes is generally in the vicinity of 20 per cent. A mean of some eighteen total white blood cell counts approximated four thousand. Reduction of glycine concentrations by sodium benzoate led to an elevation to about eight thousand and dietary control to approximately seven thousand, each with neutrophil counts in the vicinity of 40 per cent.

It has also been possible to document the fact that recurrent episodes of ketosis and acidosis have nothing to do with glycine concentrations. These acidotic episodes are, however, clearly related to dietary intake of protein. Further fractionation of the syndrome has been carried out by the administration of free amino acids in the attempt to see which were responsible for the production of ketosis. Symptoms have now been produced regularly by leucine, isoleucine, valine, threonine, and methionine. The picture, then, is that of a multiple amino acid toxicity. All the other amino acids have been tested and found to be innocuous. In each case, feeding of the amino acid that reproduces the clinical manifestations of ketosis is associated with the elevation of the levels of that amino acid in the blood. Similarly, tolerance tests carried out with each of these amino acids revealed higher concentrations of the toxic amino acids in the patient than in the control; these high concentrations indicate some problem in the patient's metabolism. On this basis, a diet has been developed based on a small amount of protein, approximately 0.5 gm. per kg. In addition, free amino acids from the nontoxic group have been added in amounts which are present in 1.5 gm. per kg. of casein.

Experience with a patient diagnosed in the newborn period is indicated in Table 13. This little girl was a sibling of the first case of ketotic

TABLE 13

Case 9—A. G.

---

Born: 5/29/63    3975 gm.    Sibling of Case 1
     Plasma glycine (cord): 2.28 mg/100 ml
Day 3: Ketonuria (3–4+), lethargy, vomiting
     Plasma glycine: 4.10 mg/100 ml
Dietary Treatment: 40 Days: 0.6 g/kg protein + 3.0 g/kg nonketogenic AA mixture
          2 Months: 0.6 g/kg protein
          Thereafter: 1.3 g/kg protein
     Plasma glycine during treatment: 1.8–2.2 mg/100 ml
3 Years: Growth and development O.K.; hepatomegaly; CHD

---

hyperglycinemia. She was found to have ketonuria on the third day of life, at which time she had distinct elevation of the plasma concentration of glycine. Treatment was started with a diet that contained 0.6 gm. per kg. of protein supplemented with amino acids up to the equivalent of 3 gm. per kg. She was managed in this way for about forty days, after which the amino acid supplementation was stopped because she developed diarrhea. Thereafter, she received the low protein diet for approximately two months; then the protein content was raised judiciously to 1.3 gm. per kg. On this regimen, she has had few episodes of ketosis and few hospitalizations. At three years of age, she is a charming little girl who has undergone careful psychological examination that indicates she is normal intellectually.

In our first approach to the study of the metabolic defect, we carried out experiments in our first patient and in some control individuals using glycine, which was labeled in the 2 position with tritium (Nyhan and Childs 1964). In controls, this conversion of serine to glycine took place very rapidly. The specific activity was found to decline from peak levels as early as seven minutes after injection. The curve obtained in the patient appeared to be qualitatively different from the curve obtained in

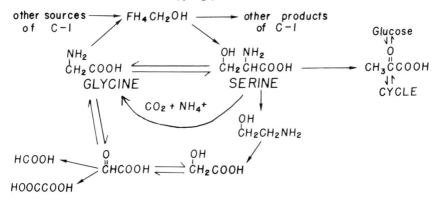

FIGURE 11. Metabolism of glycine. Interconversions of glycine and serine. (Reprinted with permission from Nyhan, Ando, and Gerritsen.)

the controls. The formation of serine from glycine was considerably slower and maximum specific activity was not reached until thirty minutes. In view of the possibility that these findings could be influenced by large pools of glycine, the experiment was repeated in the patient at a time when concentrations of glycine were lower than those of the first experiment. The curve of the specific activity of serine in the patient was even flatter. These data were interpreted to indicate a fundamental abnormality in the conversion of glycine to serine.

We have attempted, therefore, to design an experiment with greater resolving power. We have not been able to carry out these experiments in patients with ketotic hyperglycinemia, and the experiments described below have been performed in two patients with nonketotic hyperglycinemia. Our further considerations will, therefore, reflect the metabolism of glycine in control individuals and in individuals with nonketotic hyperglycinemia. Information on the interrelation of glycine and serine are given in Figure 11. In this view, glycine-serine interconversions are central. It is known that glycine is readily converted to serine and vice versa. The arrows in the center illustrate this conversion without any commitment as to mechanism. The route generally considered to be the major one involves the participation of a tetrahydrofolic acid intermediate and an enzyme most commonly referred to as serine hydroxymethyltransferase; this route is shown at the top. The hydroxymethyltetrahydrofolate can, of course, be formed from other sources of one carbon unit than glycine, and, regardless of source, can also form other products that require a

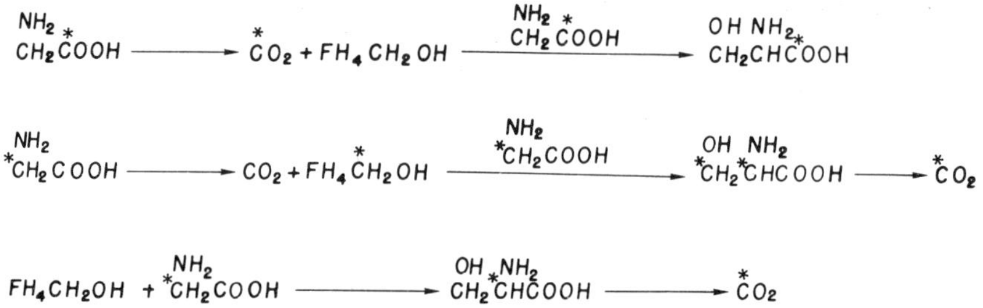

$$\overset{NH_2}{\underset{*}{CH_2}COOH} \longrightarrow \overset{*}{C}O_2 + FH_4CH_2OH \longrightarrow \overset{NH_2}{\underset{*}{CH_2}}\overset{*}{COOH} \longrightarrow \overset{OH\ NH_2}{\underset{*}{CH_2CHCOOH}}$$

$$\overset{NH_2}{\underset{*}{CH_2}COOH} \longrightarrow CO_2 + FH_4\overset{*}{C}H_2OH \longrightarrow \overset{NH_2}{\underset{*}{C}H_2COOH} \longrightarrow \overset{OH\ NH_2}{\underset{*}{C}H_2\overset{*}{C}HCOOH} \longrightarrow \overset{*}{C}O_2$$

$$FH_4CH_2OH + \overset{NH_2}{\underset{*}{C}H_2COOH} \longrightarrow \overset{OH\ NH_2}{CH_2\overset{*}{C}H\overset{*}{C}OOH} \longrightarrow \overset{*}{C}O_2$$

FIGURE 12. Elements of experimental design. Expected labeling patterns in experiments using glycine-1-$^{14}$C and glycine-2-$^{14}$C. C* represents a $^{14}$C atom. (Reprinted with permission from Nyhan, Ando, and Gerritsen.)

single carbon unit. Serine can also be converted to ethanolamine and then to glycine, and glycine can be converted to glyoxylate by glycine oxidase and ultimately to oxalate. A newly described pathway from serine to glycine illustrated just below the double arrow in the middle is probably reversible (Kawasaki, Sato, and Kikuchi 1966). It proceeds in rat liver mitochondria in nitrogen. It requires ammonia and involves a documented $CO_2$ fixation. This reaction would provide a mechanism for the production of increased quantities of glycine in hyperammonemia and would explain the findings in a patient like the one reported by J. H. Freeman and his associates (1964). Figure 12 illustrates certain aspects of the design of the experiment. The stars represent $^{14}$C-labeled glycine and its labeled products. Thus glycine-1-$^{14}$C leads directly to $^{14}CO_2$ and a hydroxymethyl derivative, which may react with another molecule of glycine-1-$^{14}$C to yield serine-1-$^{14}$C. Glycine-2-$^{14}$C, on the other hand, leads initially to unlabeled $CO_2$ and a labeled hydroxymethyl derivative, which reacts with another molecule of glycine-2-$^{14}$C to yield serine labeled in the 2 and 3 positions; this then leads to the formation of $^{14}CO_2$. We have, therefore, undertaken experiments in hyperglycinemic patients using glycine-1-$^{14}$C and glycine-2-$^{14}$C. We have collected respiratory $CO_2$ and have isolated glycine and serine from the blood. The isolated serine has been degraded with periodate to permit the trapping of the formaldehyde produced from the $\beta$-carbon and the assessment of the labeling of this carbon 3 of serine. Figure 13 illustrates the formation of $^{14}CO_2$ under these conditions. The patient T. Z. is a nonketotic hyperglycinemic boy whom we have studied in Salt Lake City in collaboration with Drs. Bray and Heiner. Similar data have now been obtained in collaboration

$^{14}CO_2$ from $^{14}C$- GLYCINE

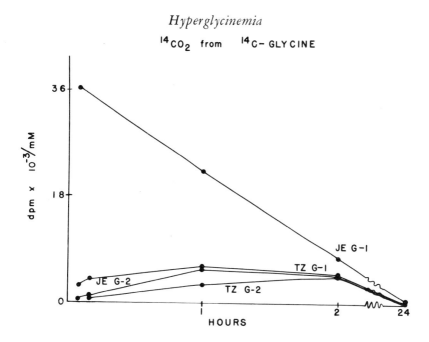

FIGURE 13. $^{14}CO_2$ formation. The data are the specific activities of respiratory $CO_2$. The curves are labeled with the initials of the subject and G-1 for glycine-1-$^{14}C$ and G-2 for glycine-2-$^{14}C$. (Reprinted with permission from Nyhan, Ando, and Gerritsen.)

with Dr. Gerritsen on his patient with nonketotic hyperglycinemia. J. E. was a control patient, and curves similar to his have now been obtained on two other control individuals. In the control, the formation of $^{14}CO_2$ from glycine-1-$^{14}C$ was very rapid. There was a linear decline from a maximum specific activity at five minutes, the earliest time point studied. The formation of $CO_2$ from glycine-2-$^{14}C$ was considerably slower as one might expect if formation of serine and oxidation through the citric acid cycle were required to release this carbon as $^{14}CO_2$. In contrast, in the patient formations of $^{14}CO_2$ from glycine-1-$^{14}C$ and from glycine-2-$^{14}C$ were very similar, suggesting that the same processes were involved in the oxidation of both carbons. The specific activity of $^{14}CO_2$ formed from glycine-1-$^{14}C$ in the control was over ten times that of the patient at five minutes. These data indicate a marked defect in the immediate oxidation of the first carbon of glycine. This would be consistent with a defect in glycine oxidase or in the first step of the process indicated in Figure 12.

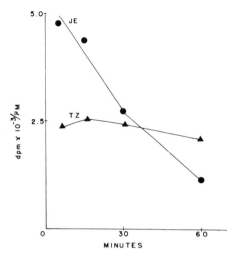

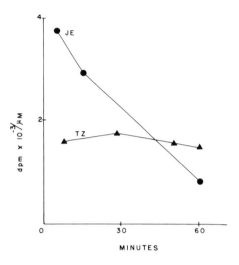

FIGURE 14. Formation of serine from glycine-1-¹⁴C. (From data reported in Nyhan, Ando, and Gerritsen.)

FIGURE 15. Formation of serine from glycine-2-¹⁴C. (From data reported in Nyhan, Ando, and Gerritsen.)

TABLE 14

Conversion of 2-¹⁴C-Glycine to $\beta$-Carbon of Serine

|  | Time (minutes) | dpm in $\beta$-C/$\mu$M Serine | % of Total Isotope in Serine |
|---|---|---|---|
| J. E. (control) | 5 | 693 | 18.4 |
|  | 15 | 776 | 26.4 |
|  | 60 | 93 | 11.3 |
|  | 78 | 31 | 3.8 |
| T. Z. | 8 | 42 | 2.6 |
|  | 28 | 19 | 1.0 |
|  | 50 | 3 | 0.2 |
|  | 60 | 3 | 0.2 |

# Hyperglycinemia

Figure 14 illustrates the specific activities of the serine isolated from the blood following the administration of glycine-1-$^{14}$C. The shapes of the curves were reminiscent of those obtained with tritium-labeled glycine in ketotic hyperglycinemia. Again these are representative experiments. We have now obtained similar results in an additional patient and in two additional controls. The curve for the patient was rather flat, while that of the control showed a linear decline from peak specific activity at the earliest time point studied. These data indicate that normally there are very rapid conversions of glycine to serine. The results obtained with glycine-2-$^{14}$C (Fig. 15) were quite similar. Peak specific activities in the control were over twice those found in the patient.

The degradation of the serine isolated is illustrated in Table 14. We show only the data from glycine-2-$^{14}$C as there was no isotope found in the $\beta$-carbon of serine in patients or the controls after the administration of glycine-1-$^{14}$C. This confirms the theory. Appreciable isotope was found in the $\beta$-carbon of the serine of the controls after glycine-2-$^{14}$C. The data obtained for the patient did not differ significantly from background counting. It is concluded that in hyperglycinemia there is virtually no conversion of the 2-carbon of glycine to the 3-carbon of serine.

These data indicate that in hypooxaluric hyperglycinemia there is a defect in the conversion of glycine to $CO_2$ and hydroxymethyltetrahydrofolic acid. These observations exclude glycine oxidase as the site of the defect. Such a defect would lead to diminished $^{14}CO_2$ formation from glycine-1-$^{14}$C but normal or increased rates of conversion of serine and unaltered metabolism of glycine-2-$^{14}$C. Possible defects in the first step of transformation of glycine to $CO_2$ and the tetrahydrofolate derivative could involve the enzyme itself, its attachment to glycine, its conversion to $CO_2$, its formation of the tetrahydrofolate derivative, or the tetrahydrofolate cofactor itself. Further exploration will have to be carried out *in vitro*, and it will be of considerable interest to apply this experimental design to the study of ketotic hyperglycinemia.

# DISCUSSION

G. DONNELL: Most of our patients have developed symptoms early. However, one of our patients did not. Since she had had a sibling who died earlier with hyperglycinemia, she was followed very closely from birth both clinically and from the standpoint of urinary ketone bodies and amino acids. She was apparently normal for four or five weeks and then began to vomit intermittently. Since this was several years ago, I cannot recall the exact sequence. She was admitted to our Clinical Research Center at seven or eight weeks of age, and by that time full-scale symptoms had developed. There was severe acidosis, ketosis, and neutropenia. A large glycine spot was found on urinary chromatograms. Since then she has done well on dietary management although there have been episodes of acidosis and neutropenia concurrent with infections. The point I wish to stress is that the condition may be missed by biochemical screening during the first three to four weeks of life in some patients. In known families, any apparently normal newborn must be followed carefully for an extended period before the diagnosis can be excluded.

W. NYHAN: Thank you very much. Those are very important observations.

N. CARSON: Dr. Nyhan, we had one patient with the ketotic type of hyperglycinemia who after a mild infection had a severe episode of metabolic acidosis associated with hyperglycemia to a level of 400 mg. per cent. A dose of insulin quickly reverted the high blood sugar levels to normal. We did not observe any further hyperglycemia after this one episode.

W. NYHAN: This one episode with ketosis was the only one with a high blood sugar?

N. CARSON: Yes, this patient had other episodes of infection which were not associated with hyperglycinemia.

W. NYHAN: I do not have a good explanation for it except to say that those of us who are dealing with very sick children are frequently mystified by the occurrence of hyperglycemia under conditions of severe stress. We had a baby on our wards approximately two weeks ago who died of what was probably an overwhelming viremia; the infant similarly had very high concentrations of sugar in the blood which then disappeared spontaneously even though the patient did not get better.

# REFERENCES

Arnstein, H. R. J., and Neuberger, A. 1953. The synthesis of glycine and serine by the rat. *Biochem. J.* 55:271.

Childs, B., and Nyhan, W. L. 1964. Further observations of a patient with hyperglycinemia. *Pediatrics* 33:403.

Childs, B., Nyhan, W. L., Borden, M., Bard, L., and Cooke, R. E. 1961. Idiopathic hyperglycinemia and hyperglycinuria, a new disorder of amino acid metabolism. *Pediatrics* 27:522.

Cleveland, W. W., Adams, W. C., Mann, J. B., and Nyhan, W. L. 1965. Acquired Fanconi syndrome following degraded tetracycline. *J. Pediat.* 66:333.

DeVries, A., Kochwa, S., Lazebnik, J., Frank, M., and Djaldetti, M. 1957. Glycinuria, a hereditary disorder associated with nephrolithiasis. *Am. J. Med.* 23:408.

Freeman, J. M., Nicholson, J. F., Masland, W. S., Rowland, L. P., and Carter, S. 1964. Ammonia intoxication due to a congenital defect in urea synthesis. *Proc. Am. Pediat. Soc.* 74:36.

Gerritsen, T., Kaveggia, E., and Waisman, H. A. 1965. A new type of idiopathic hyperglycinemia with hypooxaluria. *Pediatrics* 36:882.

Kaser, H., Cottier, P., and Antener, I. 1962. Glucoglycinuria, a new familial syndrome. *J. Pediat.* 61:386.

Kawasaki, H., Sato, T., and Kikuchi, G. 1966. A new reaction for glycine biosynthesis. *Biochem. Biophys. Res. Comm.* 23:227.

Mabry, C. C., and Karam, A. 1963. Idiopathic hyperglycinemia and hyperglycinuria. *Southern Med. J.* 56:1444.

Nyhan, W. L., Ando, T., and Gerritsen, T. 1965. *Hyperglycinemia in amino acid metabolism and genetic variation,* edited by W. L. Nyhan. New York: Mc-Graw-Hill.

Nyhan, W. L., and Childs, B. 1964. Hyperglycinemia. V: The miscible pool and turnover rate of glycine and the formation of serine. *J. Clin. Invest.* 43:2404.

Nyhan, W. L., Chisolm, J. U., Jr., and Edwards, R. O., Jr. 1963. Idiopathic hyperglycinuria. III: Report of a second case. *J. Pediat.* 62:540.

Prader, A. 1967. Discussion of papers on hyperglycinemia and sarcosinemia. *Am. J. Dis. Child.* 113:137.

Sass-Kortsak, A., Choitz, H. C., Balfe, J. W., Levinson, H., Handley, W. B., Jackson, S. H. 1965. Neonatal hyperglycinemia. *Proc. Soc. Pediat. Res.* 35:32.

Schreier, K., and Muller, W. 1964. Idiopathische hyperglycinamie (glycinose). *Deutsche Med. Wschr.* 89:1739.

Tada, K., Yoshida, T., Morikawa, T., Minakawa, A., Wada, Y., Ando, T., and Shimura, K. 1963. Idiopathic hyperglycinemia (the first case in Japan). *Tohuku J. Exp. Med.* 80:218.

Visser, H. K. A., Veenstra, H. W., and Pik, C. 1964. Hyperglycinaemia and hyperglycinuria in a newborn infant. *Arch. Dis. Child.* 39:397.

# Abnormal Galactose Metabolism in Man[1]

GEORGE N. DONNELL, M.D., WILLIAM R. BERGREN, Ph.D.,
and RICHARD KOCH, M.D.

*Departments of Pediatrics and Biochemistry of the School of Medicine, University
of Southern California, and Children's Hospital of Los Angeles*

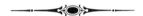

Galactosemia provides an excellent example of the progress made in the study of a genetic disease through the combined efforts of basic and medical disciplines. For many years the inability of some individuals to metabolize galactose had been recognized by physicians. The genetic character of the problem became apparent. The nature of the enzyme defect was established by H. M. Kalckar and his colleagues, who applied to man the knowledge on galactose metabolism derived from bacteria and yeast.

The term "galactosemia," which implies the presence of galactose in the blood, has been applied customarily to the inborn error of galactose metabolism resulting from a deficiency in activity of the enzyme galactose-1-phosphate uridyl transferase (transferase). However, R. Gitzelmann (1967) now has described another genetic entity (galactokinase deficiency) associated with elevation of blood galactose. In the future it will be necessary to identify particular entities associated with elevated blood galactose on the basis of the specific enzyme deficiency. In the present

[1] This work was supported by Grants AM-04135, HD-00800, and AM-04837 from the United States Public Health Service.

Appreciation is expressed to Academic Press, Inc. for permission to use Figures 16, 17, 18 and Table 15, originally published in *Biochemical Medicine*.

communication, the term "galactosemia" refers to the condition in which transferase activity is negligible or absent.

In 1908 A. Von Reuss described the first patient who can be identified retrospectively as affected by galactosemia. Earlier R. Bauer (1906) had noted an association of cirrhosis of the liver with abnormal galactose tolerance. In 1917 F. Goeppert found that urinary galactose excretion following administration of lactose could occur as a chronic familial problem. H. H. Mason and M. E. Turner (1935) used the term "chronic galactemia," and they suggested that the clinical state resulted from an inability of the liver to convert galactose to glycogen. The first clear statement that galactosemia must be considered as an inborn error of metabolism was made in 1951 by E. Gorter.

### Galactose Metabolism

The pathway for the utilization of galactose in yeast had been worked out by H. W. Kosterlitz (1943) and L. F. Leloir and others (Caputto *et al.* 1950), and it was later found that the same sequence of reactions was applicable to man. An important contribution was made by V. Schwarz and his colleagues (1956), who observed that galactose-1-phosphate accumulated in erythrocytes of untreated galactosemic patients. This finding suggested that the metabolic defect in the disease might be in the step in which galactose-1-phosphate is converted to the next intermediate in the pathway. K. J. Isselbacher and his associates (1956) identified the defect as being absence of transferase activity.

The principal pathways of galactose metabolism are shown in Figure 16. The phosphorylation of galactose to galactose-1-phosphate (Gal-1-P) is catalyzed by the enzyme galactokinase. In the second step, the formation of the nucleotide sugar uridine diphosphate galactose (UDPGal) from Gal-1-P and uridine diphosphate glucose (UDPG) is catalyzed by transferase, and at this point glucose-1-phosphate (G-1-P) appears. Finally, UDPGal is transformed to UDPG by the action of the enzyme UDPGal-4-epimerase (epimerase). It is in this third step that the conversion of the original galactose molecule to the glucose structure (in UDPG) occurs. The UDPG formed can be thought of as joining the pool of this compound for continuing use.

It will be noted that when transferase activity is absent, as in the case of galactosemia, galactose-1-phosphate will accumulate in tissues.

Recent investigations have indicated that galactitol, the product of a secondary pathway of galactose metabolism, may also be damaging to

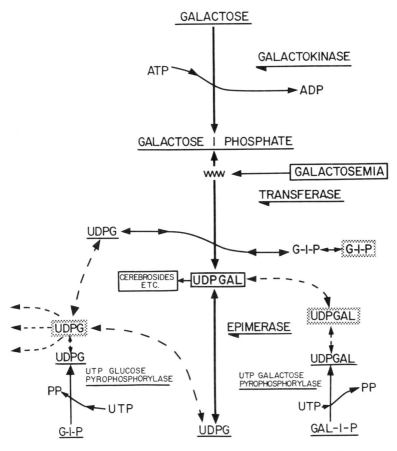

FIGURE 16.  Principal pathways of galactose metabolism.

tissues. W. W. Wells and his associates (1964, 1965) have shown that this sugar alcohol is present in the urine and tissues of untreated galactosemics. In the patients with a galactokinase defect described by Gitzelmann (1967), excretion of both galactose and galactitol occurred on diets containing sources of galactose, but accumulation of Gal-1-P in erythrocytes did not occur. In these patients cataracts were present, but none of the other manifestations of galactosemia were observed.

In addition to reduction to galactitol, other suggested alternate pathways for metabolism of galactose include formation of UDPGal from

ORAL GALACTOSE TOLERANCE TESTS

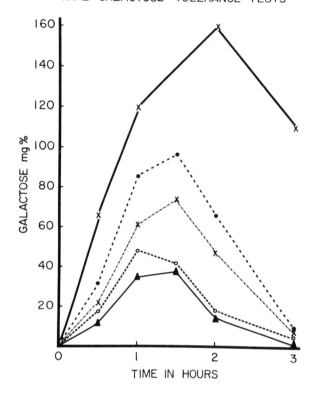

FIGURE 17.    Oral galactose tolerance tests.

Gal-1-P by the enzyme UDPGal pyrophosphorylase (Isselbacher 1957), formation of Gal-6-P from Gal-1-P and subsequent oxidation (Inouye, Tannenbaum, and Hsia 1962), and direct oxidation of galactose with ultimate formation of D-xylulose (Cuatrecasas and Segal 1966). The importance of these pathways remains to be assessed, but alternate metabolic routes may have a bearing upon variability in clinical manifestations of the disease.

## Genetics

Familial occurrence, involvement of siblings of both sexes, and the apparent normality of parents suggests autosomal recessive inheritance of galactosemia. The oral galactose tolerance test has been evaluated as a means of detecting the carrier state (Holzel and Komrower 1955; Donnell *et al.* 1959). The test discriminated between groups of individuals representing the three genotypes (Fig. 17), but it was not found to be reliable for establishing heterozygosity in any particular individual.

The use of enzymatic methods has proven useful in distinguishing between heterozygotes and normal individuals. D.Y.-Y. Hsia and his associates (1958) used the original UDPG consumption method of E. P. Anderson and her co-workers (1957), and found decreased hemolysate transferase values for parents of galactosemic patients. However, there was overlap with normal values. N. H. Kirkman and E. Bynum (1959)

TABLE 15

Erythrocyte Galactose-1-Phosphate
Uridyl Transferase Activity in Galactosemic
Families and Normal Controls

| Subjects | No. | Range | Mean | SD |
|---|---|---|---|---|
| Normal controls | 310 | 4.1–8.4 | 5.42 | ±0.934 |
| Galactosemic Children | 45 | 0–0.1 | 0 | — |
| Parents | | | | |
|   Fathers | 29 | 1.2–3.8 | 2.6 | ±0.83 |
|   Mothers | 34 | 0.9–3.8 | 2.6 | ±0.73 |
| Normal siblings | 12 | 5.0–7.0 | 5.7 | ±0.53 |
| Heterozygote presumed | 21 | 1.1–3.6 | 2.6 | ±0.81 |
| Normal relatives | 78 | 4.1–8.5 | 5.8 | ±0.99 |
| Heterozygote presumed | 39 | 1.4–3.9 | 2.8 | ±0.70 |

($\mu$M UDPG consumed per ml. packed RBC per hour)

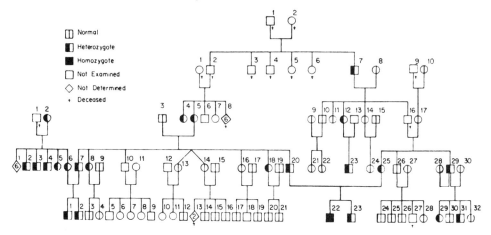

FIGURE 18.   Pedigree of a galactosemic family.

showed clear distinction between normals and parents of patients by a manometric method. R. K. Bretthauer and others (1959) modified the transferase assay of Anderson and her co-workers to provide conditions that broadened the range of discrimination sufficiently to permit recognition of the heterozygote state. We applied this modified UDPG consumption procedure to measure erythrocyte transferase activity in members of affected families. Including normal controls, 568 individuals were studied (Table 15). This data substantiated the conclusion that galactosemia is transmitted by autosomal Mendelian inheritance. An example of a pedigree is shown in Figure 18.

In view of the polymorphism described for a number of enzymes, it could be anticipated that variant forms of transferase might exist. E. Beutler and his associates (1965) have reported a transferase variant (Duarte variant) for which homozygotes are asymptomatic. Homozygotes have about 50 per cent of normal erythrocyte transferase activity, whereas heterozygotes average 75 per cent of normal. Starch gel electrophoresis has substantiated that a different transferase is present in the Duarte variant (Mathai and Beutler 1966).

W. J. Mellman and his associates (1965) have presented evidence for a different kind of variant. Two Negro families, each having one child with typical galactosemia, were studied. In both parents of one child and in the single surviving parent of the other, the expected reduction of hemolysate transferase activity was found, but leucocyte transferase activity was normal. In contrast, heterozygote activity values were demonstrated both for hemolysates and for leucocytes of parents in two galactosemic families of European origin. However, among our own patients, the two Negro families have reduced values of transferase both in leucocytes and in hemolysates.

S. Segal and his associates (1962) have described Negro patients who, despite absent erythrocyte transferase activity, were able to convert substantial amounts of intravenously administered carbon-labeled galactose to radioactive carbon dioxide. A. N. Weinberg (1961) showed that both whole blood and leucocytes from one of these individuals were able to convert galactose-1-$C^{14}$ *in vitro* to labeled carbon dioxide at a greater rate (12 to 15 fold) than observed with other galactosemics, although the amount of galactose oxidized *in vitro* was only 5 to 8 per cent of that found for normal individuals. Isselbacher (1966) also has found substantial *in vitro* production of carbon dioxide from labeled galactose by erythrocytes from galactosemic individuals.

The question of an incomplete block of transferase activity has been raised by a number of investigators. Utilizing a UDPG consumption assay, Hsia and his associates (1960) concluded that some activity was present in a few patients. Schwarz and others (1961) found by a manometric procedure that there was no demonstrable erythrocyte transferase activity in ten of twenty-three galactosemic children but that in the remainder the activity averaged 7 per cent of normal value. In our own clinic an increased *in vitro* production of labeled carbon dioxide by red blood cells was observed for three patients, and a chromatographic study of intermediates indicated that labeled nucleotide was formed (Ng, Bergren, and Donnell 1964). The conclusion was reached that some degree of transferase activity was present in the erythrocytes of these particular patients.

## Clinical Findings

Our own experience with galactosemia encompasses fifty-four cases in thirty-three families. Of the fifty-four patients, forty-one are living. In only two of the thirteen who died during early infancy was a diagnosis made prior to death: in the remaining eleven, the diagnosis was made retrospectively on the basis of history, autopsy information, and the presence in the family of a known galactosemic sibling. Twenty-seven were male and twenty-seven female. Two were Negro. Consanguinity was present in one family.

In Table 16 are summarized the signs and symptoms recorded for

TABLE 16

Signs and Symptoms among Forty-three Cases of Galactosemia

| System | Sign or Symptom | Incidence |
| --- | --- | --- |
| General | Anorexia and weight loss | 53 per cent |
| | Pallor | 7 |
| | Lethargy | 16 |
| | Cyanosis | 7 |
| Hepatic | Hepatomegaly | 90 |
| | Jaundice | 76 |
| | Ascites | 14 |
| | Edema of extremities | 2 |
| | Hemorrhagic phenomenon | 5 |
| Gastrointestinal | Vomiting | 37 |
| | Abdominal distention | 20 |
| | Diarrhea | 7 |
| | Light stool | 2 |
| Ophthalmologic | Cataract | 42 |
| Spleen | Splenomegaly | 14 |
| Genitourinary | Dysuria and frequency | 2 |
| | Dark urine | 14 |
| Central Nervous System | Bulging anterior fontanel | 9 |

forty-three children diagnosed after onset of symptoms. Eleven of the total group are omitted, since these patients were diagnosed at birth, prior to any milk feedings, because of the presence of a known galactosemic in the family. The only abnormality noted in this group was the presence of cataracts in one patient.

The clinical manifestations occurred following milk feedings, with hepatic, ophthalmologic, and gastrointestinal symptoms predominating. Hepatomegaly was the most constant physical finding. Weight loss due to vomiting was frequent. Jaundice developed within two to three days after milk feedings were begun and persisted in varying degree until institution of dietary treatment. Exchange transfusion was carried out in one infant.

Cataracts were noted in some patients as early as a few days of age. Cataracts were detected in eighteen of the affected children, but this figure may be a minimal one due to difficulty in detecting small lenticular opacities in the young infant. In two children who were diagnosed late, the cataracts were denser, and iridectomy was required in one.

A bulging anterior fontanel was noted in four patients; this sign led to an initial impression of hydrocephalus in one infant.

As is evident in Table 16, no single patient exhibited all the symptoms listed. The clinical course of seven patients was fulminant and associated with sepsis. One of these cases presented gangrenous toes associated with *E. coli sepsis*; osteomyelitis occurred in another; and meningitis was present in a third. In a few cases, the overt manifestations were less severe, and the true nature of the disease escaped immediate recognition.

### Pathology

The histologic changes in the liver of patients with galactosemia are of interest. In the younger infants, perhaps because of inanition and infection, the prominent feature is an extremely severe fatty change of the liver. In our experience, in patients under four to six months of age the liver often showed evidence of an active process of cell damage and repair. Hepatic cells were swollen and distorted. Fat and/or glycogen deposition could be demonstrated to a varying degree, bile duct proliferation was extensive and there was mild to moderate fibrosis. After four to six months of age, severe hepatic cellular damage was not as evident. Lobules were distorted and rimmed by connective tissue, giving a picture of inactive cirrhosis. As in the younger group, glycogen storage may be present to a varying degree. The one feature common to specimens of liver in this disease, particularly in patients between three weeks and four months of age, was the alveolar pattern illustrated in Figure 19. This pattern consisted of a rosette-like arrangement of liver cells about a dilated canaliculus that was frequently filled with bile pigment. Similar pigment was present to a greater or lesser degree in hepatic cells, canaliculi, and small intrahepatic ducts. The significance of this lesion is not clear, but its presence should arouse suspicion of galactosemia.

95

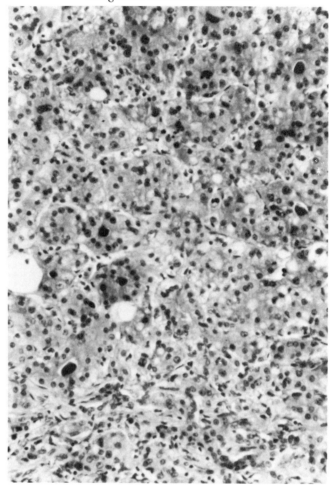

FIGURE 19.    Photomicrograph of a liver biopsy of a galactosemic patient.

## Laboratory Aspects

The diagnosis of galactosemia can be suspected on clinical grounds, but laboratory confirmation is essential. Although galactosuria and proteinuria are usually found in the symptomatic patient, their presence depends upon ingestion of galactose. Galactosuria may be differentiated from glucosuria by using the glucose oxidase test in addition to a copper-reducing method. Galactose may be positively identified by chromatography.

The method of choice for laboratory confirmation of diagnosis is estimation of transferase activity in erythrocytes. A number of procedures are available. It has been our practice, when diagnosis is suspected, to institute dietary treatment pending definitive enzyme studies.

The oral galactose tolerance test could be applied, but there are dangers associated with its use in infants. As the concentration of blood galactose increases, that of glucose declines, sometimes to hypoglycemia levels.

## Dietary Treatment

The treatment of galactosemia involves exclusion of galactose from the diet to prevent accumulation of galactose metabolites in body tissues. Supplementary means may be required initially to correct infection, hypoglycemia, hyperbilirubinemia, hypoprothrombinemia, and anemia. However, concomitant dietary therapy is essential.

The largest contributors of galactose to the diet are milk and foods containing milk. The basis for a restricted diet is a milk substitute formula substantially free of galactose. In our clinic a casein hydrolysate (Nutramigen) has been employed, and soybean formulas also have been used. Galactose is known to be present in small amounts in other foods, especially in legumes. The problems associated with establishing a suitable dietary pattern have been discussed in detail elsewhere (Koch *et al.* 1963).

Adherence to the restricted diet is of prime importance in treatment of an affected infant. Problems can arise through carelessness of a parent, actions of the child as he grows older, or intake of foodstuffs with an unsuspected galactose content. Education of the parent and child, together with careful interim dietary histories, have been helpful. In addition, we have found erythrocyte galactose-1-phosphate assay to be of value as a means of detecting consistent deviation from dietary galactose restriction. It has been our practice to determine the galactose-1-phosphate concentration in erythrocytes of galactosemic patients at each clinic visit. Values up to 4 mg. per 100 ml. of packed red cells are commonly seen in the treated galactosemic patient. It is not known whether these result from small amounts of galactose in the restricted diet or from endogenous sources. Values above 4 mg. per cent can be attributed in most instances to dietary breaks. However, the assay is of limited usefulness in detecting single violations of diet since elevations of erythrocyte galactose-1-phosphate following ingestion of galactose return to baseline by 24 to 48 hours (Donnell 1963).

## Results of Treatment

It is generally agreed that dietary treatment of the infant with galactosemia saves the child's life. The long-term effects of treatment are difficult to evaluate, but partial answers are provided by the longitudinal observations we have made over the past eighteen years on our group of patients.

With the exception of eleven infants diagnosed at birth, all the children initially were moderately or severely ill. Weight loss, hepatomegaly, and jaundice were seen in the majority of patients. After treatment was initiated, most clinical features of the disorder were reversed in a few weeks or months. Jaundice disappeared in a few days, and weight gain was restored within a week or two. In most patients, the liver diminished in size relatively soon, but in a number it did not return to normal for several months or more. About half of the patients had lenticular lesions, primarily of the punctate variety. Only two patients, each treated relatively late, had mature cataracts. There was no progression in any of the patients after institution of treatment. Most improved, but in some there were residual lesions visible by slit lamp examinations.

Birth weights of the affected children were normal, with the exception of one premature infant. Excluding infants diagnosed at birth, the weights in symptomatic children at time of diagnosis ($\frac{1}{2}$ to 17 months of age) were markedly less than expected for their age. Physical growth improved following institution of dietary therapy, and after twelve to 18 months the increments of height and weight followed a normal pattern (Donnell, Koch, and Bergren 1968). Skeletal maturation, assessed at periodic intervals, did not differ from that expected for normal children.

Intellectual status of our galactosemic children was assessed at regular intervals. Under three years of age, the Gesell Developmental Scales (D.Q.) were used. Over three years of age, evaluation was made according to the Stanford-Binet Scale (I.Q.), and in the teen-age period the Wechsler Intelligence Scale for Children was employed. The results of the latest intellectual achievement tests on forty-one patients may be summarized as follows: twenty-nine fall within the normal range (I.Q. 85 or greater), seven are within the borderline range (I.Q. 70 to 84), two are mildly retarded (I.Q. 55 to 69), three are severely retarded.

Of the severely retarded, two have been essentially untreated, and it is suspected that the retardation in the third is from some cause other than galactosemia. Our observations on intellectual development have recently been presented in detail (Donnell, Koch, and Bergren 1968).

Of the group of forty-one children, twenty-five now are enrolled in school, fifteen in regular classes. Ten children, six boys and four girls, attend special education classes. Two children have mature, dense cataracts and attend sight-saving classes. The other eight children require special attention because of an intellectual, emotional, or social problem. Some degree of visual-perceptual difficulty has been noted in many of the children tested, and in some cases this problem may have contributed to difficulty in learning under formal school conditions (Donnell *et al.* 1968; Fishler *et al.* 1966).

To date, there is nothing definitive in the literature to support the view that galactosemic children might adapt to galactose with increasing age (Donnell, Koch, and Bergren 1968). We have allowed relaxation of dietary restriction only to a limited extent and only with older children of school age. Before prescribing a completely uncontrolled diet, a carefully planned prospective study is indicated.

# DISCUSSION

H. B. ANSTALL: I would like to thank Dr. Donnell very sincerely for an excellent and comprehensive clinical presentation of this problem. I would like also now to throw open this meeting to discussion. I might begin by asking one question myself. With regard to the apparent improvement in the tolerance to galactose in the older galactosemic, there has been some data accumulated where if $C^{14}$-labeled galactose in one position is given intravenously to a normal individual and the amount of activity as $CO_2$ recovered is monitored over a five- or six-hour period, about 35 or 40 per cent of the initial radioactivity can be recovered. In the classical galactosemic, I believe recovered $CO_2$ is some 6 or 7 per cent by contrast (or even lower). However, there are a number of these individuals who have been studied who have shown recoveries somewhat approaching the normal, particularly in the adult, and I wondered whether you think that these represent a rather specific type of the disorder? Can one talk about subgroups with this condition? This is a rather interesting finding and somewhat difficult to explain.

G. DONNELL: I do not have a satisfactory answer. The patients to which you refer were reported by Segal. Members of this group demonstrated the classical clinical manifestations of galactosemia as infants, and galactose-1-phosphate uridyl transferase activity was absent in erythrocytes. Despite this, they had a capability of converting labeled galactose to labeled $CO_2$ *in vivo* more efficiently than other galactosemics. It is of interest that all of these exceptional individuals have been Negro. As far as I know, this phenomenon has not been described in galactosemic children of European extraction. These examples suggest that the individuals described may represent a different genetic grouping. Whether the D-xylulose pathway recently described by Cuatrecasas and Segal may be a contributing factor in the differences observed is still not known.

H. B. ANSTALL: I think there have been one or two people who have talked about the possibility of accumulation of galactose-6-phosphate in erythrocytes. In some of these cases, there is partial metabolism by the hexose monophosphate shunt.

G. DONNELL: Inouye and Hsia have demonstrated accumulation of galactose-6-phosphate in erythrocytes of galactosemic individuals when these cells were exposed to galactose. Dr. Ng of our own laboratory has not yet been able to confirm these findings. Further work is necessary to determine with certainty whether conversion of galactose to galactose-6-phosphate does occur in galactosemics and, if so, by what mechanism.

R. HILL: What is the incidence of galactosemia in Los Angeles? Second question: Your feelings in reference to screening newborn infants for galactosemia.

G. DONNELL: I cannot give you an incidence figure of galactosemia for the Los Angeles area. We have not screened for heterozygotes nor have we made any effort to ascertain the number of galactosemic children born in this area. What I can say is that we see on the average of two new patients per year at our hospital. The incidence of galactosemia has been variably reported as 1 in 10,000 to 1 in 68,000. The true figure is somewhere in between. I would hesitate to offer a figure at this time. The method of ascertainment, either by identification of heterozygotes in a population or by survey for affected children is important. As I have indicated, Duarte variant homozygotes have transferase values in the galactosemic heterozygote range, and this must be taken into account in studies utilizing heterozygote detections as a means of determining the incidence of galactosemia. The frequency with which the Duarte variant is seen may in part be responsible for the high incidence figures reported by some.

I am sure my feelings on screening of newborn infants for galactosemia are no different from the feelings of most of us here with regard to PKU. The methods now employed for detection of affected infants have been in use only for a short time, and it is too early to tell how effective they will be. One of the large hospitals in the Los Angeles area has been screening for galactosemia for some time by the Guthrie method. Although I cannot quote the total number of infants screened to date, we do know that at least two infants with galactosemia were part of the population screened.

D. KEELE: If any of your patients gets pregnant, how do you plan to manage them during pregnancy? Do nongalactosemic infants of galactosemic mothers have mental retardation?

G. DONNELL: The mothers of our galactosemic children do not have problems with the handling of galactose. It has been our practice to recommend a restricted galactose intake during the whole pregnancy. The indication for restriction of lactose during pregnancy is suggested by reports of a few galactosemic infants being born with clinical manifestations and by the experiments of Segal and his group with rats which have shown that ingestion of large amounts of lactose during pregnancy results in damage to the offspring.

D. KEELE: What about the mothers who are galactosemic?

G. DONNELL: I am sorry I missed the sense of your question. I thought that you were referring to galactosemic heterozygotes not to the pregnant galactosemic homozygote. I do not know of any female galactosemic individuals who have given birth to children. However, in view of the maternal PKU problem, one would have to be concerned about possible damage to the offspring. Were I to be faced with the problem at the present time, I would recommend rigid restriction of lactose and galactose intake throughout pregnancy.

T. WILSON: Do heterozygotes or Duarte variants have any difficulty in handling galactose per se?

G. DONNELL: It has been reported that heterozygotes for clinical galactosemia have occasionally had intolerance to milk. Whether this intolerance is to galactose or lactose has not been indicated.

T. WILSON: Have any of the heterozygotes or Duarte variants had elevated fasting levels?

G. DONNELL: I have not studied patients who are homozygote for the Duarte variant but have been told by Dr. Beutler that they do not have elevated blood galactose levels. Dr. Beutler has carried out galactose tolerance tests on homozygote individuals for the Duarte variant, with findings similar to those for classical galactosemia heterozygotes. None of the Duarte variants have been clinically symptomatic.

T. WILSON: Have any of your galactosemics not had early symptoms such as jaundice?

G. DONNELL: All our patients, with the exception of those diagnosed at birth, have been moderately to severely ill. More than 60 per cent of the untreated galactosemic infants developed jaundice.

E. AIRAKSINEN: I was wondering about the sex difference in your galactose loading, both in normal controls and in parents. We have had the same experience with galactose loading so that we may have higher values in females even in healthy controls without any history of disease. What might be the reason for that?

G. DONNELL: It is true that mean values for galactose tolerance tests tended to be higher for females, but we could not demonstrate in our sample any statistically significant difference between the sexes. Some workers have stated that there may be some sex difference in the incidence of galactosemia, but this has not been our experience. It may be fortuitous, but our group of affected individuals consists of twenty-seven boys and twenty-seven girls.

N. CARSON: What is the routine method used for transport of blood samples for galactosemic enzyme studies?

G. DONNELL: The best method of transport of blood for enzyme studies depends upon the assay method to be used. In our laboratories the Bretthauer modification of the UDPG consumption method, or the radioactive assay described by Ng, is used. In order to insure that activity of the enzyme is preserved, it has been our practice to request that hemolysates be prepared, quick frozen, and shipped in the frozen state within a few days. In the frozen state, transferase activity changes very little over a two-week period. I understand that heparinized blood can be shipped unrefrigerated with little loss of activity. If one is concerned with recognition of the carrier state, loss in activity may lead to erroneous assignment of genotype. We request that a control be sent along to insure that sample preparation and shipment have not affected the activity of the enzyme of the sample sent.

N. CARSON: One of our galactosemics has very poor hair growth. The hair itself appears to be of normal texture. She is about three years of age and is normal physically and mentally. Any cases with very short hair?

G. DONNELL: No, they have perfectly normal hair growth.

H. LEVY: Just one quick question, Dr. Donnell. Have you had any experience with the Beutler test, and by this I mean the most recent Beutler test.

G. DONNELL: You mean the fluorescent method?

H. LEVY: Right.

G. DONNELL: I have not had any personal experience with this method for mass screening.

# REFERENCES

Anderson, E. P., Kalckar, H. M., Kurahashi, K., and Isselbacher, K. J. 1957. A specific enzymatic assay for the diagnosis of congenital galactosemia. I: The consumption test. *J. Lab. Clin. Med.* 50:469.

Bauer, R. 1906. Weitere untersuchungen über alimentäre galaktosurie. *Wien. Med. Wochschr.* 56:2538.

Beutler, E., Baluda, M. C., Sturgeon, P., and Day, R. 1965. A new genetic abnormality resulting in galactose-1-phosphate uridyltransferase deficiency. *Lancet* 1:353.

Bretthauer, R. K., Hansen, R. G., Donnell, G. N., and Bergren, W. R. 1959. A procedure for detecting carriers of galactosemia. *Proc. Natl. Acad. Sci.* 45:328.

Caputto, R., Leloir, L. F., Cardini, C. E., and Paladini, A. C. 1950. Isolation of the coenzyme of the galactose phosphate-glucose phosphate transformation. *J. Biol. Chem.* 184:333.

Cuatrecasas, P., and Segal, S. 1966. Galactose conversion to D-xylulose: An alternate route of galactose metabolism. *Science* 153:549.

Donnell, G. N., Bergren, W. R., and Roldan, M. 1959. Genetic studies in galactosemia. I: The oral galactose tolerance test and the heterozygous state. *Pediatrics* 24:418.

Donnell, G. N., Bergren, W. R., Perry, G., and Koch, R. 1963. Galactose-1-phosphate in galactosemia. *Pediatrics* 31:802.

Donnell, G. N., Koch, R., and Bergren, W. R. 1968. In *Galactosemia*, ed. David Hsia. Springfield, Ill.: Charles Thomas.

Fishler, K., Koch, R., Donnell, G. N., and Graliker, B. V. 1966. Psychological correlates in galactosemia. *Am. J. Ment. Def.* 71:116.

Gitzelmann, R. 1967. Hereditary galactokinase deficiency, a newly recognized cause of juvenile cataracts. *Pediat. Res.* 1:14.

Goeppert, F. 1917. Galaktosurie nach Milchzuckergabe bei angeborenem, familiarem, chronischem leberleiden. *Berlin. Klin. Wochschr.* 54:473.

Gorter, E. 1951. Familial galactosuria. *Arch. Dis. Child.* 26:271.

Holzel, A., and Komrower, G. M. 1955. A study of the genetics of galactosaemia. *Arch. Dis. Child.* 30:155.

Hsia, D. Y.-Y., Huang, I., and Driscoll, S. G. 1958. The heterozygous carrier in galactosemia. *Nature* 182:1389.

Hsia, D. Y.-Y., Tannenbaum, M., Schneider, J. A., Huang, I., and Simpson, K. 1960. Further studies on the heterozygous carrier in galactosemia. *J. Lab. Clin. Med.* 56:368.

Inouye, T., Tannenbaum, M., and Hsia, D. Y.-Y. 1962. Identification of galactose-6-phosphate in galactosemic erythrocytes. *Nature* 193:67.

## Abnormal Galactose Metabolism

Isselbacher, K. J.
1957. Evidence for an accessary pathway of galactose metabolism in mammalian liver. *Science* 126:652.
1966. In *The metabolic basis of inherited disease*, eds. J. B. Stanbury, J. G. Wyngaarden, and D. S. Fredrickson. New York: McGraw-Hill.

Isselbacher, K. J., Anderson, E. P., Kurahashi, K., and Kalckar, H. M. 1956. Congenital galactosemia, a single enzymatic block in galactose metabolism. *Science* 123:635.

Kirkman, H. N., and Bynum, E. 1959. Enzymatic evidence of a galactosemic trait in parents of galactosemic children. *Ann. Hum. Genet.* 23:117.

Koch, R., Acosta, P., Ragsdale, N., and Donnell, G. N. 1963. Nutrition in the treatment of galactosemia. *J. Am. Dietetic Assoc.* 43:216.

Kosterlitz, H. W. 1943. The fermentation of galactose and galactose-1-phosphate. *Biochem. J.* 37:322.

Mason, H. H., and Turner, M. E. 1935. Chronic galactemia. *Am. J. Dis. Child.* 50:359.

Mathai, C. K., and Beutler, E. 1966. Electrophoretic variation of galactose-1-phosphate uridyl transferase. *Science* 154:1179.

Mellman, W. J., Tedesco, T. A., and Baker, L. 1965. A new genetic abnormality. *Lancet* 1:1395.

Ng, W. G., Bergren, W. R., and Donnell, G. N. 1964. Galactose-1-phosphate uridyl transferase activity in galactosaemia. *Nature* 203:845.

Schwarz, V., Goldberg, L., Komrower, G. M., and Holzel, A. 1956. Some disturbances of erythrocyte metabolism in galactosemia. *Biochem. J.* 62:34.

Schwarz, V., Wells, A. R., Holzel, A., Komrower, G. M., and Simpson, I. M. N. 1961. A study of the genetics of galactosemia. *Ann. Hum. Genet.* 25:179.

Segal, S., Blair, A., and Topper, Y. J. 1962. Oxidation of carbon-14 labeled galactose by subjects with congenital galactosemia. *Science* 136:150.

Von Reuss, A. 1908. Zukerausscheidung im säuglingsalter. *Wien. Med. Wochschr.* 58:799.

Weinberg, A. N. 1961. Detection of congenital galactosemia and the carrier state using galactose $C^{14}$ and blood cells. *Metabolism* 10:728.

Wells, W. W., Pittman, T. A., and Egan, T. J. 1964. The isolation and identification of galactitol from the urine of patients with galactosemia. *J. Biol. Chem.* 239:3192.

Wells, W. W., Pittman, T. A., Wells, H. J., and Egan, T. J. 1965. The isolation and identification of galactitol from the brains of galactosemic patients. *J. Biol. Chem.* 240:1002.

# Familial Hyperuricemia in
# a Negro Family

DOMAN K. KEELE, M.D., JAMES F. MARKS, M.D.,
and JACOB L. KAY, M.D.

*Department of Pediatrics, Southwestern Medical School of The University
of Texas, Dallas, Texas, and the Medical Department
of the Denton State School, Denton, Texas*

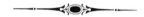

In 1964 H. Lesch and W. L. Nyhan described a familial neurological disorder consisting of choreoathetosis, spasticity, mental retardation, aggressive behavior, and compulsive biting, resulting in mutilation of the lips and fingers. These findings were first described in two young brothers associated with hyperuricemia and excessive uric acid synthesis. Subsequently other cases have been described.[1] The original patients excrete in their daily urine, three to six times the amount of uric acid found in the urine from control subjects of similar body size and age. Studies indicate that this is an X-linked recessive disorder of the male (Shapir *et al.* 1966; Nyhan *et al.* 1967). J. E. Seegmiller and his associates (1967) have demonstrated deficient activity of the enzyme, hypoxanthineguanine phosphoribosyltransferase, in this disease. The purpose of this paper is to present the pedigree in a Negro family with special emphasis on a newborn infant with this entity.

The propositus in this pedigree was the oldest boy in the family, who

[1] Holfnagel 1965; Holfnagel *et al.* 1965; Nyhan *et al.* 1967; Partington and Hermen 1967; Reed and Fish 1966; Sass, Itabashi, and Dexter 1965; Shapir *et al.* 1966.

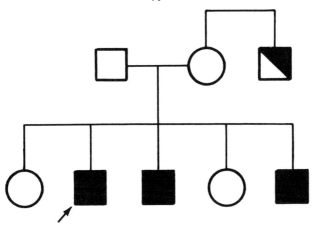

■ Clinical findings of familial hyperuricemia.

■ Clinical and biochemical findings of familial hyperuricemia.

□ Male.

○ Female.

↗ Propositus.

FIGURE 20.   Family pedigree, present report.

was admitted on November 5, 1964, to the Denton State School, an institution for mentally retarded individuals at Denton, Texas. He was B. J. F., a seven-year-old male. He was rather thin, was mentally retarded, and had a Social Quotient on the Vineland Social Maturity Scale of 10. His mother reported that he had chewed off his lower lip. He was nonambulatory and had spasticity of all extremities. Choreoathetosis was present. He was restless and irritable, and his lower lip was partially missing. He also had compulsive biting of his fingers. Urinary uric acid excretion was 0.746 gm. per 24 hours; the serum uric acid level was 7.6 to 6.9 mg. per cent; and the blood urea nitrogen was normal, being 5.4 mg. per cent. The urinalysis was normal except for the presence of uric acid crystals. The patient was treated with allopurinol, 100 mg. three times per day. On this dosage, the serum uric acid has been maintained near normal levels. The nurses who provide his care feel that his aggressiveness and restlessness are much less on allopurinol, and for this reason the drug has been continued. There have been no control studies with placebos to confirm this observation. The drug has been stopped on two occasions, each lasting two weeks, with resulting increase in restlessness and irritability. On resumption of the same dosage the irritability and restlessness decreased.

A. F., the brother of B. J. F., was born on April 13, 1962. On admission to the Denton State School in April 1967, he had marked developmental retardation, was nonambulatory, and was not toilet trained. The mother had wrapped his hands in boxing gloves fashion to prevent him from biting them. On the Vineland Social Maturity Scale, the Social Quotient was 25. On physical examination, the lower lip was missing. Spasticity and choreoathetosis was evident in all extremities. The serum uric acid was 7.9 mg. per cent. His present therapy consists of 500 mg. of allopurinol per day. The care personnel feel this dosage is helpful for controlling irritability and restlessness. The present serum uric acid levels are in normal range.

Family history revealed that there are two normal female siblings (Fig. 20). The mother's brother died at Children's Medical Center in Dallas, Texas, in 1951; he had mental retardation, poor growth, spasticity, choreoathetosis, and self-mutilation consisting of self-destruction of the lower lip.

During hospitalization of these brothers at the Denton State School, it was observed that the mother was again pregnant. The mother was receiving prenatal care at Parkland Memorial Hospital in Dallas, Texas. The medical staff was advised prior to the birth of her fifth child on April 17, 1966.

The physical examination of this male infant at birth was essentially normal. The following laboratory studies were accomplished on the first day of life: umbilical cord uric level was 8 mg. per cent (normal being 4.36 +0.95). The maternal uric acid level was 5.5 mg. per cent. The infant's first voided urine was normal; no uric acid crystals were seen. Shortly after twenty-four hours, the infant's blood uric acid level was 18.9 mg. per cent. At ninety-four hours, the blood uric acid was 14.5 mg. per cent. At this time the infant was started on a regimen of allopurinol.

The patient's dose of allopurinol was gradually increased, and the dosage was adjusted to maintain the serum uric acid in the near normal range (Marks *et al.* unpublished). The clinical course is summarized as follows. The infant was evaluated at eight weeks of age and was thought to be normal physically and developmentally. He was also thought to be

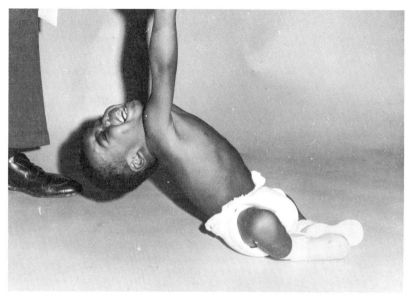

FIGURE 21. Hypotonia, at fourteen months of age.

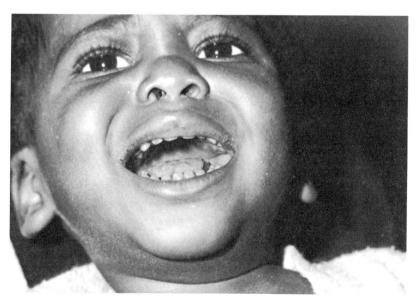

FIGURE 22. Tongue lesion due to self-destructive biting.

developmentally normal at ten weeks of age, except for possible hypotonia. At twenty-four weeks of age, his developmental age was estimated to be sixteen weeks and hypotonia was definite. At fourteen months of age, the developmental age was estimated to be at the six months level and hypotonia was marked (Fig. 21). At seventeen months of age, tension athetosis was observed, and at nineteen months of age, self-mutilation involving the tongue was first observed during a febrile illness (Fig. 22).

## Summary

1. A pedigree in a Negro family compatible with the X-linked form of familial hyperuricemia has been presented.

2. A tentative diagnosis was made in a newborn male infant in this family based on an elevated cord serum uric acid level and subsequently confirmed by a rapid rise of the infant's serum uric acid. Despite allopurinol treatment, the infant developed the typical clinical syndrome of hyperuricemia.

# DISCUSSION

W. NYHAN: Dr. Keele has presented a very interesting documentation of the syndrome and illustrated its salient features very well. I would like to emphasize some aspects of his presentation. One of the striking features that this family illustrates is that the diagnosis is readily made in the newborn period. The patient presented is one of two known patients in this country who were born into families in which it was known ahead of time that there were hyperuricemic siblings. In each instance it has been possible within the first twenty-four hours of life to make a specific diagnosis. Evidence suggests, therefore, that this is a condition in which very early diagnosis is going to be possible. In fact, the concentrations of uric acid in the plasma of these newborns have generally been higher than we have seen at any other period of life.

The patient is also interesting genetically. A Negro family is particularly interesting from the point of view of the study of gene linkages. We are interested, for instance, in the possibility of linkage between types of glucose-6-phosphate dehydrogenase, which are located on the X chromosome and are common in Negroes, and this disorder, which is also located on the X chromosome. Such information might contribute to the mapping of the X chromosome in which there is a certain amount of genetic interest. Glucose-6-phosphate dehydrogenase has already been studied in this family, and there is no evidence of deficiency. There are, to my knowledge, two other Negro boys with the syndrome in the United States, and one of them has so far not been studied for glucose-6-phosphate dehydrogenase deficiency. The syndrome has been seen with considerable regularity throughout the world, and I think it is probably a relatively common inborn error of metabolism—as one might expect for an X-linked trait. One might expect that an X-linked disease would be more common than diseases that are autosomal recessive. Investigation of the isozymes of glucose-6-phosphate dehydrogenase is now in progress.

The experience with allopurinol is of some interest. When we undertook allopurinol treatment in patients with this disorder, we were not sanguine about the possibility of influencing the central nervous system manifestations. As you know, allopurinol is a xanthine oxidase inhibitor; it inhibits the overproduction of purine at the very last step before the formation of uric acid. In this sense, it is a mode of therapy that is very well-designed for the treatment of gout. Manifestations of disease in these patients and in adults with gout are related to uric acid itself and are effectively managed by use of allopurinol. On the other hand, we have known for some time that there is practically no uric acid in the central nervous system. Concentrations in the cerebrospinal fluid are quite low. In fact, in these patients the levels of the oxypurines, particularly hypoxanthine, are quite high in the cerebrospinal fluid even in the untreated state. One might postulate, as Seegmiller and colleagues have done, that allopurinol treatment could make the patient worse because it should raise the levels of oxypurine. If oxypurine were the toxic element responsible for the central nervous system manifestations, this would certainly be true. I think that there is evidence that hypoxanthine and xanthine, like uric acid, are not responsible for the central nervous system manifestation of the disease. We have now studied a number of children with the established disease during treatment with allopurinol. The experience Dr. Keele has described and the other patient diagnosed in the newborn period are very important in this respect. The other patient was diagnosed with Michener of Cleveland and was also treated from the first days of life with allopurinol. One can see that allopurinol does not prevent the development of the central nervous system manifestations of the disease; on the other hand, it certainly does not make them worse.

I would now like to discuss some other aspects of the syndrome. We now know that there is a spectrum of clinical manifestations in the disorder. The fundamental abnormalities that make up the syndrome are hyperuricemia, mental retardation, spastic cerebral palsy, choreoathetosis, and behavioral abnormalities. Some children may not have all these features. Choreoathetosis may be one of the key features, present in all patients after infancy. Most of us who have taken care of children with this disorder have felt that these children have been more intelligent than their test results would suggest. This may well relate to the extreme severity of their motor defect which is reflected not only in the way they move their extremities, but also in the way they move their mouths. They are dysarthric; they have trouble communicating; and they test very poorly. Yet, by and large, they have a much brighter eye than the average patient you find bedridden in the institutions for the retarded. When one learns to communicate with them, many of them communicate very efficiently. Self-mutilating behavior is probably the most striking manifestation of the syndrome. Most of these children bite their lips. They also damage themselves in other ways and demonstrate an overall pattern of aggressive behavior. Some boys pick at themselves, lacerate themselves with braces, or catch themselves in the spokes of wheelchairs. In addition, they are aggressive to others. If you get close to them they will bite you, hit you, and kick you. These actions are a kind of compulsive behavior which is not associated with an unpleasant personality. These boys cannot help what they do. If they are old enough, they apologize if they are fairly successful at doing something like knocking off your glasses; they usually laugh if your glasses do not break. They are very complex personalities, and this is one of the most interesting features of the problem. This is the first disease I know of in which a biochemical defect is associated with a stereotyped pattern of behavior. I think it may be one of the few handles one has on behavior. Certainly, if we could understand more about aggressive behavior, we could understand a lot more about our society.

One of the latest chapters in this story was introduced by the observations of Sorensen that the immunosuppressive agent, azathioprine, is effective in inhibiting the formation of uric acid in adults with gout. Figure 23 illustrates an experiment we performed on an adult patient with gout. The initial uric acid concentration was in the vicinity of 10 mg. per 100 ml. After a week or so of azathioprine treatment, the patient had a normal level of uric acid; these results could certainly confirm what Sorensen had reported. We turned then to an assessment of the response to the drug in a patient with the syndrome. In the experiment illustrated in Figure 24, we started out again with a patient with a uric acid in the vicinity of 10 mg. per 100 ml. and treated him with a similar dose of azathioprine. In this patient and in two others, there was no decrease in uric acid production in response to azathioprine. We felt that this was an important observation. A significant extension of these findings was made by the work of Drs. Seegmiller, Rosenbloom, and Kelly of the National Institutes of Health. They realized that for azathioprine to be active it must first be converted to its parent compound, 6-mercaptopurine, and then to its nucleotide. The enzyme that converts 6-mercaptopurine to its nucleotide is known as inosinic acid (IMP) pyrophosphorylase and now more commonly known as hypoxanthineguanine phosphoribosyltransferase. It is a nonspecific enzyme. It converts either

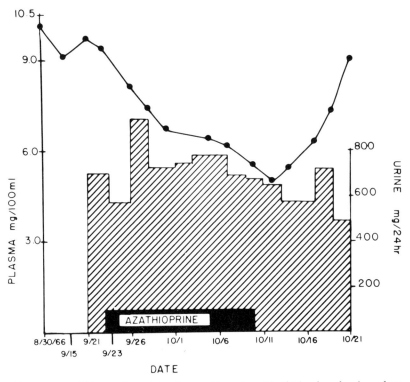

FIGURE 23. Effects of azathioprine on the uric acid of blood and urine of an adult with gout. (Reprinted with permission from Nyhan *et al.*, 1968, *J. Pediat.* 72:111.)

guanine or hypoxanthine by reaction with phosphoribosyl-pyrophosphate (PRPP) to guanylic acid (GMP) or inosinic acid (IMP). If one started with 6-mercaptopurine (6-MP) the product would be its nucleotide, 6-MPP. The fact that azathioprine did not work in these patients suggested that this enzyme might be missing. In fact, it was so documented. Seegmiller and colleagues first reported the absence of this enzyme. We have confirmed these findings both in fibroblasts grown in cell culture and in erythrocytes. We have studied control children ranging in age from nine months to fifteen years, and they have a tremendous amount of activity as measured from hypoxanthine. The patient has a level of flat zero for the activity of this enzyme.

As one looks at the synthesis of uric acid, it certainly reflects an increase in the *de novo* synthesis of purine starting from the first committed step in which PRPP and glutamine react (Fig. 25) ultimately to form IMP.

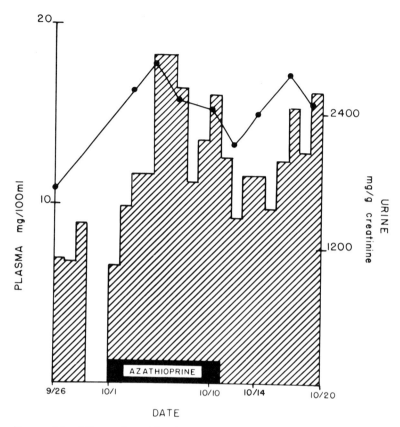

FIGURE 24. Effects of azathioprine on the uric acid of blood and urine of a boy with a disorder of uric acid metabolism and cerebral function. (Reprinted with permission from Nyhan *et al.*, 1968, *J. Pediat.* 72:111.)

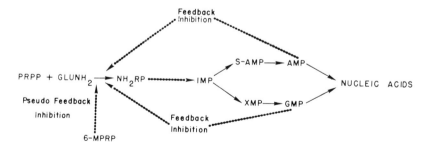

FIGURE 25. Interrelations of purine metabolism and the mechanisms of feedback inhibition of purine synthesis. (Reprinted with permission from Nyhan *et al.*, 1968, *J. Pediat.* 72: 111.)

This then forms nucleic acid, but it also can be degraded to uric acid. Too much purine is being made in this syndrome. The normal control mechanism is the feedback inhibition of the very first step by the nucleotides, AMP and GMP. It is also true that 6-MP inhibits because its nucleotide inhibits at this step. It can be concluded, therefore, that these patients overproduce purine because they do not have a normal feedback inhibition mechanism. We are further basing our analysis on the concept that the central nervous system manifestations of this disease are related to the purine that is overproduced.

H. GHADIMI: The patients under treatment get a great deal of attention. How would you evaluate the effect of attention they get in comparison to the effect of the specific therapy?

W. NYHAN: Many of our children who have grown up during the period in which there was no treatment have gotten equally careful attention from the parents. One of the problems is that this is a degenerative disease. These children almost invariably start out normal. Therefore, you are dealing with a family that brings up a little boy who starts sitting and doing things normally until about eight months. Then he begins to develop athetosis and goes downhill. Most of these patients have developed their worst symptoms somewhere between one and three years. Such a boy has usually received quite a lot of attention from his parents, and I cannot distinguish in this respect between the allopurinol-treated and the untreated. The renal disease that one sees in these patients is among the most severe of gouty nephropathies. If these patients live long enough, they develop a very distressing gouty disease, which is completely preventable by the use of allopurinol. I think that one sometimes runs into philosophical problems with the treatment of children who have very severe central nervous system disease. Certainly, treatment means prolonging life in a patient with serious problems. Obviously, the parents must participate in these decisions. The parents of our patients have uniformly favored the treatment of the disease with allopurinol.

P. DOYLE: What about sodium metabolism using allopurinol in Dr. Keele's third case? Was the prolonged seizure due to hyponatremia?

D. KEELE: The serum sodium was normal.

G. DONNELL: Dr. Nyhan, as you know, Dr. Kogut and I are studying a phenocopy of the Lesch-Nyhan syndrome. Our patient is a girl with overt manifestations of the self-mutilating syndrome. However, the large majority of blood uric acid determinations have been in the normal range, although she did excrete more uric acid than one would expect for her age (8 mg. per kg. per day to 29 mg. per kg. per day). I understand that other such phenocopies have been recognized. It is interesting that similar clinical pictures with gross retardation are seen in individuals with different biochemical findings. This child's retardation, when contrasted with reports that high intelligence has been associated with hyperuricemia, casts some doubt that uric acid per se is responsible for the clinical manifestations. Would you like to comment on this?

W. NYHAN: I agree that your patient is a very exciting one. Dr. Keele also has a male who may be a phenocopy, and there is a girl we have been studying in Orlando who mutilates and has choreoathetosis but has normal levels of urate in the blood. I think that the spectrum of phenocopies has probably not yet been defined. Some of them do seem to have borderline or high amounts of uric acid in the urine. So far, none have had persistent hyperuricemia. We have felt, inasmuch as the evidence today suggests that it is some product of purine metabolism other than uric acid, that these patients may very well provide a real clue to the mechanisms of the central nervous system defect. If these patients have different inborn errors of metabolism, and these errors are discovered to involve purines, common biochemical features may point more strongly to what causes the behavioral and neurological abnormalities. We are currently pursuing this problem using methods for the fractionation of purines in urine and cerebrospinal fluid.

# REFERENCES

Holfnagel, D. 1965. Syndrome of athetoid cerebral palsy, mental deficiency, self mutilation and hyperuricemia. *J. Ment. Def. Res.* 9:69.

Holfnagel, D., Andrew, E. D., Mireault, M. G., and Berndit, W. O. 1965. Hereditary choreoathetosis, self mutilation and hyperuricemia in young males. *New Eng. J. Med.* 273:130.

Lesch, M., and Nyhan, W. L. 1964. A familial disorder of uric acid metabolism and central nervous system function. *Am. J. Med.* 36:561.

Marks, J. F., Baum, J., Keele, D. K., Day, J. L., and McFarlen, A. The Lesch-Nyhan syndrome treated from the early neonatal period. To be submitted for publication.

Nyhan, W. L., Pesek, J., Sweetman, L., Carpenter, D. G., and Carter, C. H. 1967. Genetics of an X-linked disorder of uric acid metabolism and cerebral function. *Pediat. Res.* 1:5.

Partington, M. W., and Hermen, B. K. E. 1967. The Lesch-Nyhan syndrome: Self-destructive biting, mental retardation, neurological disorder and hyperuricemia. *Devel. Med. and Child Neurol.* 9:563.

Reed, W. B., and Fish, C. H. 1966. Hyperuricemia with self mutilation and choreoathetosis. Lesch-Nyhan syndrome. *Arch. Derm.* 94:194.

Sass, S. K., Itabashi, H. H., Dexter, R. A. 1965. Juvenile gout with brain involvement. *Arch. Neurol.* (Chic.) 13:639.

Seegmiller, J. E., Rosenbloom, F. M., and Kelly, W. M. 1967. Enzyme defect associated with a sex-linked human neurological disorder and excessive purine synthesis. *Science* 155:1682.

Shapir, S. L., Sheppard, G. L., Jr., Dreifuss, F. E., and Newcombe, D. S. 1966. X-linked recessive inheritance of a syndrome of mental retardation with hyperuricemia. *Proc. Soc. Exp. Biol.* (N.Y.) 122:609.

# Chromosomal Anomalies and Mental Retardation[1]

JOSÉ M. TRUJILLO, M.D.

*Cytogenetic Laboratory, Department of Pathology, The University of Texas M. D. Anderson Hospital and Tumor Institute, Houston, Texas*

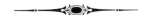

The study of human chromosomes, known as human cytogenetics, is a relatively new field. As in several other scientific disciplines, much of the basic knowledge was acquired many years ago (Wilson 1928). Many of us still remember when it was an accepted teaching that the correct chromosome number of man was forty-eight. This mistaken figure persisted until recently because the classical cytologist of older times could only study the chromosomes of higher organisms on fine tissue sections where it was virtually impossible to obtain an accurate count (Ford and Hamerton 1956).

The modern discoveries in cytogenetics became possible due to a few rather simple technical improvements, one of the most fundamental, perhaps, being hypotonic treatment to spread the chromosomes (Makino and Nishimura 1952). Parallel advances in tissue-culture techniques made the attainment of dividing cells a simpler procedure within reach of the common hospital laboratory (Moorehead *et al.* 1960). It should also be mentioned that almost at the same time concurrent developments in molecular biology have significantly broadened the scope of the biological sciences and added new perspectives to the field of genetics. Thus,

1 This work was supported by the Public Health Service Research Grant # CA 06939 from the National Cancer Institute.

simultaneous advances in biochemical genetics and cytology definitely established the following facts:

1. The desoxyribonucleic acid (DNA) constitutes the basic chemical substance of inheritance and carries within its molecular structure the genetic code that appears to be universal and common to most forms of life known to man (Crick 1958).

2. The genetic code results from the linear arrangement of four purine and pyrimidine bases (adenine, thymine, guanine, and cytosine), one of which is invariably present in each nucleotide of the DNA molecule. Although this sequence of four bases determines the code, the key unit is a triplet of bases (codon) which codifies for each specific amino acid (Nirenberg *et al.* 1963).

3. The DNA molecule thus forms a large strand composed of many nucleotides. Each nucleotide contains, besides the bases, a pentose sugar (ribose) and a phosphate group. These nucleotides are kept together by bonding of the phosphates with the C-3 and C-5 of the pentose. In this way, almost limitless numbers of different sequences of base triplets can be assured. According to the model of J. D. Watson and F. H. C. Crick, this genetic material is organized in a double-coiled spiral with the DNA strands facing each other at the base level and linked by bonds of hydrogen atoms (Watson and Crick 1953). The fundamental code is able to replicate itself and operates by transcribing its sequence of bases in a complementary manner through another nucleic acid, messenger ribonucleic acid (RNA). This messenger RNA proceeds then to the cytoplasm and at the ribosome level acts as a template for protein biosynthesis by establishing the sequence of amino acids in the nascent polypeptides (Watson 1965).

4. The chromosomes carry the genetic material or DNA, but the structural organization of this genetic substance within the chromosomes is still unknown. With the exception of the sex chromosomes, the chromosomal elements are present in homologous pairs that segregate independently during cell division in accordance with the fundamental laws of Mendel (Swanson 1957). Although the cytogenetic techniques are fairly simple and are based on the attainment of sufficient numbers of dividing cells with well-spread chromosomes, a qualified cytogeneticist must be well acquainted with the fundamental laws of genetics and with these new developments in biochemical genetics. Otherwise, interpretation of structural changes becomes an almost impossible task. The fact that each chromosomal unit carries a large number of genes, which in turn are

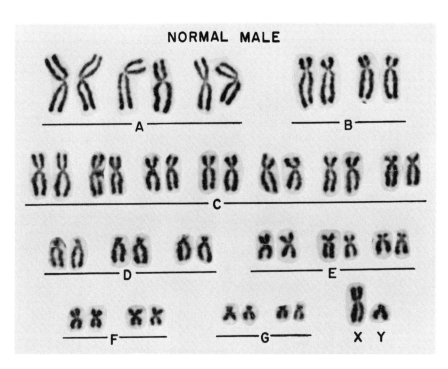

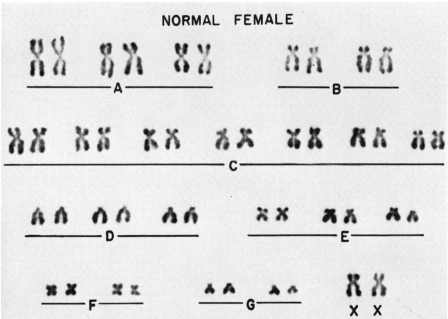

FIGURE 26. Human male and female karyotypes.

composed of hundreds of code units or base triplets, must be considered while doing chromosomal analyses and, especially, while trying to interpret chromosomal aberrations in terms of phenotypic alterations.

J. H. Tjio and A. Levan first demonstrated that the human cell contains forty-six chromosomes, which can be arranged into twenty-two pairs of homologous autosomes and one pair of sex chromosomes, XX for the female and XY for the male (Tjio and Levan 1956). Simple observation of the human chromosomes reveals morphological similarities and differences that permit the arrangement of the elements into groups of similar pairs. This is the basis for the classification established in Denver in 1960 and known as the Denver-Patau System (Report of a study group 1960). Although arbitrary, this system is a very useful method for chromosomal analysis. The human autosomes can then be classified in the groups A through G with the sex chromosomes as a separate pair, permitting immediate recognition of numerical abnormalities as well as of gross alterations in length and morphology (Fig. 26). It is also evident that the determination of sex is entirely dependent upon the chromosomal formula. A normal human female carries two X chromosomes while a male individual carries one X and one Y chromosome. The female, therefore, produces two similar gametes, each one with an X chromosome and the male, two dissimilar gametes, one with an X chromosome and one with a Y chromosome. Thus the sex of the zygote is dependent upon the chromosomal make-up of the male gamete involved in fertilization.

For many years, it has been known that chromosomes of animals and plants can present different types of numerical aberrations as well as complex structural changes. Similar abnormalities have recently been demonstrated in the human chromosomes. Obviously, we cannot deal in this presentation with the entire gamut of aberrations affecting human chromosomes. However, in brief, numerical alterations involve the loss or gain of chromosomal elements and are known as monosomies, trisomies, tetrasomies, and so on. Some of the more common structural changes are: deletion (loss of chromosomal material), translocation (attachment of a broken portion of a chromosome to the broken end of another chromosome), inversion (reverse attachment of a chromosomal segment between two breaks), and duplication (doubling of a chromosomal segment). These structural aberrations are, in almost all instances, preceded by chromosomal breaks and could also result in the formation of aberrant elements such as ring chromosomes, dicentrics, isochromosomes, and so on (Fig. 27; Swanson 1957).

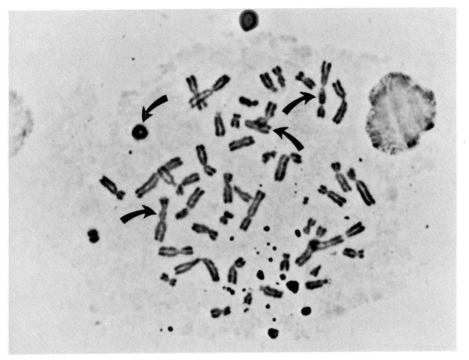

FIGURE 27. Chromosome damage in human leukocytes induced by ionizing radiation resulting in the occurrence of abnormal elements (ring chromosome, dicentric chromosomes, and acentric fragments indicated by arrows).

The aberrations of human chromosomes can be subdivided into two main groups: 1. sex chromosome anomalies and 2. autosomal anomalies.

### Sex Chromosome Anomalies

Due to special circumstances involving the inactivation and alternatively the genetic expression of the individual sex chromosomes, aberrations involving these elements seem to be more viable and better tolerated (Ohno and Makino 1961; Lyon 1962; Russell 1963). Some of the more common sex chromosome anomalies are (Miller 1964):

1. XO syndrome known as Turner's syndrome: These individuals usually have a female phenotype with only forty-five chromosomes due to the absence of one of the X chromosomes.

2. XXY syndrome or Klinefelter's syndrome: This syndrome is charac-

terized by a male phenotype with forty-seven chromosomes due to the presence of the extra X chromosome. Several cytogenetic variants of this latter syndrome have been described such as XXYY (double male), XXXY, XXXXY, XXXXXY.

Other types of sex chromosome aberrations include the XXX females (super-females) and the XYY males.

In general, all these individuals present abnormal sexual development and are often sterile. Physical malformations involve mainly the reproductive system. Mental retardation may or may not be a feature of these conditions. For instance, some studies among institutionalized mentally defective individuals revealed an incidence of about 1 per cent being XXY (Maclean *et al.* 1962). In general, it appears that the larger the number of X chromosomes present, the more severe the degree of mental retardation. On the other hand, it is interesting to note that some XYY males may have average and even superior intelligence. Psychopathic traits, especially excessive aggressiveness toward the opposite sex, seem to be common in these individuals. They are often tall, usually more than 6 feet, have normal development of the sexual organs, and are able to reproduce (Price *et al.* 1966).

Numerous cases have also been reported of individuals carrying populations of cells with different chromosome number which resulted from either the loss or gain of one of the sex chromosomes. These individuals are called mosaics and may present mild or severe alterations of sexual development depending upon the proportions maintained between the different cell lines. Their intelligence varies accordingly. In general, it can be assumed that the higher the proportion of cells with normal genetic constitution in these individuals, the more normal they are (Maclean *et al.* 1962).

## Autosomal Anomalies

Aberrations in the number of autosomes are, as a rule, much more damaging to the individual than the sex chromosome anomalies. From the point of view of mental retardation, one of the most important chromosomal defects involves one of the small autosomes. This condition is commonly referred to as mongolism but is also called Down's syndrome. The earliest description was made by Sequin in 1846. However, Down's name was associated with the disease following his report on the classification of idiots in a London hospital in 1866 (Oster 1953). It is commonly used in the English literature and should perhaps be preferred

## DOWN'S SYNDROME - G2I TRISOMY ( ♀ )

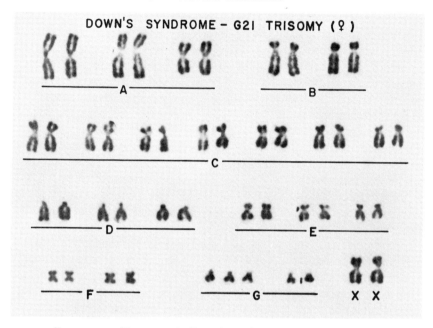

FIGURE 28. Karyotype in Down's syndrome with G21 trisomy.

to the unfortunate term of mongolism which incorrectly suggests a non-existent racial association with the disease.

It is worth mentioning that until a few years ago, the etiology of the Down's syndrome was completely obscure. J. Warkany remarked that before 1959, at least thirty-nine theories had been offered as a possible explanation for the disease (Warkany 1960). One of the more complete studies on this condition, performed in Denmark by Jakob Oster in 1953, involved a clinicogenealogical investigation of 526 mongoloid children. In one of his final remarks, Oster stated: "Finally, it is concluded that mongolism is no hereditary disease, but probably has its cause in exogenous factors related to the mother's depressed reproductive faculty" (Oster 1953). It is fair to mention, too, that several investigators, such as Waardenberg (1932), Bleyer (1934), Fanconi (1939), and Penrose (1939) had suggested that a chromosomal defect might be associated with this condition (Warkany 1960). In 1959, through the utilization of the new cytological techniques, J. Lejeune and his associates reported that, indeed, mongoloid individuals had forty-seven chromosomes with the extra element belonging to the small group of acrocentrics (Lejeune, Gautier, and Turpin 1959). This finding was rapidly confirmed by other investigators in this country and in Europe. The condition accounts for approximately 10 per cent of all institutionalized mentally retarded patients (McIntire, Menolasino, and Wiley 1965). According to Reed, in over four million newborns per year in the United States more than eight thousand infants will have Down's syndrome (Reed 1963). These figures alone demonstrate the significance of the chromosomal breakthrough and illustrate the important role that human genetics, as a whole, and cytogenetics, in particular, should play in any investigation concerning mental retardation.

The extra chromosomal element in Down's syndrome is generally identified as a member of the twenty-first pair (Fig. 28). The disease is characterized by several physical features, none of which alone has a total diagnostic value. Oster emphasized ten "cardinal" signs for the clinical diagnosis of mongolism. These include: "simian crease; short crook of the fifth finger; short, broad hands; hyperflexibility of the joints; oblique palpebral fissures; epicanthus; furrowed tongue; irregular, abnormal sets of teeth; narrow, high palate; and flat occiput" (Oster 1953). The one common symptom is mental deficiency. According to some investigators, the degree of mental retardation varies somewhat with an I.Q. ranging between 25 and 50, although Oster, in his series, reported that a small percentage of patients could read or even write. There is also a variable degree of retardation in physical development in these children. The internal organs may be normal, but congenital anomalies, which include heart and brain defects, hypoplastic thyroid, hypoplastic adrenals, and abnormal thymus, have been reported (Oster 1953).

Although the most common cytogenetic finding is the presence of the extra chromosome or G21 trisomy, a group of mongoloid children with forty-six chromosomes and four small acrocentrics instead of the suspected five have been found. Their karyotypes contained five elements in the D group with an additional submetacentric chromosome in the C group. This chromosomal variation was first reported by Polani in 1960 and has since been confirmed by many different investigators (Polani *et al.* 1960). In fact, these children are still trisomic for the greater part of the G21 since their karyotype is only the reflection of a translocation of most of the long arms of this chromosome to a member of the D group. Children with this type of translocation-mongolism are clinically identical to those with the standard trisomy. It has been shown that this type of chromo-

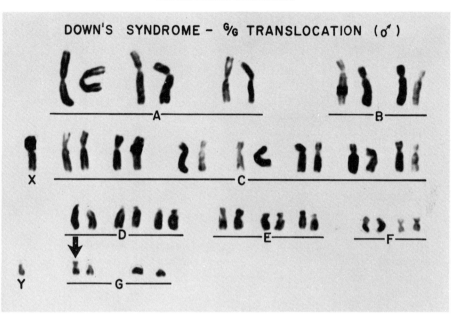

FIGURE 29. Karyotype in Down's syndrome with 46 chromosomes and G/G translocation. (Courtesy of Dr. Sinha, Cytogenetics Laboratory, Texas Children's Hospital, Houston, Texas.)

somal aberration can occur *de novo* or be the result of a balanced translocation in one of the parents. In the latter case, we speak of familial translocation. The parent with the balanced translocation is referred to as a "carrier" and has a karyotype with forty-five chromosomes due to the apparent loss of two elements, one from the D group and one from the G group, which have fused together (translocated) and resulted in one extra element in the C group. This type of familial condition has been observed by different investigators and found to be transmitted though several generations (Polani 1963; Bartalos and Baramki 1967). The chromosomes in the germ cells of the "carrier" will undergo defective pairing during the first meiotic prophase. The random segregation of these abnormally paired elements results in four main types of gametes even though, theoretically, eight different forms are possible. In the event of fertilization, these four gametes can produce individuals with four different types of chromosomal constitutions: a "carrier" with forty-five chromosomes and balanced translocation; a mongoloid child with forty-six chromosomes; a normal individual; and an individual monosomic for the G21 chromosome. The familial transmission of mongolism can also be the result of other types of translocations between the G21 chromosome and other elements of the G group, such as G21/G22 and G21/G21 (Fraccaro, Kayser, and Lindsten 1960; see Fig. 29). In the case of a familial translocation of the G21/G22 type, the meiotic segregation occurs in a way similar to that described in the D/G21 type. If the translocation is G21/G21, only two gametes can be formed, one carrying the translocation and one lacking the G21 chromosome. The chance of transmitting mongolism in this case is approximately 50 per cent, thus mimicking an autosomal dominant mode of inheritance.

Mosaic forms of mongolism have been reported with two populations of cells, one having a normal karyotype and the other having a G21 trisomy. The clinical picture in these cases seems to be more variable. Some of these mosaic individuals in which the majority of the cells possess a normal chromosomal constitution have shown none or only a few physical features of mongolism and were not mentally retarded (Bartalos and Baramki 1967).

From the series of cases reported in this country and in Europe, the average incidence of the disease is approximately one child in every six hundred live births (Oster 1953; McIntire, Menolasino, and Wiley 1965; Reed 1963; Bartalos and Baramki 1967; Carter and MacCarthy 1951). According to Reed, if one could include the loss of undiagnosed affected babies, the frequency would increase to about one per five hundred births (Reed 1963). For years it has been known that the risk of having a child with Down's syndrome rises steeply with the age of the mother. Below the age of twenty-nine years, the risk is 1 to 3,000, and between thirty and forty years, it is 1 in 600. When the mother's age ranges from forty to forty-four years, the risk increases to around 1 in 70 (Carter and MacCarthy 1951). In the case of familial mongolism, with D/G21 or G21/G22 translocation, the risk exceeds 25 per cent. Some investigators believe that even when the parents are cytologically normal, regardless of maternal age, the risk of recurrence, after the birth of one child with G21 trisomy, is higher than in the general population and fluctuates between 1 and 4 per cent (Hamerton *et al.* 1961; Book and Reed 1950).

Other known types of autosomal aberrations involving an extra chromosome are the E and D trisomies (Fig. 30). The former is also known as "Edwards' syndrome" since this investigator and his associates first described it in 1960 (Edwards *et al.* 1960). The general consensus is that the

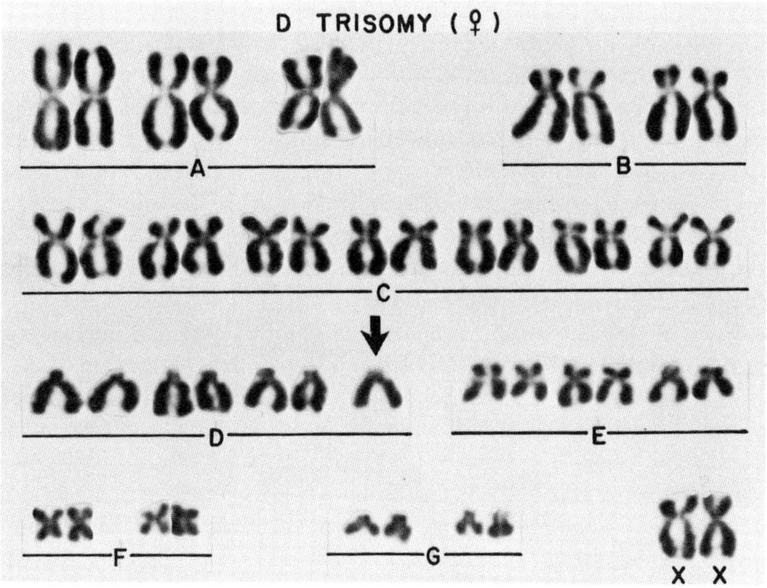

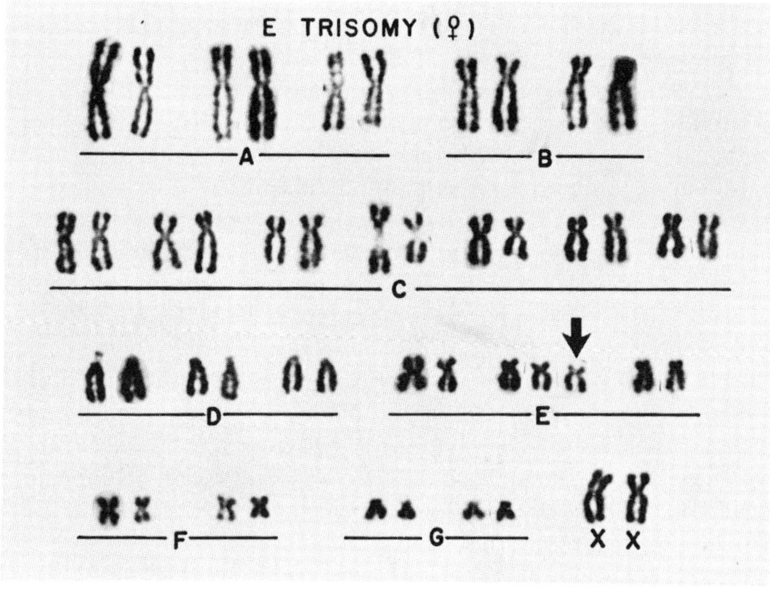

FIGURE 30. Karyotypes of children with E and D trisomy.

chromosomal pair involved is the eighteenth pair of the E group, however, this has not been definitely established (Bartalos and Baramki 1967). Children with this chromosomal aberration present multiple congenital defects. Again, the one common feature is mental retardation. Some of the most common clinical findings are hypertonicity, micrognathia, low-set malformed ears, ventricular septal defects, patent *ductus arteriosus* and renal anomalies. A characteristic hand deformity consisting of flexion and overlapping of the index and the fifth fingers over the third and the fourth fingers is often encountered. As in other chromosomal trisomy syndromes there appears to be a maternal age effect. The incidence of this chromosomal aberration is rather low and fluctuates between 1 in 3,000 and 1 in 5,000 births. The majority of these malformed children dies during the first year of life. One of the oldest living patients reported is a fifteen-year-old mentally retarded female (Bartalos and Baramki 1967).

The D trisomy was described by Patau in 1960 (Patau *et al.*), although the congenital anomalies characteristic of the syndrome were already known and had been reported as "prosencephaly" by Kundrat in 1886 (Smith 1964). The malformations of this syndrome are multiple and often overlap those found in the E trisomy, although, as a rule, they are more severe. Various developmental defects on the central nervous system such as microcephaly, absence of the olfactory tracts, interhemispheral fissures, absence of trigone and *corpus callosum*, and cerebellar hypoplasia are often found. Other common malformations are cleft palate, microphthalmia, simian crease, polydactyly, intraventricular septal defects, dextroposition of the heart, and absence of the auditory canals. Again, the one common defect is mental retardation. As the name implies, the karyotype of these children shows the presence of an extra chromosome in the D group. A few clinical cases of D trisomy with forty-six chromosomes and a D/D translocation have also been reported (Bartalos and Baramki 1967; Smith 1964).

The E and D trisomies can also appear in mosaic form, where populations of cells with both normal and abnormal karyotypes are present. While the children affected by the full trisomies usually die before the first six months, the mosaic babies, often with less severe malformations, have shown better survival rates. Even in these cases, however, mental retardation is present (Bartalos and Baramki 1967; Smith 1964).

Another group of autosomal anomalies are those which present structural aberrations. The cases reported in the literature have increased

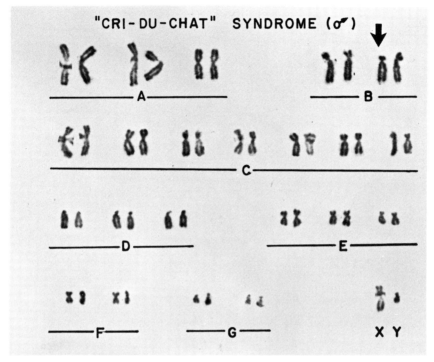

FIGURE 31. Karyotype of child with "Cri-du-Chat" syndrome (short arm deletion in member of B group indicated by arrow).

markedly in the last few years. From the point of view of both the persistence of the phenotypic alterations and the cytogenetic picture, only a few of them conform to a specific pattern and can be classified as a particular syndrome. Perhaps the one that has recently become better known is the "Cri-du-Chat" or "Cat-Cry" syndrome, which is associated with a chromosomal deletion of the short arm of a member of the B group. This anomaly was described by Lejeune and associates in 1963. The most characteristic clinical feature in these patients is their cry which resembles the mewing of a cat. Already more than fifty cases have been recognized and all of them seem to present similar phenotypes (McGavin *et al.* 1967). In all instances, the karyotype has shown the deletion of the short arm of one member of the B group (Fig. 31). Most interesting is the fact that, with the exception of a few mosaics, all variants of auto-

## MITOSIS

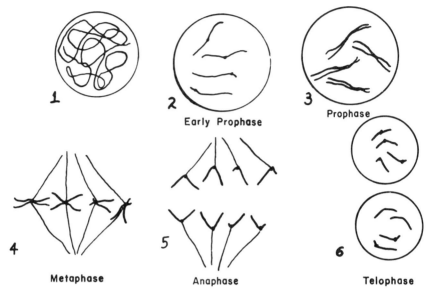

FIGURE 32. Schematic representation of the different stages of mitosis.

somal anomalies which have been reported have as a common denominator mental retardation.

### Origin of Chromosomal Aberrations

The numerical chromosomal aberrations are the result of abnormal segregation or nondisjunction of the chromosomes during cell division. The phenomenon of nondisjunction may occur during mitosis or meiosis and may affect the somatic cells and the germ cells, respectively.

The genetic material or DNA is duplicated during the so-called S period, part of the long interval of the cell cycle preceding mitosis known as interphase. It is only during mitosis that the chromosomes condense sufficiently to become visible. The mitotic period takes only one to two hours of the cell cycle and is divided into four stages known as prophase, metaphase, anaphase, and telophase. These successive stages lead to random segregation and equal distribution of the chromosomes to the two daughter cells (Swanson 1957; see Fig. 32).

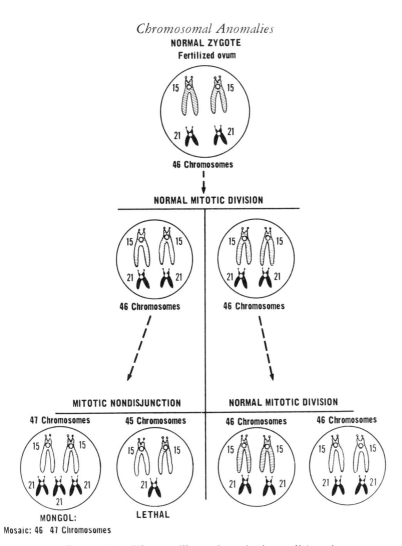

FIGURE 33. Diagram illustrating mitotic nondisjunction.

When mitotic nondisjunction occurs, a pair of chromosomes fails to segregate, and both elements migrate to the same pole. This migration results in one daughter cell having an extra element and in the other lacking one element. The mistake may also consist of a simple failure to migrate, "lag," during the anaphase period so that one chromosome will be excluded from one of the two daughter cells. The phenomenon of mitotic nondisjunction is important in the production of chromosomal anomalies when it occurs during the first few divisions of the zygotic cells (Fig. 33). As suggested by Ford, selective forces of some kind may play a definite role in influencing the rate of division of the aberrant cells. It is possible that most of the mosaic forms originate through this process. However, others prefer the reverse mechanism, which implies that the zygote has an abnormal chromosomal constitution to begin with. Thereafter, a few of these cells would undergo mitotic nondisjunction and produce normal diploid cells that, on the basis of selective advantage, will also establish themselves and thus give rise to a mosaic (Ford 1961).

Meiosis is a specialized type of cell division that occurs only in the germ cells. The entire meiotic cycle involves two cell divisions: the first division in which the number of diploid chromosomes is reduced to half and the second division, which is similar to any other mitotic process. The prophase of the first meiotic division is a long process in which five separate states can be differentiated: leptotene, zygotene, pachytene, diplotene, and diakinesis (Rhoades 1961). Leptotene is characterized by the appearance of long, loose chromosomal strands. It is uncertain whether DNA synthesis takes place during this stage or prior to it. During zygotene, small condensations along the chromosomal strands, chromomeres, become evident and the homologues start "pairing" along the entire length of the chromosome. This is called synapsis, and interchange of chromosomal material may occur at this stage. In pachytene, the two sister strands of each chromosome become distinct as they condense and shorten. The resulting structure is thus composed of four chromatids and is called a "bivalent" to reflect the synapsis of the maternal and paternal chromosomes. These bivalents become more clearly defined during diplotene when the double units begin to separate, starting at the centromeres. Interchange or crossing-over is now quite evident, and the points of occurrence are called "chiasmata." Diakinesis is characterized by marked separation of the bivalents with migration, "terminalization," of the chiasmata toward the end of the chromosomes. After this long, meiotic prophase has occurred, the metaphase and the anaphase stages merely continue the cell division toward completion with the arranging of the bivalents along the equatorial plate and later segregation of the pairs. The telophase and the final separation of the two daughter cells complete the first meiotic division. After a short resting period, which involves no DNA synthesis, the second meiotic division occurs in the usual fashion, giving rise to four haploid cells (Fig. 34). It is evident,

# MEIOSIS

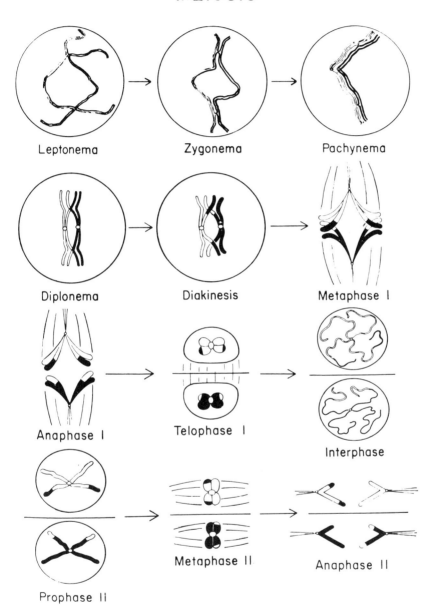

FIGURE 34.  Schematic representation of the stages in the two major divisions of meiosis. (Reprinted, with permission, from *The Cell*, II, eds. Jean Brachet and Alfred Mirsky, © 1961 Academic Press.)

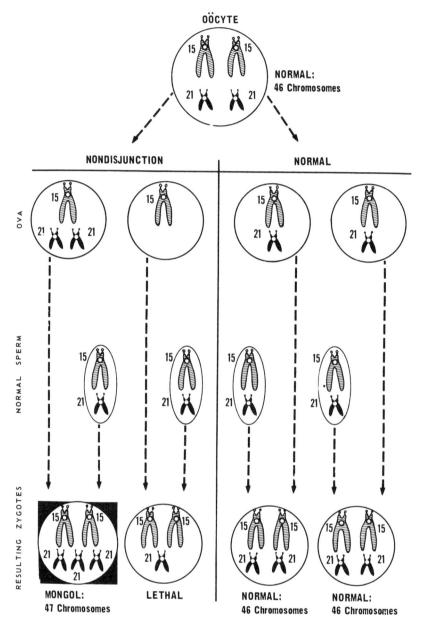

FIGURE 35. Diagram illustrating meiotic nondisjunction.

therefore, that every germ cell can produce four gametes by undertaking these two successive meiotic divisions. This process occurs in spermatogenesis. On the other hand during oögenesis, one daughter cell, "polar body," is excluded after each of the two meiotic divisions, thus resulting in one gamete being produced for every germ cell (Rhoades 1961).

It may well be that interference with this orderly process of meiosis, particularly during the complex stages of the first meiotic prophase, will cause nondisjunction with the production of gametes carrying abnormal numbers of chromosomes (Patau 1963; see Fig. 35). E. Witschi has shown that in amphibia "aging" or overripeness of the egg may induce congenital malformations and chromosomal abnormalities (Witschi and Laguens 1963). In view of the fact that the first meiotic prophase takes place in the female during her embryonic life of two to seven months (Ohno, Klinger, and Atkin 1962), "aging" may indeed have something to do with meiotic nondisjunction during oögenesis. Certainly the direct relationship that exists between the occurrence of chromosomal trisomies and the age of the mother adds to this theory. However, it should be pointed out that the phenomenon of cell "aging" in terms of metabolic and biochemical parameters is still not understood. On the other hand, since many chromosomal aberrations occur independently of the parent's age, other factors of a physical, chemical, or biological nature may be equally important in inducing meiotic nondisjunction. It is also conceivable that small balanced translocations, undetected by the usual cytogenetic techniques, could induce nondisjunction due to abnormal meiotic pairing. Crossing-over under those circumstances is a complicating factor and would give rise to more complex aberrations (Trujillo *et al.* 1966). As some investigators have lately postulated, viruses might also be influential in human nondisjunction (Bartalos and Baramki 1967; Stoller and Collmann 1965). In addition, in lower species there is evidence that nondisjunction can be genetically controlled (Swanson 1957; Spieler 1963). Therefore, the familial occurrence of multiple aneuploid states in man has led some investigators to suggest a "genetic predisposition" to nondisjunction (Hamerton *et al.* 1961; Hecht *et al.* 1964).

Structural aberrations may result from damage to the chromosomes by physical, chemical, and biological agents. Of the physical agents, the most important are the ionizing radiations (Bartalos and Baramki 1967; Bender and Gooch 1962). Several chemicals, including the one of recent interest, LSD (lysergic acid diethylamide), seem to be able to damage human chromosomes and induce structural aberrations (Bartalos and

Baramki 1967; Cohen *et al.* 1966). The same is true of several biological agents, such as viruses (Nichols *et al.* 1963; Moorehead and Saksela 1963). The precise mode of action of these agents is still obscure, and it may vary from actual chemical derangement of the molecular structure of the chromosomes to interference with the synthesis of the DNA and the nuclear proteins.

### Prevention of Chromosomal Aberrations

The old fatalistic idea that nothing can be done about a genetic defect is long disregarded due to the continued advances of the biological sciences. As with any pathological condition, the medical solution lies in one of two possibilities: prevention or cure. With genetic diseases a successful treatment requires a precise knowledge of the nature and *modus operandi* of the defective gene, resulting in the adoption of appropriate measures to counteract its action. This is the conduct followed with considerable success in the management of patients with known inborn metabolic errors, such as phenylketonuria, galactosemia, and so forth. It is based on the well-established genetic fact that it is occasionally possible to bypass the genotype and obtain a more desirable phenocopy by changing environmental factors—diet or temperature (Sinott, Dunn, and Dobzhansky 1958). However, in the case of patients with chromosomal defects, this therapeutic approach may be hindered by the fact that frequently there are many genes involved in the aberrations. Knowledge of the genetic loci in man is very incomplete; a reason for the deleterious effects of the partial or total trisomies and an understanding of why the monosomies more often appear to be lethal are still unknown. From this point of view, chromosomal anomalies may become valuable tools in learning about the precise location of human genes. In the case of trisomies, some investigators have suggested that more damaging than the extra dose of genes is the regulatory imbalance created by the excessive genetic material (Bartalos and Baramki 1967; Trujillo *et al.* 1966). Others think that the presence of harmful recessive genes is the more important contributing factor (Bartalos and Baramki 1967). Whatever the reason, it is interesting to know that a large number of these chromosomal aberrations, and practically all when only the autosomes are involved, carry mental retardation as a common stigma. Possibly the common denominator of mental retardation results from a nonspecific chromosomal effect since any agent able to interfere with the orderly process of embryogenesis may, and often does, result in such a defect. Conversely, it may be argued that normal mental development is a slow, gradual, extremely sensitive process that requires the expression at different times of many diverse genetic loci involving practically all the chromosomal units. In the case of the more common autosomal defect, the G21 trisomy associated with Down's syndrome, there is frequently a lack of gross interference with the normal embryogenesis of the central nervous system, and it may well be that only one or a few biochemical mistakes are directly involved in the impairment of intelligence observed in these patients.

Consequently, to date the best solution for the medical problem created by the chromosomal anomalies lies in the preventive approach. Public education and genetic counseling could be very helpful, particularly in cases of familial translocation. The relationship of the mother's age to mongolism and other chromosomal anomalies must be emphasized. It is worth mentioning that a procedure has been devised which can ascertain beyond any doubt the karyotype of the human embryo. The method requires the aspiration of amniotic fluid for culturing and karyotype analysis of the fetal cells present in the fluid. Since the amniotic cells grow very fast, the chromosomal formula can be obtained in a period of between one and two weeks. Although still experimental, this procedure could prove to be of significant value in cases of selected genetic risk (Jacobson).

The ideal solution, of course, would be the prevention of the occurrence of chromosomal aberrations. Minimizing the exposure to those exogenous agents that can damage the human chromosomes is the first step. Much more research is needed, however, to clarify the mechanism of such cellular mistakes as nondisjunction. Since human cytogenetics is still a young discipline, we have every good reason to be optimistic for the future.

# REFERENCES

Bartalos, M., and Baramki, T. A. 1967. *Medical cytogenetics.* Baltimore: The Williams & Wilkins Co.

Bender, M. A., and Gooch, P. C. 1962. Persistent chromosome aberrations in irradiated human subjects. *Rad. Res.* 16:44.

Book, J. A., and Reed, S. C. 1950. Empiric risk figures in mongolism. *J. A. M. A.* 143:730.

Carter, C. O., and MacCarthy, D. 1951. Incidence of mongolism and its diagnosis in the newborn. *Brit. J. Soc. Med.* 5:83.

Cohen, M. M., Marinello, M. J., and Back, N. 1966. Chromosomal damage in human leukocytes induced by lysergic acid diethylamide. *Science* 155:1417.

Crick, F. H. C. 1958. On protein synthesis. *Symp. Soc. Exptl. Biol.* 12:138.

Edwards, J. H., Harnden, D. G., Cameron, A. G., Crosse, V. M., and Wolff, O. H. 1960. A new trisomic syndrome. *Lancet* 1:787.

Ford, C. E. 1961. Human chromosome mosaics. In *Proceedings of the conference on human chromosomal abnormalities*, ed. W. M. Davidson and R. Smith. Springfield, Ill.: Charles C. Thomas.

Ford, C. E., and Hamerton, J. L. 1956. The chromosomes of man. *Nature* 178: 1020.

Fraccaro, M., Kayser, K., and Lindsten, J. 1960. Chromosomal abnormalities in father and mongol child. *Lancet* 1:724.

Hamerton, J. L., Briggs, J. M., Gianelli, F., and Carter, C. O. 1961. Chromosome studies in detection of parents with high risk of second child with Down's syndrome. *Lancet* 2:788.

Hecht, F., Bryant, J. S., Bruber, D., and Townes, P. L. 1964. The non-randomness of chromosomal abnormalities: Association of trisomy 18 and Down's syndrome. *New Eng. J. Med.* 271:1081.

Jacobson, C. B. Personal communication.

Lejeune, J., Gautier, M., and Turpin, R. 1959. Etude des chromosomes somatiques des neuf enfants mongoliens. *C. R. Acad. Sci.* (Paris) 248:1721.

Lejeune, J., Lafourcade, J., Berger, R., Vialette, J., Baeswillwald, M., Seringe, P., and Turpin, R. 1963. Trois cas de deletion partielle des bras courts d'un chromosome 5. *C. R. Acad. Sci.* (Paris) 257:3098.

Lyon, M. F. 1962. Sex chromatin and gene action in the mammalian X-chromosome. *Am. J. Hum. Genet.* 14:135.

McGavin, D. D. M., Cant, J. S., Ferguson-Smith, M. A., and Ellis, P. M. 1967. The cri-du-chat syndrome with apparently normal karyotype. *Lancet* 2:326.

McIntire, M. S., Menolasino, F. J., and Wiley, J. H. 1965. Mongolism—some clinical aspects. *Am. J. Ment. Def.* 69:794.

Maclean, N., Mitchell, J. M., Harnden, D. G., Williams, I., Jacobs, P. A., Buckton, K. A., Baikie, A. G., Court Brown, W. M., McBride, J. A., Strong, J. A., Close, H. G., and Jones, D. C. 1962. A survey of sex chromosome abnormalities among 4514 mental defectives. *Lancet* 1:293.

Makino, S., and Nishimura, I. 1952. Water pre-treatment squash technique. A new and simple method for the chromosome study of animals. *Stain Tech.* 27:1.

Miller, O. J. 1964. The sex chromosome anomalies. *Am. J. Obst. & Gynec.* 90:1079.

Moorehead, P. S., Nowell, P. C., Mellman, W. J., Battips, D. M., and Hungerford, D. A. 1960. Chromosome preparations of leukocytes cultured from human peripheral blood. *Exptl. Cell Res.* 20:613.

Moorehead, P. S., and Saksela, E. 1963. Non-random chromosomal aberrations in $SV_{40}$ transformed human cells. *J. Cell Comp. Physiol.* 62:57.

Nichols, W. W., Levan, A., Hall, B., and Ostergren, G. 1963. Measles associated with chromosome breakage. *Hereditas* 50:53.

Nirenberg, N. W., Jones, O. W., Leder, P., Clark, B. F. C., Sly, W. S., and Pestka, S. 1963. On coding of genetic information. *Cold Spring Harbor Symp. Quant. Biol.* 28:549.

Ohno, S., and Makino, S. 1961. The single-X nature of sex chromatin in man. *Lancet* 1:78.

Ohno, S., Klinger, H. P., and Atkin, N. B. 1962. Human oogenesis. *Cytogenet.* 1:42.

Oster, J. 1953. *Mongolism.* Copenhagen: Danish Science Press, Ltd.

Patau, K. 1963. The origin of chromosomal abnormalities. *Path. Biol.* 11:1163.

Patau, K., Smith, D. W., Therman, E., Inhorn, S. L., and Wagner, H. P. 1960. Multiple congenital anomaly caused by an extra autosome. *Lancet* 1:790.

Polani, P. E. 1963. Cytogenetics of Down's syndrome (mongolism). *Pediat. Clin., North America* 10:423.

Polani, P. E., Briggs, J. H., Ford, C. E., Clarke, C. M., and Berg, J. M. 1960. A mongol girl with 46 chromosomes. *Lancet* 1:721.

Price, W. H., Strong, J. A., Whatmore, P. B., and McClement, W. F. 1966. Criminal patients with XYY sex-chromosome complement. *Lancet* 1:565.

Reed, S. C. 1963. *Counseling in medical genetics.* Philadelphia: W. B. Saunders Co.

Report of a study group: A proposed standard system of individual chromosomes, especially in man. 1960. *Am. J. Hum. Genet.* 12:250.

Rhoades, M. M. 1961. Meiosis. In *The Cell, III,* ed. J. Brachet and A. Mirsky. New York, Academic Press.

Russell, L. B. 1963. Mammalian X-chromosome action: Inactivation limited in spread and in region of origin. *Science* 140:976.

Sinott, E. W., Dunn, L. C., and Dobzhansky, T. 1958. *Principles of genetics.* 5th ed. New York: McGraw-Hill Book Co.

Smith, D. W. 1964. Autosomal abnormalities. *Am. J. Obst. & Gynec.* 9:1055.

Spieler, R. A. 1963. Genetic control of chromosome loss and nondisjunction in drosophila melanogaster. *Genet.* 48:73.

Stoller, A., and Collmann, R. D. 1965. Virus aetiology for Down's syndrome (mongolism). *Nature* 208:903.

Swanson, C. P. 1957. *Cytology and cytogenetics.* Englewood Cliffs, N. J.: Prentice-Hall, Inc.

Tjio, J. H., and Levan, A. 1956. The chromosome number of man. *Hereditas* 42:1.

Trujillo, J. M., Zeller, R. S., Plessala, R. A., and List-Young, B. 1966. Translocation heterozygosis in man. *Am. J. Hum. Genet.* 18:215.

Warkany, J. 1960. Etiology of mongolism. *J. Pediat.* 56:412.

Watson, J. D. 1965. *Molecular biology of the gene.* New York: W. A. Benjamin.

Watson, J. D., and Crick, F. H. C. 1953. Molecular structure of nucleic acids: Structure of deoxyribonucleic acid. *Nature* 171:737.

Wilson, E. B. 1928. *The cell in development and heredity,* 3rd ed. New York. The Macmillan Co.

Witschi, E., and Laguens, R. 1963. Chromosomal aberrations in embryos from overripe eggs. *Develop. Biol.* 7:605.

# Nondisjunction of Chromosome Number 21 in Siblings[1]

ANIL K. SINHA, Ph.D., GLORIA G. COCHRAN, M.D.,
and WINSTON E. COCHRAN, M.D.

*Departments of Pathology, Pediatrics, and the Division of Experimental Biology,
Baylor University College of Medicine, Houston, Texas*

In general, patients with mongolism (Down's syndrome) possess an extra chromosome number 21[2] or a portion of it in addition to the usual homologous pair of this chromosome. It is speculated that such trisomic individuals are the result of nondisjunction of a chromosome of pair 21 that failed to reach the opposite pole of its partner during anaphase movement of nuclear division. Such irregularities in chromosome distribution may occur during early embryogenesis or during a parental gametogenesis. Since this mishap happens to be the consequence of anomalies in pre-embryonic or postembryonic stages of development, this condition has been considered a sporadic event without familial significance.

At the child development clinics of Texas Children's Hospital, three

[1] This study was financed in part by grants from the Texas Heart Association, Baylor University College of Medicine General Research Support Grant (P-68-4), and a grant from the U.S. Children's Bureau (P-4-36). We wish to express our indebtedness to Drs. Harvey S. Rosenberg and Margery W. Shaw for their helpful suggestions.

[2] Although the chromosome pairs 21 and 22 are morphologically indistinguishable, it is conventionally understood that chromosome 21 in triplicate is responsible for mongolism.

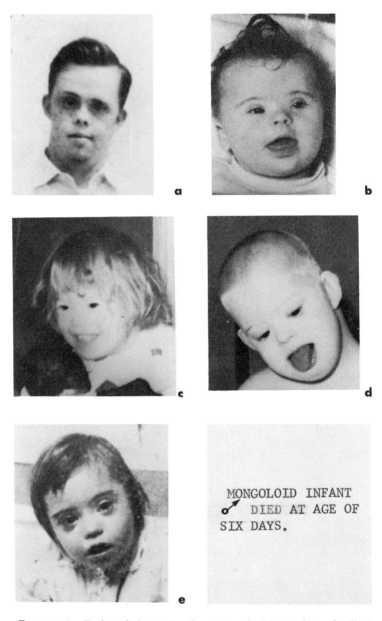

MONGOLOID INFANT
⚲ DIED AT AGE OF
SIX DAYS.

FIGURE 36. Facies of the probands: (a) and (b) are from family I, the male at twenty-four years of age and the younger sister when six months old. (c) and (d) are from family II, both when four years old. (e) is the surviving proband of family III, at two years of age.

families have been seen where more than one sibling had Down's pheno-type. The karyotypes of the patients exhibited a modal aneuploid number forty-seven with an extra 21 chromosome.

## Observations

All but one of the probands were referred by the Harris County Center for the Retarded to the Texas Children's Hospital clinics. They represent-ed three unrelated Caucasian families. In each family two siblings had the Down's phenotype (Fig. 36). There were no consanguineous mar-riages between the respective parents. All available parents were pheno-typically normal.

### Family I

The probands, on physical examination, exhibited typical phenotypic characteristics of Down's syndrome. The male and female were 24 and 16 and 2/12 years old respectively. Between their births, the parents had one normal son. Before the birth of the first affected child, the parents had five children. Of these, the eldest was a fertile female but had surgery for uterine carcinoma. Others were enjoying normal health except one who was suffering from arthritis.

When the first child with Down's was born, the mother was thirty-five and the father was thirty-four years old. Eight years later at age forty-three, the mother gave birth, with the same father, to the other child with Down's syndrome. The father's family history was not significant in re-gard to the occurrence of cancer or Down's syndrome. The mother had seven siblings. Her sibs had large families with no history of Down's syndrome.

### Family II

The two probands, a female aged 5 and 6/12 and a male aged 4 and 6/12, were the last children of the parents.

The mother had two spontaneous abortions during the first three months of pregnancy. Two years later she delivered a normal boy with a gestation period of forty-two weeks. After this delivery, a pregnancy of forty-two weeks ended in the birth of a female with Down's syndrome. At that time the mother was twenty-four years old and the father was twenty-six years old. A year later, the parents had the second child with Down's syndrome.

There was no known history of Down's syndrome on either side of the

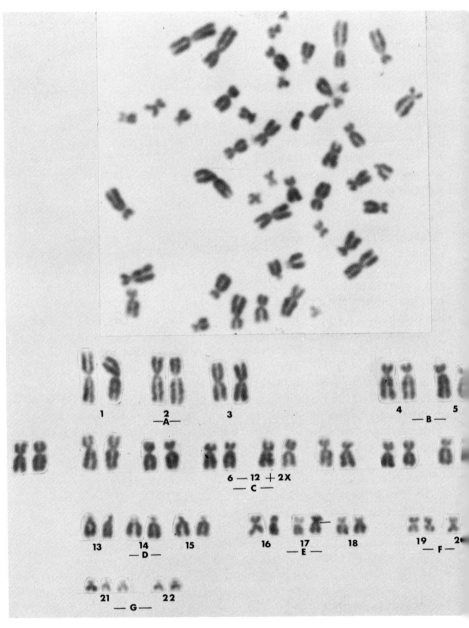

FIGURE 37.  A representative karyotype of the patients showing forty-seven chromosomes; trisomy-21.

patients' family. The mother had one brother, aged 30, living and well. He had one normal girl three years old. The father had two siblings and three half-siblings. They were married and had normal children. The paternal grandmother was fifty-nine years old.

### Family III

The proband, a two-year-old girl, was born with the stigmata of Down's syndrome after ten months gestation, a pregnancy complicated by fainting spells and a urinary infection. At the time of the birth of the patient, the mother was twenty-three years old and the father was twenty-seven years old. The mother's immediate prior pregnancy had terminated at eight months with the birth of a male child with Down's syndrome who died at six days of age. The gestation period in other pregnancies was likewise abnormal. Her last pregnancy with a different father was relatively uncomplicated except for occasional "fainting spells."

The patient had two normal sisters six and seven years old and a normal half-sister two months old. Family histories of the parents were noncontributory.

## Chromosome Findings

Chromosomes of the patients and of their normal relatives who made themselves available were studied by utilizing the peripheral blood culture technique of P. S. Moorehead and his associates (1960).

### Family I

The brother and sister with Down's syndrome had a modal aneuploid number of forty-seven with an extra 21 chromosome (Fig. 37). There were no obvious structural aberrations in the chromosome complements of the patients. The father refused to give a blood sample for chromosome studies. The chromosome preparation of a normal sibling conformed with the usual pattern of forty-six.

### Family II

The parents, their children with Down's, and the normal child were evaluated for their chromosome patterns. The normal child and the parents were considered chromosomally normal. The patients with Down's were found as trisomics for 21 chromosome. There were no other chromosomal aberrations in the probands.

*Family III*

The father of the proband with Down's was not located for chromosome analysis. Karyotypic studies were done on the mother, the proband with Down's and the half-sister of the proband. The mother and her phenotypically normal child had the usual mode of chromosome distribution. The proband had forty-seven chromosomes with number 21 in triplicate.

## Comments

Nondisjunction of chromosome number 21 in association with Down's phenotype involving more than one sibling is a rare phenomenon. That repeated nondisjunction occurs, nonetheless, is illustrated by the present families. M. W. Shaw (1962) has reported three trisomy-21 mongols born to a phenotypically normal couple. Their other two children were normal. K. H. Gustavson and his co-workers (1962) and Vislie and his associates (1962) observed siblings with five G-group chromosomes. Since these siblings had nonmongoloid features it was considered that chromosome number 21 was not involved in these cases.

Recurrence of nondisjunction of a 21 chromosome is difficult to explain, and there has been considerable discussion of reasons for such familial disjunctional errors. Late maternal age seems to act as a major factor in the production of mongoloid siblings (Carter and Evans 1961; Lejeune 1964). It has also been suggested that chromosomal rearrangements in the parents may induce irregular meiosis leading to repeated missegregation of the homologs in the offspring (Shaw 1962; Lejeune 1964).

The first family was probably a maternal age-related example of repeated Down's syndrome in successive pregnancies. Since the mothers involved in the other two families were fairly young, the age factor does not seem very significant in the production of their mongoloid children.

Parental karyotypic abnormalities were also considered. Although the parents who were not available for chromosome studies might have had some alterations, the chances are small since the normal close relatives of the patients exhibited no obvious aberration. It remains possible, however, that submicroscopic defects in the parental genotypes lead to repeated disjunctional errors.

# DISCUSSION

N. CARSON: Would either Dr. Sinha or Dr. Trujillo care to elaborate on the testing of amniotic fluid in the detection of inborn errors of metabolism?

J. TRUJILLO: Unfortunately, as far as I know, this work has not yet been published. However, about two weeks ago, I attended the last meeting of Mammalian Cytology and Somatic Cell Genetics in Monterrey and talked with Dr. Jacobson of George Washington University who has been performing these tests. He is a gynecologist interested in studying chromosomes, and he assured me that the method is practically harmless. It consists of the insertion of a needle through the dome of the pregnant uterus and the aspiration of a few milliliters of amniotic fluid. The fluid, which contains cells, is then placed directly into a tissue culture flask. According to him, there is no need to wash the cells since apparently they grow even better under these conditions. In his words, one or two weeks later they are able to obtain the karyotype of the conceptus. They are performing these tests in cases like those mentioned by Dr. Sinha which involve young mothers who have a mongoloid child and, being pregnant again, want to be reassured that the expected child is not also similarly affected. Of course, they are also studying, in the same manner, cases of translocation mongolism and other similar types involving high genetic risk. Apparently they have become very experienced in this test since, according to Dr. Jacobson, they have performed approximately three hundred amniocenteses without ill effects to the mother or the fetus. I do not know for sure how early in the pregnancy they can perform these tests, but I think it has to be at least at the end of the second or third month, since the first month is obviously too early.

G. DONNELL: Would you like to comment on the many studies in patients with Down's syndrome which attempt to place various gene loci on chromosome 21?

M. SHAW: Well, chromosome number 21 is getting quite crowded with genes. The general consensus at the present time is that a chromosomal imbalance will affect enzyme activity in a general way rather than by specific gene dosage. The most telling evidence is in the case of glucose-6-phosphate dehydrogenase activity, which is changed or increased in mongolism. Since we know that the glucose-6-phosphate dehydrogenase locus is on the X chromosome, it cannot be due to three doses of the gene on chromosome 21—and this puts a damper on the problem for the moment. We still do not understand the regulation of the enzyme activity or the effect nonspecific imbalance of the genes has on the cell or the organism. In addition to the biochemical or enzymatic assay and the chromosomal assay, amniocentesis for karyotyping can be used to determine sex in the case of sex-linked lethal diseases. The syndrome with hyperuricemia with self-mutilation would be an excellent example of an application in that case. If the woman is known to be carrying a male fetus, there would be one chance in two that the child would have received the abnormal gene. In the case of a female fetus, only a carrier or heterozygote state could result. The same would be true, of course, for hemophilia.

D. KEELE: Does Turner's syndrome have a higher incidence of mental retardation? I was not aware that this was so.

J. TRUJILLO: No, I did not mention Turner's.

D. KEELE: We had a child at Denton who should have had the cat-cry syndrome; she had all of the morphological features of the cat-cry syndrome, but I could not elicit exhibition of the cat-cry sound from the mother in any aspect. I just finally flat asked her and she said. "No, not like a cat." Well, we did a chromosome analysis; it was a ring chromosome instead of the deletion.

M. SHAW: Was it in the B group?

D. KEELE: Yes. And, then we went to the literature and found that somebody was ahead of us. Somebody from California reported the ring chromosome in the B group in a child with the cat-cry syndrome. It certainly appears that maybe there is a spectrum of syndromes involving abnormalities in the B group.

M. SHAW: Well, there are two pairs in the B group: chromosome 4 and chromosome 5, and there are known cases of deletion of the short arm in both pairs. The deletion in chromosome 5 is believed to be more commonly associated with cat-cry and the deletion in chromosome 4 without the cat-cry. This is a generalization and not always true. There is some overlapping, but the difference could explain your particular case.

It could be a ring chromosome number 4 rather than a number 5 and you cannot separate these two pairs morphologically or cytologically.

J. TRUJILLO: There are many cases studied so far. A friend of mine in the Children's Hospital in Los Angeles, who has been studying about fifty cases of mental retardation a month has collected, I think, five cases of "cri-du-chat" up to now and one of them is a twin.

# REFERENCES

Carter, D. O., and Evans, K. A. 1961. Risk of parents who have had one child with Down's syndrome (mongolism) having another child similarly affected. *Lancet* 2:785.

Gustavson, K. H., Hagberg, B., Finley, S. C., and Finley, W. H. 1962. An apparently identical extra autosome in two severely retarded sisters with multiple malformations. *Cytogenet.* 1:32.

Lejeune, J. 1964. The 21 trisomy—current stage of chromosomal research. *Prog. in Med. Genet.* 3:144.

Moorehead, P. S., Nowell, P. C., Mellman, W. J., Battips, D. M., and Hungerford, D. A. 1960. Chromosome preparations of leukocytes cultured for human peripheral blood. *Exp. Cell Res.* 20:613.

Shaw, M. W. 1962. Familial mongolism. *Cytogenet.* 1:141.

Vislie, H., Wehn, M., Brogger, A., and Mohr, J. 1962. Chromosome abnormalities in a mother and two mentally retarded children. *Lancet* 2:76.

# Large-Scale Studies in Massachusetts

HARVEY L. LEVY, M.D.

*Department of Neurology, Massachusetts General Hospital, Boston, Massachusetts*

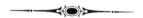

Large-scale studies presently being conducted in Massachusetts are predicated on two basic concepts:

1. That many inborn errors of metabolism are potentially treatable and that the earlier in life such therapy begins the more likely will damage (such as brain damage) be prevented.

2. That inborn errors of metabolism are rare diseases that can be studied in relatively large numbers only if large segments of the population are screened.

It is with these concepts in mind that Massachusetts embarked upon a program in 1962 to screen all newborns in the state for phenylketonuria. The program was conducted by the Massachusetts Department of Public Health under the direction of Dr. Robert A. MacCready and utilized the newly developed Guthrie bacterial inhibition assay as the means of detecting elevated levels of phenylalanine in blood-impregnated filter paper spots.

My purpose is not to dwell on the phenylketonuria detection program. Much has been published regarding these results (Kennedy *et al.* 1967). I will summarize such results in Table 17.

As the table depicts, the total number of hyperphenylalaninemics so far discovered is seventy-three. It is difficult to say how many represent the so-called typical PKU. But approximately thirty-four meet requirements for "typicality" in that the tolerance for phenylalanine has continued to

TABLE 17

Results of PKU Screening in Massachusetts
1962–November, 1967

| | | |
|---|---|---|
| Total births | 550,413 | |
| Number screened | 517,206 (94)% | |
| Hyperphenylalaninemia | 73 | |
| | 34 | "Classical" PKU |
| | 11 | "Atypical" PKU |
| | 28 | Others |

be very low. It is interesting that when this group was reevaluated it was discovered that all members had phenylalanine blood levels within the first ten days of life that exceeded 20 mg. per cent, and most were very high (over 35 mg. per cent. The normal blood phenylalanine level is about 2 mg. per cent.) The second group of eleven "atypical" members has been so classified because the phenylalanine dietary requirement in these children has been greater than the requirement in the "classical" type but not as high as that in the normal child. The newborn phenylalanine blood levels of these infants were usually 12 to 20 mg. per cent, and no one in this group had a phenylalanine level greater than 35 mg. per cent. The third group of "others" includes those children whose phenylalanine tolerance has become normal; most of these children initially had relatively low blood phenylalanine levels within the hyperphenylalaninemia classification, but all levels were greater than 4 mg. per cent.

In 1964 Dr. Efron and others published a simple, inexpensive, and convenient technique for the analysis of amino acids in whole blood which enabled screening programs to be greatly expanded (Efron *et al.* 1964). This technique utilizes the whole-blood–impregnated-filter-paper spot that is used in the Guthrie Test (Fig. 38). The filter paper is autoclaved and dried. A portion of the spot is then punched out and inserted into a punch hole in Whatman 3MM chromatography paper. Duplicate papers are chromatographed overnight in butanol:acetic acid:water (12:3:5) solvent. In the morning the papers are dried. One paper is stained with 0.1 per cent ninhydrin for amino acids. After this stained paper is inspected, it is overstained with diazotized sulfanilic acid for imidazole compounds, histidine being the most common of these compounds present in blood. The duplicate paper is stained with 0.2 per cent isatin for proline and overstained with Ehrlich's reagent for hydroxyproline. This

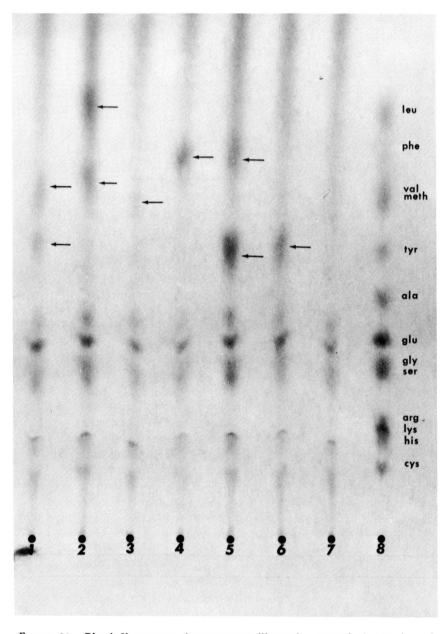

FIGURE 38. Blood filter paper chromatogram illustrating several abnormal specimens. 1. Neonatal homocystinuria with elevated methionine. 2. Maple syrup urine
disease. 3. Transient hypermethioninemia. 4. Phenylketonuria. 5. Tyrosinemia with
hyperphenylalaninemia. 6. Tyrosinemia. 7. Normal blood. 8. Amino acid mixture.

(Reproduced from *Clinical Biochemistry* 1:203, 1968, and with permission of the
Canadian Society of Clinical Chemists and the University of Toronto Press.)

combination of techniques should then identify most of the amino acid and imino acid disorders that are identifiable in blood.

Since 1964 this system has been used in the amino acid laboratory at the Massachusetts General Hospital. In 1966 it was incorporated into the Massachusetts screening program. We currently have data on almost 100,000 specimens representing between 96,000 and 97,000 individuals. About 95 per cent of these specimens have been obtained through the Massachusetts screening program.

I wish to discuss some of these findings.

1. The first disease diagnosed by this method is a newly discovered condition, which is soon to be reported and which has been given the name of *ornithinemia* and is characterized by an elevation of blood ornithine, ammonia intoxication, myoclonic seizures, and mental retardation. One little fellow was diagnosed at the Massachusetts General Hospital at the age of sixteen months where he was under investigation for the myoclonic seizures and developmental retardation. Treatment with a low-protein diet has succeeded in controlling the ammonia intoxication and the myoclonic seizures.

2. *Homocystinuria.* About seven months ago a four-day blood specimen from a newborn in the Massachusetts Screening Program was noted to contain a large quantity of methionine (Fig. 38). Investigation of the family revealed that the sister was retarded and that both the sister and the newborn brother had methionine elevations in the blood and the presence of homocystine in the blood and urine. After the diagnosis of homocystinuria was made, both of the children were placed on a low-methionine diet. The brother has progressed normally and at the age of eight months is perfectly normal in growth and development. The sister has also shown marked improvement in development although she is still mildly retarded. This case is similar to one reported by Dr. Perry and his colleagues in 1966. Of further interest, we were able to locate the original blood spot taken for the PKU Guthrie Test on the sister two and one-half years ago. This blood specimen clearly revealed an elevation of methionine in the sister at that time.

3. *MSUD.* A four and one-half–month-old male was hospitalized at the Massachusetts General Hospital for failure to thrive and developmental retardation. The blood amino acid chromatogram revealed an elevation of leucine, isoleucine, and valine (Fig. 38). Subsequent study revealed the typical biochemical features of maple syrup urine disease. He is now under treatment but is still developmentally retarded. An interesting side-

TABLE 18

Blood Amino Acid Abnormalities in Massachusetts

| Condition | Blood AA Elevations |
|---|---|
| Homocystinuria | Methionine |
|  | Homocystine |
| Maple syrup urine disease | Leucine |
|  | Isoleucine |
|  | Allo-isoleucine |
|  | Valine |
| Ornithinemia | Ornithine |
| Transient tyrosinemia | Tyrosine |
|  | ? Phenylalanine |
| Transient hypermethioninemia | Methionine |
| Transient hyperaminoacidemia | Many AA |
|  | Mostly essential |
| ? Dietary |  |

light to this problem is that the parents moved from Massachusetts to a neighboring state one month before he was born. Presumably, he would have been diagnosed during the first days of life had they remained in Massachusetts.

A second baby was born in Massachusetts with maple syrup urine disease. Since he was a premature he was not discharged from the hospital at the age of four days and inadvertently his blood was not sent to the Massachusetts Metabolic Screening Laboratory until he had been ill with opisthotonus and vomiting for over a month. Just prior to the time of submission of this blood specimen to the state laboratory the diagnosis of maple syrup urine disease was made by the local hospital. His blood showed the same findings as the blood of the previous baby. He was treated with the synthetic diet for maple syrup urine disease but died of complications at the age of six months. He also would have been diagnosed in the early days of life had his blood been analyzed at that time.

4. *Transient neonatal tyrosinemia.* This condition, a common one (Avery *et al.* 1967), has been diagnosed with the Massachusetts screening method. Actually about 0.5 per cent of all the newborn blood samples analyzed have shown the condition. Our policy has been to check all such elevations after 100 to 150 mg. of vitamin C has been given and so far, all such elevations have regressed. Such a check is necessary because the condition of tyrosinosis will otherwise be overlooked. This condition, charac-

terized by an elevation of tyrosine in the blood and the presence of tyrosine metabolites in the urine, is associated with liver and renal damage, both of which may be treated with a low-phenylalanine and low-tyrosine diet (Gentz *et al.* 1967).

5. Whenever a high phenylalanine level is noted in the blood by the Guthrie bacterial inhibition assay test, this same blood specimen is chromatographed by the method previously described (Fig. 38). Frequently this test reveals a high level of tyrosine so we then know that this represents some form of tyrosinemia and not phenylketonuria.

6. An interesting addendum to PKU testing has resulted from the practice of testing the mothers of all infants with elevated phenylalanine levels. One case of maternal phenylketonuria has been discovered in this manner. Such a finding might be expected because the mother with PKU would transfer her phenylalanine elevation to the baby. This elevated blood phenylalanine can perisist in the baby for several days following birth.

Table 18 summarizes the findings in Massachusetts by paper chromatography of newborn bloods.

Another category of the general metabolic screening program in Massachusetts consists of urine amino acid screening by paper chromatography.

About one-third of the hospitals in Massachusetts have been selected for this study. The parents of each infant born in these hospitals are asked to obtain a urine-impregnated filter paper on the infant when he is four to six weeks old. Generally the filter paper is inserted within the diaper and removed when wet. The filter paper is then sent to the State Public Health Laboratory where a disc is punched out and tested with cyanide and nitroprusside for cystinuria and homocystinuria. Another disc of each filter paper is then subjected to unidimensional chromatography in the same manner as described for the whole blood samples.

Figure 39 depicts a chromatogram with many of the abnormal urine samples.

This category of the Massachusetts screening program has been active since January 1966, and at present about 17,000 samples have been analyzed. This represents about 30 per cent of the eligible infants.

In closing, I wish briefly to present the results.

1. Ten infants with cystinuria have been identified (Fig. 39). Two of these have been homozygous for Type I; they have had large amounts of cystine, lysine, ornithine, and arginine in the urine, normal blood amino acids, and parents with normal urine amino acids. One of these cases has

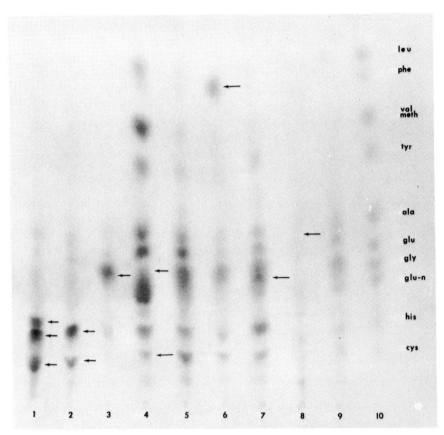

FIGURE 39. Urine filter paper chromatogram illustrating several abnormal specimens. 1. Cystinuria. Upper arrows point to lysine, ornithine, and arginine elevations.
2. Histidinemia. 3. Hyperglycinuria. 4. Hartnup disease. Note the elevation of
many amino acids but no elevation in glycine, cystine, lysine-ornithine, and arginine
areas. 5. Generalized hyperaminoaciduria. 6. Maternal phenylketonuria. 7. Transient
hydroxyprolinuria. 8. Dilute urine. 9. Normal urine. 10. Amino acid mixture.

(Reproduced from *Clinical Biochemistry* 1:212, 1968, and with permission of the
Canadian Society of Clinical Chemists and the University of Toronto Press.)

a sibling with the same findings who in addition has coarctation of the
aorta and mental retardation. The other eight infants have had increased
cystine and lysine in the urine, typical of the heterozygous form of Type
II or Type III cystinuria (Bartter *et al.* 1965). All ten infants are clinically normal.

2. A single infant has been found who has the urine amino acid pattern of Hartnup disease (Fig. 39; see Baron *et al.* 1956). Family study revealed that he has three siblings with the identical pattern. All these children are clinically normal. Further study of this family is still in progress.

3. One infant was found to have a very large amount of hydroxyproline in the urine. Though this amino acid is normally excreted in large amounts in early infancy, the amount manifested by this infant was far in excess of normal and much greater than the amount of proline and glycine excreted. Blood hydroxyproline was normal. By the age of three months, hydroxyproline excretion had become normal. This infant is clinically normal.

4. A specimen was sent to the state Laboratory by Dr. Maurice Kibel of Rhodesia on a fourteen-year-old girl with mental retardation and arachnodactyly. She was believed clinically to have homocystinuria. Much to everyone's surprise, she had histidinemia (Fig. 39; see Ghadimi, Partington, and Hunter 1961). She is currently under investigation.

5. In an attempt to detect metabolic disorders in the parents of institutionalized retarded children, the urine screening program has included the parents of all such children. Although far from completion, this program has already resulted in the discovery of a mother with phenylketonuria. She is the parent of three institutionalized retarded children, none of whom has phenylketonuria. Figure 39 depicts her urine pattern.

Table 19 summarizes those conditions detected by the urine screening program.

TABLE 19

Urine Amino Acid Abnormalities in Massachusetts

| Condition | Urine AA Elevations |
| --- | --- |
| Cystinuria | Cystine |
| | Lysine |
| | Ornithine |
| | Arginine |
| Hartnup disease | "Neutral" AA |
| Histidinemia | Histidine |
| | (metabolites) |
| Hyperglycinuria | Glycine |
| Transient hydroxyprolinuria | Hydroxyproline |

We feel that the entire program has been a success in terms of cooperation from physicians and parents and the detection of amino acid disorders. Such a comprehensive program is only now beginning to yield dividends that in the future may help to answer many of the questions raised by these conditions.

# DISCUSSION

D. TAUSCH: Dr. Levy, the state laboratory here requests repeat tests on initial Guthrie results considered "elevated but *less* than 4 mg. per cent." If a chromatogram procedure were to be set up and we were to check the results that are considered elevated, should that be at a level of only 4 mg. or only 6 mg. or something like that?

H. LEVY: Did you say you request repeat samples on Guthrie tests that are elevated above 4 or below 4?

D. TAUSCH: They are considered "elevated but less than 4." The normal range would be on the order of 2 mg. per cent.

H. LEVY: Well, I think one simple way of evaluating this would be to do paper chromatography on the filter paper specimen sent in for the initial Guthrie, and then you will probably see tyrosine elevations in 90 per cent of these cases. If you wish to investigate this further for the detection of tyrosinosis, you should then suggest that ascorbic acid be given and obtain another specimen in a week or so. I do think that on the basis of your seeing the very high elevation of tyrosine I have illustrated, you can reassure both the parents and the physician that the child does not have phenylketonuria. We have yet to see an infant with a true elevation of tyrosine who turned out to be phenylketonuric.

G. DONNELL: How long does it take you to get the results back into the hands of the referring physician from the time that you receive the sample? Rapid communication between laboratory and clinician is a great problem. With some of the metabolic conditions that are not lethal in the first few days of life this may not be catastrophic, but, as you know, with disorders such as maple syrup urine disease, hyperglycinemia, and galactosemia, the infant may well be dead before the report reaches the clinician.

H. LEVY. Well, in answer to your question, Dr. Donnell, I cannot say exactly how long it does take to get these results back because the time lags are variable. It might depend on what disease is suspected. If we discovered a child with maple syrup urine disease or suspected maple syrup urine disease, we would try to get that information to the pediatrician immediately in the hope that he could get it to the parent within a few hours. This would mean a telephone call, which we commonly employ, to tell the pediatrician what has been found in hopes that the child will then be seen, that the child is still well, and that the necessary blood samples will then be sent to us so that further investigation could be done in the next day or two to define whether this child truly has maple syrup urine disease or not. If the suspicion were very strong, we might recommend a temporary diet in the interim. In cases in which we have found urinary abnormalities, as in the heterozygotic form of cystinuria (which we think is benign in most cases, if not in all), we have been considerably more relaxed. We contact the pediatrician a day or two or even a week later. But, again, on cases such as phenylketonuria, suspected maple syrup urine disease, hyperglycinemia, or problems similar to these, we try to get the information and explanations to those involved as soon as possible. We have been burned on this in the past as you know.

G. Donnell: I know.

H. Levy: So have others.

G. Donnell: How long does it take from receipt of the blood sample to get a result in your own hands?

H. Levy: I am sorry. Maybe I did not make this clear. The chromatography screening is done at the Massachusetts Public Health Laboratories. It is not done at the Massachusetts General Hospital. Almost all of what I have discussed has been done as part of the Massachusetts State Public Health Laboratory metabolic screening program under the direction of Dr. MacCready.

E. Airaksinen: Who is reading those chromatogram slides—is it always the same person? There might be some question of interpretation sometimes?

H. Levy: Well, let me say this. The technicians and chemists at the Public Health Laboratory are very good and have been there for some time. The individual directly responsible for the chromatography, Miss Phyllis Madigan, has been there for a few years now and has seen tens of thousands of chromatograms. She is very good at interpretation. When there are any questions regarding any of the chromatograms, I or Dr. Shih will go down to the state laboratory and personally look at these chromatograms. In actuality, one of us is at the state laboratory on a regular consulting basis. Generally, if there is any question in interpretation, a repeat sample is requested.

H. BERRY: Have you followed up any of the infants with cystinuria—not the homozygous form? Is it permanent or transient?

H. LEVY: That is a good question. I must admit that we have not followed many of them. We have followed some of them—you mean the heterozygote or presumed heterozygous form?

H. BERRY: Whatever you are excepting from the homozygous form. The cystine-lysinuria without ornithine and arginine.

H. LEVY: We have followed some of these children. Most of them have been picked up within very recent months, and I would say that most of them are only about six to nine months of age now. We have two who are over a year of age. We have followed both of them, and we find that the condition in these infants is essentially unchanged at approximately a year of age in one and, I think, about fourteen months of age in the other. There is another question that has been asked by one of the chemists at the state Public Health Laboratory. "How do we know these infants do not have a condition like Wilson's disease?" You know the first renal amino acid defect that one may find in Wilson's disease is cystine lysinuria. This finding may be very striking. Some of Dr. Dent's original cases of cystine lysinuria were later found by him to have Wilson's disease. We have not looked carefully for this sort of thing.

H. BERRY: I inquired because we find the incidence of cystine-lysinuria without arginine and ornithine, without cystine stones, and usually with no evidence of abnormality in the family to be much higher in a mentally retarded population than in the normal population.

H. LEVY: Yes, I know you have reported this.

H. BERRY: Have you a comparable screening of retarded children?

H. LEVY: We have now screened the populations of three institutions for the retarded with a total population of about seven thousand and we have found three cases of homozygotic cystinuria and probably about ten heterozygotic cystinurics. I do not know what that would mean in terms of the general population. I would guess that would be a bit higher than what has been reported to be true of the general population, but I do not think it is much higher. Besides, the incidence of cystinuria in the normal population varies markedly from one study to another. Our feeling at the moment is that there is probably no etiologic relationship between cystinuria and mental retardation. Certainly, most of the children with cystinuria who are known have so far been clinically normal.

K. LEWIS: Do you have any estimate of the increased cost of this type of screening over the Guthrie Test alone?

H. LEVY: Well, I have been asked that question several times, and I do not have any absolute figures. The Public Health Laboratory does not have accurate figures because so many costs are interrelated with other programs. The most recent figure I obtained from Miss Valerie Karolkewicz, who is in charge of the laboratory staff, was something like $40,000 per year. By what percentage does the screening increase the program costs over the cost for doing only the Guthrie Test for PKU? I cannot really answer that except to say that it might increase the cost of Guthrie testing by maybe 25 per cent—something like that. Some of the personnel, of course, can be used interchangeably. The expense, therefore, would not be doubled, but it would certainly be increased.

G. DONNELL: I have one more question. You have limited your discussion to screening for disorders of amino acid metabolism. I would like to ask what your experience has been with screening for galactosemia in Massachusetts. I believe that you have been employing the Guthrie screening method. Is this not correct?

H. LEVY: Well, it is embarrassing to comment on that, Dr. Donnell, because we are either simply missing them all, or people with galactosemia all live in California. The state laboratory has screened over 100,000 newborns, and only one case of galactosemia has been found. This case was discovered by means of the Guthrie Test. We are now using the Beutler test (the second Beutler test about which I asked the question —the one in which oxidized TPN is reduced and therefore becomes fluorescent in ultraviolet light). We have found a large number of false positives. Dr. Beutler's 10 per cent false-positive incidence may be a little higher than ours, but I suspect that our false-positive incidence runs about 2 per cent or something like that. That is a lot when you are screening so many children every day, and the figure has presented a number of problems. I do not know how many children we have screened with the Beutler test now (I suppose it is in the several tens of thousands), and we have yet to recognize a case of galactosemia with this test.

L. HILL: Dr. Donnell, would you want to comment on the apparent difference in incidence between California and Massachusetts?

G. DONNELL: As I indicated before, I am not involved in mass screening. The only screening we do is in selected populations such as in children with idiopathic cataracts. In the Los Angeles area, one hospital is using the Guthrie screening method for detection of inborn errors of galactose metabolism. To the best of my knowledge, two patients with galactosemia have been part of the population screened. One of the patients was not recognized on the initial test. The subsequent test was positive after the pediatrician became suspicious on the basis of clinical manifestations. The second infant was picked up on the initial test.

H. LEVY: Of course, the Beutler test will only pick up Gal-1-P uridyl transferase deficiency. It would not pick up the galactokinase deficiency.

G. DONNELL: This is correct for the Beutler fluorescent technique.

H. LEVY: And would that be true of the Guthrie as well?

G. DONNELL: The Guthrie Test for galactosemia can recognize both transferase and galactokinase deficiencies since in both these conditions galactose is elevated in the blood. The Beutler fluorescent spot method, on the other hand, utilizes galactose-1-phosphate as a substrate so that the first enzymatic step (galactokinase) is bypassed. With this method only the transferase defect can be recognized.

H. LEVY: When Dr. Gittzlemann was in Massachusetts, we talked about this problem. We thought that perhaps we could add galactose and ATP rather than galactose-1-phosphate to the assay medium and that in this manner we could detect the galactokinase deficiencies as well with this modification. Unfortunately, this does not work because if you add ATP, you get fluorescence even if Gal-1-P uridyl transferase is not present, presumably because the ATP is used in reactions with glucose to form compounds that will eventually participate in TPN reducing reactions.

# REFERENCES

Avery, M. E., Clow, C. L., Menkes, J. H., Ramos, A., Scriver, C. R., Stern, L., and Wasserman, B. P. 1967. Transient tyrosinemia of the newborn: Dietary and clinical aspects. *Pediatrics* 39:378.

Baron, D. N., Dent, C. E., Harris, H., Hart, E. W., and Jepson, J. B. 1956. Hereditary pellagra-like skin rash with temporary cerebellar ataxia. Constant renal amino-aciduria, and other bizarre biochemical features. *Lancet* 2:421.

Bartter, F. C., Lotz, M., Thier, S., Rosenberg, L. E., and Potts, J. T., Jr. 1965. Cystinuria. *Ann. Int. Med.* 64:796.

Efron, M. L., Young, D., Moser, H. W., and MacCready, R. A. 1964. A simple chromatographic screening test for the detection of disorders of amino acid metabolism. *New Eng. J. Med.* 270:1378.

Gentz, J., Lindblad, B., Lindstedt, S., Levy, L., Shasteen, W., and Zetterstrom, R. 1967. Dietary treatment in tyrosinemia (tyrosinosis). *Am. J. Dis. Child.* 113:31.

Ghadimi, H., Partington, M. W., and Hunter, A. 1961. A familial disturbance of histidine metabolism. *New Eng. J. Med.* 265:221.

Kennedy, J. L., Wertelecki, W., Gates, L., Sperry, B. P. and Cass, V. M. 1967. The early treatment of phenylketonuria. *Am. J. Dis. Child.* 113:16.

# The Chemical Detection
# of Inherited Disorders That Result
# in Mental Deficiency[1]

PAUL M. TOCCI, Ph.D., EVA RUIZ, R.Ph.,
and GRACIELLA AQUERO, R.Ph.

*Departments of Pediatrics and Biochemistry, University
of Miami School of Medicine, Miami, Florida*

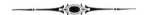

A screening program was instituted at the University of Miami in January of 1965. The objective of this program was to examine large numbers of patients suspected of having disorders of metabolism. The screening is provided on a demand service basis to the community. Acquired disorders, for instance those of renal tubular transport and tumors of the sympathetic nervous system, as well as genetic diseases, are of interest. The availability of therapy or of methodology for further intensive study has not been considered a criterion for inclusion of disorders in the screening battery. On the other hand, it is a further objective of the Biochemical Genetics Laboratory to undertake studies in depth on certain of the individuals detected in the screening program.

Because the program aims to provide a service and to be extensive both in numbers of individuals studied and in the number of conditions tested, attempts were made to use the simplest and fastest method available. The nature of the screening program, therefore, has been in a process of evo-

[1] This work was supported by H. E. W. Project #408.

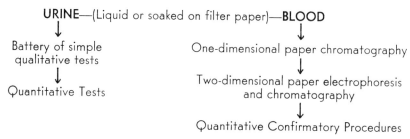

FIGURE 40. Design of routine screening workup carried out by the Biochemical Genetics Laboratory on urine and blood samples.

lution. It will inevitably change as further research and development of screening methods provide better knowledge of current and future problems. This program has crystallized sufficiently to provide an efficient diagnostic process. It is interesting to outline the screening program in its present form and to provide details of the present methods to permit their use in other communities.

A battery of simple qualitative tests are used in conjunction with one-dimensional paper chromatography (Fig. 40). The compounds currently tested for include amino acids, sugars, mucopolysaccharides, purines, pyrimidines, phenolic acids, simple organic acids, $\alpha$-keto acids, peptides, indoles, and imidazoles. Lipid, protein, and hemoglobin disorders are examined only when specifically requested. To date, over 7,000 individuals, mostly children, have been screened by this laboratory. A mass screening of newborns was not attempted. The population screened has, for the most part, been prescreened clinically and does not in any way represent the general population. Table 20 indicates the extent and variety of reasons for requesting a biochemical screening of the blood and/or urine. The reactions and possible diseases, if they are positive, are listed in Table 21.

I. Qualitative Screening Tests on Urine

Most tests can be performed on urine that is soaked on filter paper cards. The cards used for the Guthrie inhibition test for phenylketonuria are suitable or they may be hand cut from sheets of Whatman 3MM paper in three- by two-inch rectangles. In the case of infants, the card may be inserted in the diaper, and care should be taken that it not be left in for more than one micturition or that it not be contaminated with feces.

TABLE 20

Reasons for Requesting Biochemical Screening of the Blood and/or Urine

| | |
|---|---|
| Abnormal EEG | Hypotonia |
| Acidosis | Irritability |
| Alkalosis | Jaundice |
| Ataxia | Ketosis |
| Behavioral problem | Lethargy |
| Cataracts | Mental retardation |
| Cirrhosis | Muscle weakness |
| Coma | Nystagmus |
| Diarrhea | Odd facies (*FLK) |
| Dislocated lens | Odd hair |
| Dyslexia | Odd nails |
| Eczema | Odd odor |
| Failure to thrive | Photosensitivity |
| Feeding difficulty | Renal calculii |
| Flushing | Rickets |
| Gingivitis | Sibling of affected child |
| Glycosuria | Skin rash |
| Hepatomegaly | Slow speech |
| Hyperactive | Thromboembolic disease |
| Hyperpigmentation | Vomiting |
| Hypoglycemia | Wide gait |

(*Funny looking kid)

When the card or a portion of it is saturated, it is hung up to dry, and the name of the patient and the date are written at the top in pencil. It can then be mailed or stored for months in a refrigerator and is ready for analysis at any time. Liquid specimens are examined as quickly as possible and are also saturated onto the filter paper.

A. Primary Considerations

1. *Odor and Color* are examined carefully by observation. This procedure is not always pleasant but can be helpful in the interpretation of further tests.

2. *Density* is measured with a urinometer. Diabetes insipidus may be revealed by a specific gravity less than 1.006. This can be confirmed by the Hickey-Hare and Pitressin tests. Abnormally concentrated specimens are also detected.

## TABLE 21

Qualitative Screening Tests

| Reaction | Fresh Urine | Urine on Filter Paper | Substance Detected | Possible Diseases if Reaction is Positive |
|---|---|---|---|---|
| Odor and color | + | | | Phenylketonuria<br>Maple syrup urine disease<br>Oast house disease<br>Alkaptonuria |
| Density | + | | | Diabetes insipidus |
| Clinitest Tablets® (Benedict test) | + | | Reducing sugars | Diabetes mellitus<br>Essential fructosuria<br>Fructose intolerance<br>Congenital lactosuria<br>Galactosemia<br>Essential pentosuria |
| Clinistix® | + | | Glucose | Diabetes mellitus<br>Renal glycosuria |
| Cyanide-nitroprusside or Iodine-azide | + | + | Homocystine<br>Cystine | Homocystinuria<br>Cystinuria<br>Fanconi syndrome<br>Wilson's disease |
| Ferric chloride | + | + | Phenylpyruvic acid<br>Imidazole-pyruvic acid | Phenylketonuria<br>Smith-Strang syndrome<br>Histidinemia |
| 2,4-Dinitrophenyl-hydrazine | + | | Keto acids | Phenylketonuria<br>Smith-Strang syndrome<br>Histidinemia<br>Maple syrup urine disease<br>Tyrosinosis of the newborn |
| o-Tolidine | + | + | Copper | Wilson's disease |
| Azure A | + | + | Mucopoly-saccharides | Gargoylism<br>Marfan's disease<br>Morquio's disease |
| Tolidine blue | + | | Intracellular sulfatides | Metachromatic leucodystrophy |
| Millon's test | + | + | Tyrosine p-hydroxy-phenylpyruvic acid | Tyrosinosis<br>Tyrosinemia<br>Wilson's disease<br>Hartnup disease<br>Galactosemia |
| Isatin | + | + | Proline | Hyperprolinemia<br>Fanconi syndrome<br>Wilson's disease<br>Joseph's disease |

+ denotes positive reaction
® Ames Company, 1127 Myrtle Street, Elkhart, Indiana 46514

3. *Reducing Substances* are detected using Clinitest Tablets (Ames Company). Specimens giving positive reactions should be examined by paper chromatography.

4. *pH, Protein, Glucose, and Ketones* are estimated by the use of Labstix (Ames Company). The glucose strip is impregnated with glucose oxidase.

5. *Microscopic Inspection* is made of the urinary sediment after ten minutes centrifugation. The information gained by this can aid in the interpretation of further tests.

B. Specific Tests

1. *Ferric Chloride Test*

Reagent: FeCl$_3$, 5%

Procedure: To 10 drops urine, add five drops of 5% ferric chloride. A dark green color is positive.

Phenylpyruvic acid and imidazole pyruvic acid give a positive reaction. Therefore, the classic green color is indicative of histidinemia as well as of phenylketonuria.

Ames Company markets a paper strip impregnated with buffered FeCl$_3$ called Phenistix. It compares satisfactorily with the liquid reagent and has a sensitivity of 5 to 10 mg. per cent (Rupe and Free 1959; Gibbs and Woolf 1959).

2. *Keto Acids* are estimated using 2,4-dinitrophenylhydrazine (Menkes 1960).

To five drops of urine in a small test tube, add twenty drops 0.2 per cent 2,4-dinitrophenylhydrazine in 2N HCl. Wait ten minutes. Then add an equal volume of ether and shake. Remove the top layer and put it into a clean test tube. To this, add an equal volume of 10 per cent Na$_2$CO$_3$ and shake. A positive test is a yellow (or orange) color in the lower layer in the tube. Positive reactions were estimated on a 0 to 4+ scale. Thin layer chromatography may be used to identify the compounds (Tocci 1967).

3. *Cystine and Homocystine* are tested for by a modification of Brand's Test (Brand, Harris, and Biloon 1930).

To five drops of urine in a depression or spot plate, add one drop of concentrated NH$_4$OH and two drops of sodium cyanide (5% solution). Mix and wait ten minutes. Then add freshly prepared 5 per cent sodium nitroprusside drop by drop. If a deep red appears after several drops, the reaction is positive. The color fades in a few minutes. Argininosuccinic acid anhydride reacts weakly with this reagent.

4. *Cystine* may also be determined in urine that is dried on filter paper (Berry 1962). 1.5 gm. sodium azide in 50 ml. of 0.1N iodine solution. Dilute with 50 ml. of 95 per cent ethanol and store in brown bottle in refrigerator. Decolorization of reagent within five minutes indicates cystine or homocystine. Minimum detectable cystine is 200 $\mu$g per ml. (Argininosuccinic acid anhydride does not react.)

5. *Tyrosine* is estimated with Millon's reagent (Hsia 1959). 10 gm. of mercury in 11 ml. of fuming nitric acid. Pour slowly into 22 ml. of water.

To one drop of fresh urine dried on filter paper, apply one drop of Millon's reagent; let dry at room temperature. If a bright orange color develops, the test is positive. If urine is received dried on filter paper, add a small drop of reagent to the paper. If tyrosine or p-hydroxyphenylpyruvic acid is present at 300 $\mu$g. per ml. concentration, an orange-brown ring will develop in two minutes. This should be followed by paper chromatography to identify the compound.

6. *Mucopolysaccharides* are examined by the Berry method (Berry 1962).

Wet Whatman 3MM paper in Azure A reagent (0.5% Azure A in 2% acetic acid) and let dry. These papers can be stored for several weeks and used when necessary. Their dimensions are best determined by the size of the dip trays used for washing. Add one drop of urine and let dry. Many urines can be run on a single sheet of paper. Wash the paper by dipping in 2 per cent acetic acid and let paper drain. Then wash again in a fresh tray of 2 per cent acetic acid. If the urine is dried on filter paper, add one drop Azure A reagent to the paper. Let dry and wash twice with 2 per cent acetic acid. A deep, shiny purple spot, otherwise known as a metachromatic spot, which persists after the blue background has been washed out is evidence of a high concentration of mucopolysaccharides. A standard of chrondroitin sulfate A is usually spotted as well as the unknown(s). A level of 2 mg. per ml. gives a 4+ reaction. The urine of a patient known to have gargoylism may also be used as a control. A reaction of 2+ or more is considered enough to go further to identify the compound by paper chromatography.

7. *Proline* is estimated by the Berry method (Berry 1962).

Dip Whatman 3MM paper in isatin solution (20 mg. isatin in 96 ml. acetone and 4 ml. glacial acetic acid). This reagent is stable for several weeks if refrigerated. Allow the paper to dry at room temperature. Add one drop of urine and dry in oven 100° C. for ten minutes. Then, dip into 1N HCl and finally, wash with distilled water.

If the urine is dried on filter paper, add one drop of the isatin solution and proceed with HCl and water wash.

Interpretation

| Deep blue | — | Proline |
|---|---|---|
| Blue grey | — | Phenylalanine |
| Brown | — | Tryptophan |
| Purple | — | Several amino acids (Depth of color indicates the concentration of amino acids) |

Minimum concentration for a positive reaction is 0.1 mg. per ml. of proline. The guilty compound should be identified by paper chromatography.

8. *Increased α-Amino Nitrogen Excretion* is estimated by the ninhydrin method (Hyanek and Cafourkova 1965).

A drop of urine is applied to filter paper that was previously impregnated with a 3 per cent solution of KOH and dried at room temperature. The spotted paper is dipped into ninhydrin reagent (15 mg. ninhydrin in 5 ml. 95 per cent ethanol mixed with 5 ml. ethylene glycol and 0.1 M acetic acid), then heated wet for five minutes to 100° C. The authors suggested 10 mg. of ninhydrin, but in our laboratory 15 mg. gave more reliable results. Urines containing increased amino acids yield a more intense and persistent blue coloration than does normal urine.

The method is not satisfactory for high levels of taurine, asparagine, proline, or hydroxyproline because their coloration is not purple with ninhydrin. If a positive result of 2 + or more was obtained, the α-amino nitrogen was determined by a modification of the method of S. Moore and W. H. Stein (1954) using an ammonia distillation as described by A. Khachadurian and W. D. Knox (1960). Paper chromatography should be done on all specimens that give a greater than 1 + reaction.

9. *Calcium* is determined by the Sulkowitch method (Ritter, Spencer, and Samachson 1960).

Calcium in urine is precipitated as the oxalate by the addition of a buffered oxalic reagent (2.5 gm. oxalic acid, 2.5 gm. $(NH_4)_2SO_4$ and 5 ml. of glacial acetic acid in water, and add water to a final volume of 150 ml.). The pH is such that phosphates do not precipitate. The degree of turbidity is noted visually. The results provide a rough estimate of the serum calcium level. To ten drops urine in a small test tube, add ten drops of Sulkowitch reagent and mix by inversion.

Observe turbidity after one to two minutes. The turbidity is graded from 0 to 4+. Serum calcium levels should be determined with results over 2+.

Interpretation: 0 to 2+ turbidity means serum calcium level of approximately 7.5 mg. per 100 ml.; 3 to 4 + turbidity means serum calcium level of approximately 10.5 mg. per 100 ml.

10. *Metachromatic Leucodystrophy* is screened for by the Lake method (Lake 1965).

Fresh urine, and preferably *not* an early morning specimen, was centrifuged at 2000 to 3000 rpm. for ten minutes, and the *supernatant* was discarded. Six microscopic smears were made from the sediment and fixed in formalin vapor at 60° C. for one hour. The slides were washed in water and stained for ten minutes at room temperature in a 1 per cent aqueous solution of cresyl fast violet, the pH of which had been adjusted to 3.5 to 3.6 with acetic acid. The smears were washed in water and mounted in glycerin jelly. They were examined microscopically under the high and dry lens. Only intracellular material stained golden brown is considered positive.

11. *Homogentisic Acid* may be suspected when the test for reducing substances (Clinitabs) ends in an atypical reaction (brown or black color) and when the ferric chloride test yields a momentary deep blue color. Its presence is confirmed by the addition of a few drops of 10 per cent NaOH to a few milliliters of urine in a test tube. A brown to black color is produced in one to two minutes.

12. *Copper Test*: Method for urine dried on filter paper (Berry 1962).

Dissolve o-tolidine 0.1 gm. and 0.5 gm. NH₄CNS in 5 ml. of acetone immediately before use. Add a small drop of this reagent to the paper. If a blue color appears in thirty seconds, it indicates a positive reaction with 10 $\mu$g. per cent or more of copper present. It notes the possibility of Wilson's disease. The serum ceruloplasmin test should be done before quantitative analysis is attempted. See Section II, Part C.

13. *Obermayer's Test for Indican* (Miller 1955)

Procedure: Add an equal volume of urine and Obermayer's reagent (0.4% FeCl₃ in concentrated HCl) in a test tube. Mix well. Add 2 or 3 ml. chloroform or carbon bisulfide and, closing the tube with the thumb or a clean cork, rock the tube back and forth gently at least ten times. Do not shake violently. The production of a blue color in the chloroform is presumptive evidence of the presence of indican. The color is probably due to indigo blue. Occasionally, indigo red appears. Iodine also gives the same red color. Pour off the urine mixture from the colored chloroform solution, and add to the latter a few drops of a 20 per cent solution of sodium hyposulfite. Mix well. If the color does not disappear, it is due to indican. Hexamethylenetetramine and formaldehyde interfere with the reaction. Bile pigments, if present, should be removed by adding about one-third volume calcium hydroxide, mixing well, and filtering before proceeding with the test.

Interpretation: The appearance of a dark blue color and occasionally of a red color in the chloroform which does not disappear on the addition of sodium hyposulfite indicates the presence of indican in the urine in abnormal quantities. Slight traces are present in many normal urines.

## II. Blood Screening Procedures

In the absence of chromatography, the number of disorders detectable in blood by screening procedures is very limited. However, there are three important genetic diseases that can be reliably ruled out by simple tests. These are Wilson's disease (hepatolenticular degeneration), glucose-6-phosphate dehydrogenase deficiency, and galactosemia.

A. Screening Procedure for Glucose-6-Phosphate Dehydrogenase (G-6-P-D) Deficiency (Beutler and Baluda 1966)

## 1. Reagents

TABLE 22 a

Reaction Mixture for Screening Test for Glucose-6-Phosphate Dehydrogenase

| Reaction Mixture Compound* | Conc. of Stock Solution | Vol. to make 6 ml. |
|---|---|---|
| Potassium phosphate buffer pH 7.4 | $2.5 \times 10^{-1}$M | 0.3 |
| Glucose-6-phosphate | $1.0 \times 10^{-2}$M | 0.1 |
| NADP† pH 6.8 | $7.5 \times 10^{-3}$M | 0.1 |
| Digitonin | sat. sol'n | 0.2 |
| Water | — | 0.3 |

* All reagents except the buffer are available from Sigma Corporation.
† Nicotinamide—adenine dinucleotide phosphate.

2. Procedure: Incubate 0.02 ml. of red-cell suspension (1:1 suspension in isotonic saline) in 0.2 ml. of substrate mixture for fifteen minutes at room temperature. A few microliters of the incubation mixture is spotted on Whatman #1 filter paper and allowed to dry.

3. Interpretation: The fluorescence is examined under long-wave ultraviolet light for the fluorescence of NADPH.[2] No fluorescence indicates a lack of the enzyme.

## B. Screening for Galactosemia (Beutler and Baluda 1966)

### 1. Reagents

TABLE 22 b

Reaction Mixture for Screening Test for Galactosemia

| Reaction Mixture Compound | Conc. of Stock Solution | Vol. to make 6 ml. |
|---|---|---|
| Uridine diphosphoglucose | $9.5 \times 10^{-3}$M | 0.40 |
| Galactose-1-phosphate | $2.7 \times 10^{-2}$M | 0.20 |
| NADP, pH 6.8 | $6.6 \times 10^{-3}$M | 0.60 |
| Tri-acetate buffer, pH 8.0 | 0.75M | 2.00 |
| Digitonin | Sat. Sol. | 0.80 |
| Di-sodium ethylenediamine tetracetate (EDTA) | $2.7 \times 10^{-2}$M | 0.03 |
| Water | — | 1.97 |

[2] Nicotinamide—adenine dinucleotide phosphate (reduced).

2. Procedure: Incubate 0.02 ml. of red-cell suspension (1:1 suspension in isotonic saline) in 0.20 ml. of substrate mixture for three hours at 37° C. A few microliters are then spotted on Whatman #1 filter paper and allowed to dry.

3. Interpretation: The test relies on the fluorescent property of NADPH when activated by long wave length ultraviolet light. A failure to develop fluorescence may be due to galactosemia or to a severe glucose-6-phosphate dehydrogenase deficiency such as may be found in association with nonspherocytic congenital hemolytic anemia. A more specific assay must, therefore, be carried out to confirm the diagnosis. The entire assay is available in a kit form that works very well. It is sold by Hyland Laboratories of Los Angeles, California.

C. Detection of Ceruloplasmin (Aisen *et al.* 1960)

1. Reagents: Ten microliters of serum are applied to specially prepared papers, incubated in a closed container in a water bath at 45 to 50° C. for five to ten minutes. The papers are prepared by briefly immersing Whatman #1 filter paper (2 x 5 cm.) in a solution of 0.5 per cent p-phenylenediamine hydrochloride in a sodium acetate buffer of pH 5.7 and 0.5 ionic strength. They are then blotted and dried in a nitrogen atmosphere at 50° C. They can be stored for three weeks at room temperature in a nitrogen atmosphere.

2. Procedure: A control serum containing between 18 and 20 mg. per cent ceruloplasmin is run on each strip. Normal serum oxidizes the p-phenylenediamine hydrochloride and a blue-purple color is formed.

3. Interpretation: Serums with less than 20 mg. per cent ceruloplasmin will give little or no color.

III. Chromatography—Blood and Urine

A. Preparation

The most awkward part of preparing a chromatogram is the application of the specimen to the paper. For good results, the spots must be small (about 0.5 cm.) and of uniform size. Normally, many small aliquots must be applied to the paper with a micropipette; drying must take place between each application. The problem of application of the specimens has been overcome by M. L. Efron and associates (1964), who use discs of filter paper which are soaked with the specimen.

Urine, plasma, serum, whole blood, or cerebrospinal fluid (C.S.F.) are soaked on a two- by three-inch card of Whatman 3MM or Schleicher-Schuell #903 paper. The patient's name and the date are written at the top of the card in pencil. The papers are dried by hanging in air and may be stored for many months in the refrigerator in plastic sandwich bags. The cards, thus prepared, are easier to handle and store than liquid specimens. Discs are cut from the cards with a common paper punch (3/16 in. diameter). Similar holes are made in sheets of Whatman 3MM chromatography paper, one inch from the bottom of the paper and one inch between discs. The sheet may be any convenient size and is cut to fit the chromatography tank both in height and width. The tank may be a gallon pickle jar with a screw top, a commercially made cabinet measuring three by four by five feet and costing hundreds of dollars, or any glass container of suitable dimensions. Two discs of each specimen are put into the holes made in the chromatography sheet and secured by pressing around the edges of the disc with a blunt-edged instrument. The paper is then made into a cylinder and sewn together with a few stitches of white thread, so it stands by itself, or it may be suspended from the top of the tank so that the bottom of the paper just touches the bottom of the tank. The paper must be perpendicular to the bottom of the tank and only touch the tank on the bottom. Two discs of each specimen and one normal specimen are chromatographed. The discs have the advantage of maintaining uniform amount and shape of each specimen applied to the paper. Whole blood saturated on paper must be autoclaved for three minutes at 25° C. to degrade the hemoglobin. This step is omitted in the case of serum, plasma, urine, and C.S.F. The solvent is n-butanol, glacial acetic acid, and water in the proportions 12:3:5 by volume. This solvent precipitates proteins on the discs and allows for a clean separation of compounds from the origin. Enough solvent is put in the tank to wet one half-inch portion of the bottom of the paper. The solvent should be made up every forty-eight hours and may be used twice. The development time will depend upon the length of the paper. Table 23 gives the Rf's of many important compounds in this solvent and their reactions with the various location reagents. A sheet fourteen inches long is sufficient for a fifteen-hour run (from 5:00 P.M. until 8:00 A.M. the next morning, for instance). When the solvent is at, or near, the top of the paper, the chromatogram is taken out of the tank and hung up to dry. When the chromatogram is developed,

# TABLE 23

## Rf of Some Compounds in Butanol : Acetic Acid : Water (12:3:5) Ascending on Whatman 3MM Paper

| Compound | Rf* | Isatin | Ninhydrin | Pauly |
|---|---|---|---|---|
| Cystathionine, 2 spots | 2, 7 | Pk–P | Dk.P | — |
| Cystine | 11 | P–B | P | — |
| Ornithine | 16 | Pk–B | P | — |
| Lysine | 17 | Pk | P | — |
| Arginine | 18 | Pk | Dk.P | — |
| Anserine | 18 | Gy.B | Gy.P | — |
| Histidine | 18 | Gy.B | P.Gy | R |
| Carnosine | 19 | Gy.B | Gy | R |
| Argininosuccinic acid | 20 | Pk | R–P | — |
| Glycine | 22 | Pk | P | — |
| 3-Methyl histidine | 22 | P.B | Dk.P | — |
| Serine | 23 | Pk.Gy | Dk.P | — |
| Hydroxyproline | 25 | G | Bn.Y | — |
| Glutamine | 26 | Pk | Ft.P | — |
| Aspartic acid | 27 | Gy.B | Dk.P | — |
| Citrulline | 27 | Pk | Dk.P | — |
| Homocystine | 27 | Gy | Dk.P | — |
| Sarcosine | 30 | Pk | Pk.P | — |
| Glutamic acid, 2 spots | 31–34 | P.B | Dk.P | — |
| Threonine | 32 | Pk | Dk.P | — |
| Alanine | 38 | P.B | Dk.P | — |
| Proline | 39 | B | Y | — |
| Ethanolamine | 44 | B | P | — |
| β-aminoisobutyric acid | 46 | Pk | P | — |
| Indican | 48 | Pk | — | — |
| Tyrosine | 48 | B | Dk.P | R.Bn |
| β-alanine | 50 | B | P.B | — |
| Methionine | 56 | P.B | P | — |
| Tryptophan | 56 | B | Ft.P | — |
| Valine | 57 | Pk | P | — |
| Xanthurenic acid | 60 | — | — | R.P |
| Phenylalanine | 65 | Pk.B | Dk.Pk | — |
| Isoleucine | 69 | Dk.Pk | Dk.P | — |
| Leucine | 71 | Pk.P | Dk.P | — |
| p-Hydroxyphenylpyruvic acid | 83 | — | — | — |
| 3-Hydroxyanthranilic acid | 88 | — | — | — |
| Ortho-hydroxyphenylacetic acid | 90 | — | — | R–Or |
| Anthranilic acid | 94 | — | — | Ft.Y |
| p-Hydroxyphenylacetic acid | 94 | — | — | Dk.R.P |

$$* \ Rf = \frac{\text{Distance of spot from origin}}{\text{Distance of solvent travel}}$$

Abbreviations:  P = Purple      Pk = Pink
             R = Red      Bn = Brown
             G = Green      Gy = Gray
             Y = Yellow      Dk = Dark
             B = Blue      Ft = Faint
             Or = Orange

Table 24

Ascending Chromatography of Sugars

| Sugars | Color | Rg* |
|---|---|---|
| Ribose | Dark pink | 1.60 |
| Xylose | Dark pink | 1.40 |
| Fructose | Yellowish-brown | 1.13 |
| Glucose | Grayish-brown | 1.00 |
| Galactose | Gray | 0.84 |
| Sucrose | Brown | 0.44 |
| Lactose | Grayish-brown | 0.24 |
| Glucoronic acid | Dark yellow | 0.15 |

Solvent: Ethyl acetate, pyridine, water (12:5:4)
Dye: 2% Aniline, 1.66% phthalate in acetone
* Rg = $\dfrac{\text{Distance compound migrates}}{\text{Distance glucose migrates}}$

it is air-dried for ten to fifteen minutes and then oven-dried for five minutes at 100° C. Any visible spots are outlined in pencil. Then the staining procedure indicated below is followed.

#1 — Ninhydrin ——————→ Ehrlich
#2 — Isatin ——————————→ Ehrlich
#3 — Pauly
#4 — Aniline-phthalate (sugars)

Compounds can be identified from their Rf and the color reactions with the various reagents. The use of normal or control fluids as a comparison on the same sheet is mandatory for good interpretation of the chromatograms. The lack of standardized temperature, atmosphere, and the variability of reagents require care in the interpretation of the results. Under no circumstances should the chromatogram be evaluated quantitatively, and any deviation from normal should be investigated further. Slight variations are best treated by chromatographing a fresh specimen before proceeding with further testing. Grossly abnormal specimens should be examined quantitatively with the appropriate test as soon as possible.

A fourth filter paper disc impregnated with urine can be used to search for abnormal sugar excretion. For this purpose, a different solvent system is used. Ethyl acetate and pyridine in water (12:5:4) is preferable for the separation of the sugars (Smith 1960). After chromatography, the chromatograms are treated with aniline-phthalate reagent. The Rg's of several sugars and their colors with the location reagent are given in Table 24.

For various other techniques involving paper or thin layer chromatography and electrophoresis, the reader is referred to the literature.[3]

It is desirable to do a creatinine determination when examining urine. The variability of concentration of this fluid makes it extremely difficult to interpret the results of chromatography. Creatinine is determined by a modified Jaffe reaction. To 0.1 ml. of urine, add 6 ml. of alkaline picrate reagent. Mix well and read at 510 m$\mu$. after fifteen minutes. The alkaline picrate reagent should be prepared just before use in the following way:

1. 15 ml. of 1 per cent picric acid (or a saturated solution).
2. 3 ml. of 10 per cent sodium hydroxide.
3. Mix and dilute to 100 ml. with water.

Standards of 0.5 and 0.2 mg. per ml. concentration are run with each determination.

B. Location Reagents for Chromatography (Smith 1960)

1. *Ninhydrin*: 0.2 per cent in acetone (w/v).

Best results are obtained with ninhydrin purchased from Pierce Chemical Company. Immediately before use, 2 per cent pyridine is incorporated directly into the reagent in the dip tray, and the paper is dipped. Paper is heated in an oven at 100° C. for three to five minutes. The colors can be preserved by dipping the dry, stained chromatogram through a solution of copper nitrate (1 ml. saturated aqueous $CuNO_3$ in 100 ml. ethanol plus 0.1 ml. 10 per cent $HNO_3$).

2. *Isatin*: 0.2 per cent in acetone (w/v).

Incorporate 2 per cent pyridine just before use. Dip, let acetone evaporate off, and dry in oven at 100° C. for three to four minutes. Proline reacts to give a blue color; phenylalanine gives a light purple color.

3. *Pauly Reagent*

9 gm. of sulphanilic acid, 90 ml. of concentrated HCl in 900 ml. of water—1 volume.

---

[3] See Scriver, Eluned, and Cullen 1964; Samuel 1964; Sackett 1964; Turner and Juster 1964; Samuels and Ward 1966; Troughton, St. Clair Brown, and Turner 1966.

5 per cent sodium nitrite, in water (freshly made each day)—1 volume.

10 per cent sodium carbonate—2 volumes.

Mix the first two stock reagents and allow to stand four minutes in the refrigerator. Add the third reagent slowly. Dip the chromatogram and place immediately on a horizontal nonabsorbent surface. The reagent may also be sprayed lightly while the chromatogram hangs suspended.

4. *Ehrlich Reagent*

p-Dimethylaminobenzaldehyde, 10 per cent in concentrated HCl (w/v)—1 volume.

Acetone—4 volumes.

Mix the above reagents just before use. Dip paper immediately and air dry. Colors develop in twenty minutes.

5. *Cyanide Nitroprusside*

a. To 2 gm. NaCN in 5 ml. of water, add 95 ml. of 95 per cent ethanol.

An immediate precipitate appears. Use the supernatant without filtration.

b. To 1.5 gm. sodium nitroprusside in 5 ml. of $H_2SO_4$, add 95 ml. of methanol.

Add 10 ml. of concentrated $NH_4OH$.

A copious precipitate occurs. Store the filtrate in the refrigerator. Equal volumes of reagents *a* and *b* are mixed as required, and the paper is dipped and laid flat. Purple spots, which fade after about thirty minutes, are obtained with cystine, cysteine, cystamine, meso-cystine, homocysteine, homocystine, and argininosuccinic acid and its anhydride.

6. *Aniline-Phthalate Reagent*: Aniline 2 per cent and phthalic acid 1.66 per cent in acetone. Dip and heat at 100° C. for twenty minutes. Hexoses and pentoses give characteristic color.

C. Chromatography of Hydrazones (Menkes 1960)
Eastman Chromatogram Sheet, Type K, 301R (Silica GEL) 20 x 20 cm.

1. Solvent: Butanol, ethanol, ammonium hydroxide (12:1:1).
The following standards were run each time:
a. α-ketoglutaric acid.

b. α-ketoisovaleric acid.

c. α-ketoisocaproic acid.

2. Procedure: To 5 to 10 ml. of urine, add one-fifth the volume of 2 per cent 2,4-dinitrophenylhydrazine in 2N HCl. Let it stand for thirty minutes at room temperature. Extract this with 15 ml. of chloroform ethanol (8:2) three times. Save the bottom layer each time. Centrifuge if an emulsion forms. Combine the above three extracts and extract them with 15 ml. of 10 per cent $Na_2CO_3$, saving the top layer. Wash the carbonate layer with 10 ml. of chloroform ethanol mixture and save the top layer. Acidify this with 5N HCl to pH 1. Then extract three times with 10-, 5-, and 5-ml. portions of the chloroform ethanol mixture and save the bottom layer. Dry with solid anhydrous $Na_2SO_4$ added from a spatula and filter. Concentrate until dry under an air stream.

Add 0.2 ml. ethanol to precipitate. Spot from one to five microliters, depending upon the results of the screening test.

See Table 25 for Rf's and colors.

Table 25

Thin Layer Chromatography of α-Keto Acids and Other Organic Acids

| Standard | Rf | Intrinsic Color |
|---|---|---|
| α-Ketoglutaric acid | 5 | Yellow |
| 3-Hydroxy-anthranilic acid | 5.5 | Faint brown |
| Ascorbic acid | 6.4 | Faint yellow |
| p-Hydroxyphenylpyruvic acid | 21, 50 | Faint brown |
| Pyruvic acid | 40, 49 | Yellow |
| Phenylpyruvic acid | 48, 54 | Yellow |
| α-Ketoisocaproic acid | 53, 60 | Yellow |
| α-Ketoisovaleric acid | 55 | Yellow |

D. Chromatography of the Urinary Acid Mucopolysaccharides (Good) This chromatography is done when indicated by the screening test (see Section I, Part A-6).

1. Procedure: Dialyze 20 ml. of urine for forty-eight hours in ice water. Precipitate with 1 ml. of hexadecyltrimethylammonium bromide 25 per cent in cold water. Using urine from a patient with gargoylism, one should add more regeant until precipitate stops forming.

Wash twice with 2 per cent sodium acetate in 95 per cent ethanol, mix and centrifuge. Wash once with 95 per cent ethanol. Mix again and centrifuge.

Redissolve the urinary precipitate in 0.5 ml. of 0.05N NaOH.

Before spotting 2 λ of the sample, spot a 1 per cent glucose solution in the same place and allow to dry. This eliminates diffusion of the mucopolysaccharides from the origin.

2. Acetate Buffer: 410 ml. 0.2M acetate acid; 90 ml. 0.2M potassium acetate.

3. Solvent System: 215 ml. of buffer; 150 ml. of 95 per cent ethanol.

Make 0.001M with "DEDTA'.' (ethylenedinitrotetraacetic acid), disodium salt, or disodium versenate, and adjust to pH 4.75.

4. Standards: Chondroitin sulfate A (Sigma) and hepratin sulfate (Upjohn) should be run using 2 and 4 λ each. Whatman 3MM paper (7" by 7") is placed in a thin layer chromatography tank at least six hours after the solvent has been put in the tank. See Table 26.

Table 26

Mucopolysaccharide Chromatography

| Standards   (2.5 mg/ml) | Rf |
| --- | --- |
| Chondroitin sulfate A | Moves with the front |
| Chondroitin sulfate B | 0.60 and 0.80 |
| Keratosulfate | Moves with the front |
| Hepratin sulfate | 0.90 |

Dip in a solution of 0.05% Azure A in 2% acetic acid and allow to dry. All compounds stain purple on a blue background.

IV. Summary

A number of apparently healthy infants, who have genetic disorders that may later result in mental deficiency or in serious or fatal illness, can be detected by the tests described above. Most of these tests are simple enough to be done in the pediatrician's office. Some of the disorders are treatable, and early diagnosis can result in a child's normal physical and mental development despite an inherited biochemical defect. Even in cases where there is now no treatment available, the tests permit intelligent, early genetic counseling of parents. It must be emphasized that the tests outlined here are screening tests, and all positive or questionable cases must be followed up with specific quantitative tests that are usually done at central laboratories like those found at large medical centers, teaching hospitals, or public health centers. The Children's Bureau of the Welfare Administration[4] has published a list of seventeen service laboratories in the United States where extensive aid in diagnosis and treatment of the disorders discussed above may be available. The Children's Bureau has also published a laboratory manual dealing with some inborn errors of metabolism (O'Brien 1965).

[4] Biochemical and Cytogenetic Laboratory Service Program (approved for the fiscal year 1967)
Department of Health, Education, and Welfare
Welfare Administration
Children's Bureau
Washington, D.C. 20201

# DISCUSSION

N. DiFerrante: Please clarify the azure A test for mucopolysaccharidoses.

P. Tocci: I believe it is 0.5 per cent in 2 per cent acetic acid. We stain the papers with the azure A and keep them in the drawer. If we get ten or twelve urine specimens, we put a drop of each on the paper and let it dry. Then we pass the paper through 2 per cent acetic acid twice. If there are increased mucopolysaccharides, a nice purple ring will emerge, and if there are not, a washed-out spot will appear. I have used Hurler's urine as a control, and it always comes out well.

H. Levy: I wonder if I could take just a moment to say something. First of all, I am glad that I spoke before Dr. Tocci. But, perhaps I can say a few words about a difference between Dr. Tocci's screening program and the screening program I discussed which is currently being conducted in Massachusetts. As I understand it, Dr. Tocci's screening program is on liquid urine, whereas the Massachusetts screening program (and I perhaps did not make this point explicit) bases its urine screening program on urine that is sent via impregnation into filter paper. In Massachusetts, where the screening program, based on population screening, is considerably larger than the program you are conducting at the University of Miami, it would be a logistical quagmire to send liquid urines across the state. The urines I have illustrated on paper chromatography are, therefore, urines that are within filter papers. In actual practice, a strip of filter paper is given to the mother as she leaves the hospital; she is told that when the baby reaches four to six weeks of age, she is either to take this filter paper, place it inside the diaper, and wait for it to get wet, or take a wet diaper (a relatively clean wet diaper) and press the diaper into the filter paper; then she should take the filter paper and place it in the envelope, which is then sent to the State Public Health Laboratory. The types of tests we would be doing would certainly be limited in relation to the types of tests you are doing at the University of Miami.

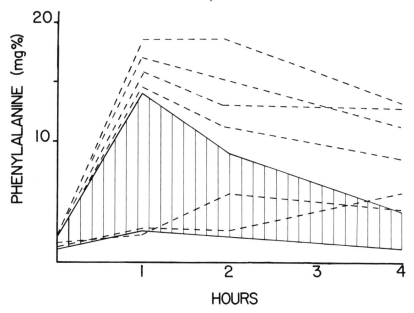

FIGURE 41. Results of phenylalanine loading tests carried out on mothers of children born with cleft palate (shown as dotted lines). The range of values from normal subjects are shown in the shaded area.

P. Tocci: Let me make a correction also. We do get about 30 to 35 per cent of our urines impregnated on paper, and the test I described to Dr. DiFerrante can be done conversely. That is, you add to the urine on a piece of filter paper a drop of 0.5 per cent azure A and allow it to dry. Then add two drops of 2 per cent acetic acid allowing the spot to dry after each drop. If the mucopolysaccharides are elevated, a ring of metachromatic stain appears. The same thing can be done with the ferric chloride test, the o-tolidine test for copper, and Millon's test for tyrosine and p-dihydroxyphenylpyruvic acid.

R. Hill: Will you please mention to the group your findings on phenylalanine levels in mothers who have given birth to infants with cleft palate and lip?

P. Tocci: I was going to do that. The information is shown in Figure 41 and represents what the government calls an offshoot of research. We have some of the pediatricians in Miami so interested in the screening program that they send us almost every patient they get—so in a way we are doing mass screening. Dr. Beber is interested in cleft palate and has a captive group of two or three hundred mothers of cleft palate children. He used to send me the urines of these women. I chromatographed about two dozen and really did not find anything unusual. After going over the results, we discovered that a lot of the women had derivatives of tyrosine in the urine, a finding that is not abnormal per se. We see these compounds in about 10 to 15 per cent of the normal adult population. However, about 60 to 70 per cent of these women had them in their urine. We decided to go ahead and do phenylalanine to tyrosine ratios since Dr. Beber was getting blood from these women for chromosome studies. The women exhibited ratios that were 1.5 and above whereas normals were about 0.5 to 0.9. On this evidence we then gave some of them phenlyalanine loading tests. The results we got were somewhat surprising. We gave loads to thirteen of these mothers, and six of them had what we call abnormal loads. As seen in Figure 41, there were three types of responses: the shaded area represents ten controls we did in our laboratory at the same time using Udenfriend's method and McKamn and Robins' method for tyrosine and phenylalanine. The mothers in question are shown as dotted lines. In four subjects the blood phenylalanine levels were high at the first hour and did not come down to normal at the fourth hour. In two instances, the blood phenylalanine levels did not go up very high in the first hours, and they continued to rise to the fourth hour. Seven others were within the shaded area. We intend to investigate this phenomenon further.

# REFERENCES

Adams, W. S., Davis, F. W., and Hansen, L. E. 1962. New method for determination of creatinine in urine by ion exchange separation and ultraviolet spectrophotometry. *Anal. Chem.* 34:845.

Aisen, P., Schorr, J. B., Morell, A. G., Gold, R. Z., and Scheinberg, I. H. 1960. A rapid screening test for deficiency of plasma ceruloplasmin and its value in the diagnosis of Wilson's disease. *Am. J. Med.* 58:550.

## Chemical Detection of Inherited Disorders

Berry, H. K. 1962. Detection of metabolic disorders among mentally retarded children by means of paper spot tests. *Am. J. Ment. Def.* 66:555.

Beutler, E., and Baluda, M. C. 1966. A simple spot screening test for galactosemia. *J. Lab. Clin. Med.* 68:137.

Brand, E., Harris, M. M., and Biloon, S. 1930. Cystinuria. The excretion of a cystine complex which decomposes in the urine with the liberation of free cystine. *J. Biol. Chem.* 86:315.

Efron, M. L., Young, D., Moser, H. W., and MacCready, R. A.. 1964. A simple chromatographic screening test for the detection of disorders of amino acids metabolism. *New Eng. J. Med.* 270:1378.

Gibbs, N. K., and Woolf, L. I. 1959. Test for phenylketonuria: Results of one-year programme for its detection in infancy and among mental defectives. *Brit. Med. J.* 12:532.

Good, T. A. Personal communication.

Hsia, D. Y.-Y. 1959. *Inborn errors of metabolism*, p. 306. Chicago: Year Book Medical Publishers.

Hyanek, J., and Cafourkova, Z. 1965. A screening test for the recognition of increased alpha amino nitrogen excretion in urine. *Clin. Chim. Acta* 12:599.

Khachadurian, A., and Knox, W. D. 1960. Colorimetric ninhydrin method for total alpha amino acids of urine. *J. Lab. Clin. Med.* 56:321.

Lake, B. D. 1965. A reliable rapid screening test for sulphatide lipidosis. *Arch. Dis. Child.* 40:284.

McEvoy-Bowe, E. 1966. Determination of creatinine in urine by separation on DEAE-Sephadex and ultraviolet spectrophotometry. *Anal. Chem.* 16:153.

Menkes, J. H. 1960. The pattern of urinary alpha keto acids in various neurologic diseases. *Am. J. Dis. Child.* 99:500.

Miller, S. E. 1955. *Textbook of clinical pathology*, p. 1037. Baltimore: The Williams and Wilkens Co.

Moore, S., and Stein, W. H. 1954. Procedures for the chromatographic determination of amino acids in 4% cross-linked sulfonated polystyrene resins. *J. Biol. Chem.* 211:893.

O'Brien, D. 1965. Rare inborn errors of metabolism in children with mental retardation. Children's Bureau of Publication, U. S. Dept. of H. E. W., publ. #429.

Ritter, S., Spencer, H., and Samachson, J. 1960. The Sulkowitch test and quantitative urinary calcium excretion. *J. Lab. Clin. Med.* 56:314.

Rupe, C. O., and Free, A. H. 1959. An improved test for phenylketonuria. *Clin. Chem.* 5:405.

Sackett, D. L. 1964. Adaptation of monodirectional high-voltage electrophoresis on long papers to the rapid qualitative identification of urinary amino acids. *J. Lab. Clin. Med.* 63:306.

Samuels, S. 1964. High-resolution screening of aminoacidurias. *Arch. Neurol.* 10:322.

Samuels, S., and Ward, S. S. 1966. Aminoaciduria screening by thin-layer high-voltage electrophoresis and chromatography on microplates. *J. Lab. Clin. Med.* 67:669.

Scriver, C. R., Eluned, D., and Cullen, A. M. 1964. Application of a simple micromethod to the screening of plasma for a variety of aminoacidopathies. *Lancet* 2:230.

Smith, I. 1960. *Aminoacids amines and related compounds, chromatographic and electrophoretic techniques*, vol. 1. New York: Interscience Publications, Inc.

Tocci, P. M. 1967. Screening for metabolic diseases. In *Amino acid metabolism and genetic variation*, ed. W. Nyhan, part 11, ch. 34. New York: McGraw-Hill.

Troughton, W. D., St. Clair Brown, R., and Turner, N. A. 1966. Separation of urinary amino acids by thin-layer high-voltage electrophoresis and chromatography. *Am. J. Clin Path.* 46:139.

Turner, B., and Juster, M. 1964. A rapid screening procedure for the identification of aminoaciduria. *Med. J. Austral.* 1:152.

# A Technique for Semiquantitative Analysis of Plasma Amino Acids[1]

EILA AIRAKSINEN, M.D., GORDON FARRELL, M.D.,
and ROBERT J. JOHNSON, Ph.D.

*Texas Research Institute of Mental Sciences, Houston, Texas*

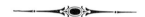

The study of plasma amino acids is critical to the diagnosis of many inborn errors of metabolism. The excellent work of M. L. Efron, Harvey Levy, and their collaborators and of Paul Tocci has already been described in this symposium. In general, preliminary screening has been carried out by paper electrophoresis or paper chromatography (Efron *et al.* 1964; Scriver *et al.* 1964), and the final workup has been done with the amino acid analyzer.

In the establishment of a screening and diagnostic facility in cooperation with the Texas State Schools for the Mentally Retarded, we were faced with the need of selecting procedures for amino acid studies. Our problems are not entirely unique, though the situation in Texas presents certain unusual difficulties because of the distances between the schools and the Institute of Mental Sciences.

First, plasma specimens had to be prepared in such a way that they could be safely transported by the mails. After some experimentation, we elected an 80 per cent ethanol solution that is readily prepared in the field. The amino acids remain in solution quantitatively; the protein precipi-

[1] The authors wish to thank Miss Erika Hopfe, Mr. Charles Rihn, and Mrs. Jeannette W. Smith for their valuable assistance in this study.

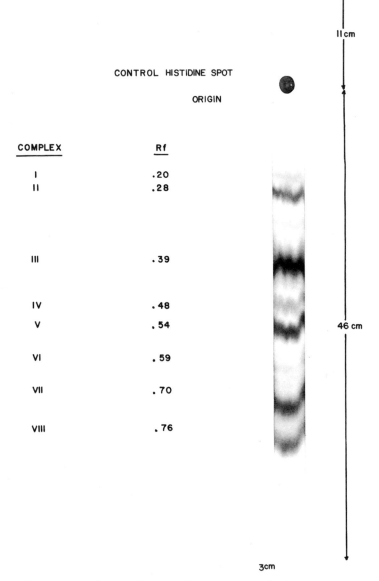

CONTROL HISTIDINE SPOT

ORIGIN

11 cm

| COMPLEX | Rf |
|---------|-----|
| I | .20 |
| II | .28 |
| III | .39 |
| IV | .48 |
| V | .54 |
| VI | .59 |
| VII | .70 |
| VIII | .76 |

46 cm

3cm

FIGURE 42. A typical paper chromatogram of plasma amino acids showing approximate Rf values of each amino acid complex.

tates. The 80 per cent ethanol preparation is stable for a week and can be mailed without difficulty. The sample can be reduced in volume conveniently under a stream of nitrogen for application to chromatograms. For the analytic technique, paper chromatography proved to be the most useful under our circumstances. However, it seemed worthwhile to introduce quantitative or semiquantitative interpretation. We hope eventually to have small screening laboratories in each of the state schools to handle their own patient load. It is desirable, therefore, to have a method that would permit the inexperienced technician to make decisions based on an objective measure.

## Methods

A fasting blood specimen is drawn in a heparinized tube. After centrifugation the red cells are discarded and 0.25 ml. of plasma is treated with 1.0 ml. of absolute ethanol to precipitate the plasma proteins. The precipitated proteins are removed by centrifugation at 1300 to 1800 xG. for fifteen minutes. The supernatant is mailed to our laboratory in a sealed tube in a self-addressed cardboard container. On receipt of the specimen, the solution is evaporated to dryness with nitrogen. The residue is dissolved in 0.05 ml. of distilled water, and the solution is applied in a horizontal line on a three-centimeter strip of Whatman 3MM paper that is prewashed with methanol. The tube is rinsed twice with 0.04 ml. of water, which is applied on the same line. The chromatogram is developed descending fourteen to sixteen hours in butanol : acetic acid : water (2:1:1). The developed strip is dried for 1.5 hours in a vented drying oven at room temperature and 200 $\mu$moles of histidine HCl in 20 $\mu$l. of solution is applied approximately 2 cm. above the origin as a control for the staining procedure. After ten minutes of drying, the strip is stained by dipping it in freshly prepared 0.2 per cent ninhydrin-acetone solution. It is then heated for thirty-five minutes at 65° C. and read with the densitometer within three hours; a blue filter at 550 m$\mu$ is used (Fig. 42).

To establish the normal ranges, amino acid chromatograms were prepared in this way from the plasma of seventy-five school-age children (six to seventeen years of age) from the Burnett-Bayland Home in Houston. The children (about the same number of boys and girls) were admitted to the hospital and placed on a standard diet. The children were given a physical examination and routine laboratory tests to exclude obvious diseases.

## 10-13 years , male

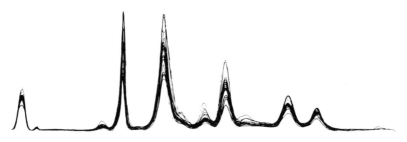

FIGURE 43.  Recording of aminograms from boys age ten to thirteen years old.

## 6-9 years , female

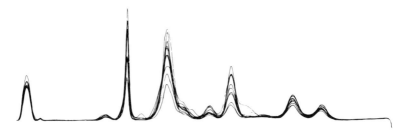

FIGURE 44.  Recording of aminograms from girls age six to nine years old. In one of the control cases note the form of Complex V which resembles hyperprolinemia. This form was found in three of seventy-five control cases.

## Results and Discussion

Figure 42 shows a typically developed and stained chromatogram. The chromatograms developed by this technique contain all the ninhydrin-positive material in deproteinized plasma, including amino acids, amines, and peptides. The ninhydrin-positive substances are distributed into a series of bands or complexes, designated Complex I to VIII. The bands on the chromatogram are interpreted by the densitometer as peaks. The resulting records resemble those reported by W. Hirsch, A. Mex, and F. Vogel (1961; 1963), who have described a similar procedure but who employ different solvent systems requiring three days chromatography time.

TABLE 27

Ratios of the Area of the Complexes to the Histidine
Control, Normal Plasma Aminograms

| Complex No. | Girls | | Boys | |
|---|---|---|---|---|
| | Mean | Max. | Mean | Max. |
| I | 0.46 | 0.70 | 0.43 | 0.70 |
| II | 1.54 | 2.12 | 1.52 | 2.07 |
| III | 3.91 | 5.81 | 3.92 | 5.50 |
| IV | 0.77 | 1.11 | 0.78 | 1.11 |
| V | 1.98 | 3.21 | 1.86 | 2.64 |
| VI | 0.94 | 1.28 | 1.09 | 1.56 |
| VII | 1.46 | 2.06 | 1.74 | 2.35 |
| VIII | 1.01 | 1.35 | 1.14 | 1.56 |

Maximum = mean + twice standard deviation

Figures 43 and 44 show typical results from control children. Although there is some variation from individual to individual, by and large the patterns are quite consistent with complexes recurring with very nearly the same Rf and with almost precisely the same configuration. Table 27 summarizes the normal values from seventy-five school-age children presented as the ratio of the area under a given complex to the control histidine stain. This mode of expression protects against chance deviation in day to day staining. On this table the maximum normal value is indicated as the mean plus two standard deviations of the population. We feel that any value from a corresponding age group which exceeds the mean plus two standard deviations differs sufficiently from the normal to warrant further investigation.

Preliminary calculations indicate that there are minor differences in the developed patterns between the age and sex groups; the differences are marginally significant and are currently being studied to see if meaningful information can be developed from the data.

Table 28 shows the position that the amino acids assume in reference to the complexes, as this position has thus far been determined. The results incorporated in Table 28 were obtained by adding extra amounts of the given amino acid to a normal plasma pool and observing the place of a new peak resulting from this amino acid.

Of critical importance is the question: "Does this technique permit the detection of the known amino acid errors?" The first approximation

# TABLE 28

Localization of Amino Acids in Complexes of Plasma Amino Acid Chromatograms

| Complex I | Cystine |
| | Cysteic acid* |
| | Cystathionine (between Complexes I and II)* |
| Complex II | Lysine |
| | Asparagine |
| | Argininosuccinic acid* |
| | Homocysteic acid* |
| | Histidine |
| | Arginine |
| | Ornithine |
| Complex III | Serine |
| | Glutamine |
| | Homocystine* |
| | Glycine |
| | Aspartic acid |
| Complex IV | Citrulline |
| | Threonine |
| | Glutamic acid |
| | Hydroxyproline |
| Complex V | Proline |
| | Alanine |
| | Sarcosine |
| Complex VI | Tyrosine |
| | Tryptophan |
| | $\gamma$-Aminobutyric acid* |
| | $\alpha$-Aminobutyric acid |
| | $\beta$-alanine |
| Complex VII | Methionine |
| | Valine |
| | $\beta$-aminoisobutyric acid* |
| | Phenylalanine (between Complexes VII and VIII) |
| | Ethanolamine |
| Complex VIII | Leucine |
| | Isoleucine |

\* not normally found in plasma

of an answer to this question was obtained as follows: Using a pooled plasma specimen from normal individuals, we prepared model amino-acidopathies by modifying the amino acid content to correspond with the published values for ten syndromes (Table 29). The models were prepared; one containing the least elevation reported in a given amino-acidopathy and the other the highest reported elevation. The plasma was processed in the usual way. The results of part of these studies are shown in Figures 45 through 54.

## PHENYLKETONURIA

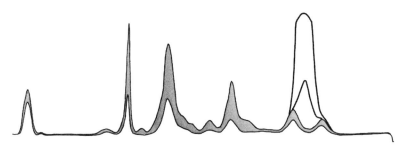

FIGURE 45. Phenylketonuria model demonstrating blood phenylalanine values of 15 mg. per cent (Berry, Sutherland, and Umbarger 1966) and 69 mg. per cent (Knox 1966). The grey area denotes the normal range.

## MAPLE SYRUP URINE DISEASE

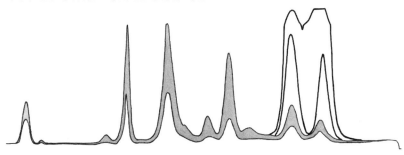

FIGURE 46. The pattern of maple syrup urine disease according to the values of J. Dancis and others (1960) and R. G. Westall (1963). Typically, Complex VII and VIII are high. The grey area is the normal variation.

## HYPERVALINEMIA

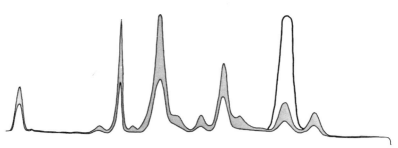

FIGURE 47.   Hypervalinemia from the case published by Y. Wada (1965). High valine concentration causes an increase of Complex VII. The grey area represents the normal variation. Note the similarity to homocystinuria.

## HYPERSARCOSINEMIA

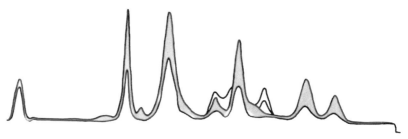

FIGURE 48.   The model of hypersarcosinemia from the case published by T. Gerritsen and H. A. Waisman (1966). Ethanolamine, which is not normally found in plasma, causes an abnormally high peak in Complex VII. Sarcosine causes the slurring of Complex IV and V. The grey area represents the normal variation.

## HYPERPROLINEMIA

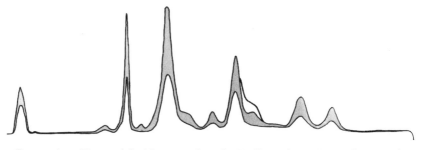

FIGURE 49.   The model of hyperprolinemia. Proline value 3.69 $\mu$moles per ml. (Efron 1966b) gives a typical slurred asymmetrical form to Complex V. The grey area is the normal variation.

## HOMOCYSTINURIA

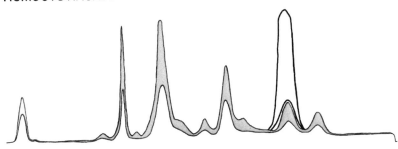

FIGURE 50. The model of homocystinuria. The methionine value for the lower curve is from Nina Carson's case (1963) and is not easily separated from the normal grey area; high values are from T. Gerritsen's case (1964). A slight amount of homocystine is found in the former case but does not cause any visible abnormality for the curve. Note the similarity to hypervalinemia.

## HYPERGLYCINEMIA

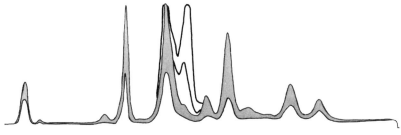

FIGURE 51. The pattern ot hyperglycinemia. Note the pattern is similar to that of citrullinemia (grey area represents normal variation).

## CITRULLINEMIA

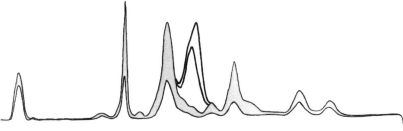

FIGURE 52. Citrullinemia pattern (Efron 1966a). The grey area represents the normal variation.

## HYPERHISTIDINEMIA

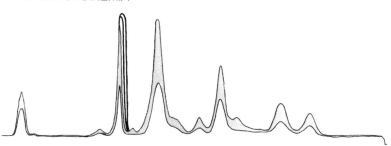

FIGURE 53. Histidinemia according to the values from the case of N. F. K. Shaw and his associates (1963) and B. N. La Du and his co-workers (1963). Observe the similarity of the curve to hyperlysinemia.

## HYPERLYSINEMIA

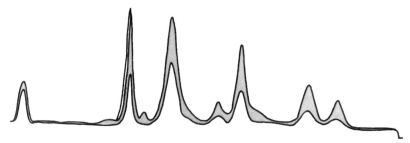

FIGURE 54. Hyperlysinemia according to the values from the case published by H. Ghadimi and his associates (1965). Observe the similarity of the curve to histidinemia.

Among those syndromes where the blood amino acid concentration is elevated, we can reliably detect phenylketonuria, maple syrup urine disease, hypervalinemia, citrullinemia, and hyperglycinemia by this method. Ehrlich's p-dimethylaminobenzaldehyde staining separates the two last mentioned. Histidinemia can be detected in most cases; hyperprolinemia may be missed if the proline concentration is relatively low unless one uses isatin or Ehrlich's p-dimethylaminobenzaldehyde staining. Homocystinuria is not easily detected by screening only the blood, if both methionine and homocystine concentrations are quite low. Urinary

## PHENYLALANINE LEVELS

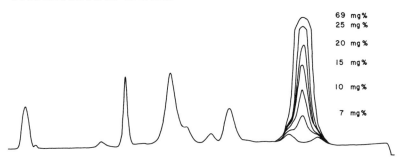

FIGURE 55.   Different plasma phenylalanine levels as seen with this method.

screening for sulfur-containing amino acids greatly increases the possibility of finding homocystinuria.

Figure 55 demonstrates that this technique may be used quite satisfactorily as the means of quantitating some amino acids (for example, phenylalanine) in the plasma. Levels varying from 7 to 69 mg. per cent can be distinguished with a fair amount of reliability. No one claims that these results are as accurate as those which might be obtained with the amino acid analyzer or fluorometric phenylalanine determination (Knox 1966); nevertheless, they appear to be sufficiently accurate for routine clinical use.

For reproducible quantitation of the ninhydrin color in the plasma, the conditions including heating time and oven temperature, must be constant during development of each chromatogram (Kay, Harris, and Entenman 1956). The pH of the chromatogram strips should be as constant as possible. Humidity is known to increase the intensity of ninhydrin color (Bull, Hahn, and Baptist 1949). If it is not possible to read the color intensity promptly after the strips are ready, it is advisable to save the strips in a vacuum desiccator. The color is stable for twenty-four hours or more in the cold room under these conditions.

This method is easy and inexpensive and tends to be more objective than screening methods in which the chromatograms are evaluated by visual comparison with control spots (Efron *et al.* 1964; Scriver *et al.* 1964).

Since September 1967 this technique has been used to study all new admissions to the Texas Schools for the Mentally Retarded. This principle is also used for urine amino acids screening. A micro method is under study for use in newborns.

## Summary

A semiquantitative method for determination of plasma amino acids is described, using one-dimensional paper chromatography of deproteinized plasma and densitometer recording. Normal blood amino acid chromatograms from seventy-five school-age children and typical patterns for some of the known hyperaminoacidemia syndromes are presented.

# DISCUSSION

K. Lewis: I was wondering if there was some special reason that was not obvious for using fasting blood samples in this chromatographic technique?

E. Airaksinen: It is known that if one eats protein diet, plasma amino acids get much higher. If one wants to compare unknown values with normal controls, the fasting state is necessary to exclude the effect of diet.

H. Levy: I really wonder to what extent the protein intake does affect the plasma amino acids? I ask that question because it seems to me that in many studies it has been suggested that a normal protein intake really does not affect plasma amino acids.

E. Airaksinen: You mean for amino acid values right after the meal, or after many days of protein ingestion?

H. Levy: No, I mean plasma amino acids following a reasonably normal protein intake. I am hesitant about this because I am not sure that one cannot induce hyperaminoacidemia with a very high protein intake. As a matter of fact, I previously alluded to a case we have in which a child may have had a hyperaminoacidemia on the basis of a very high protein intake, but I just wonder if the normal amount of protein taken into the body with the usual meal really does affect the plasma amino acids to a significant extent. Several studies of this problem have been published which to some extent have been contradictory but which have suggested rather strongly that protein intake may not measurably elevate plasma amino acids or that, if it does affect plasma amino acids in this manner, the effect is slight. Dr. Ralph Feigin of the Massachusetts General Hospital has shown that the normal circadian rhythm of the body may have greater significance in this regard and that protein intake may be less important than the circadian rhythm in terms of influencing plasma amino acids. His observation is very interesting. Dr. Feigin has found that plasma amino acids normally are much higher at 4 P.M. and 8 P.M.

than they are in the morning. This effect on plasma amino acid concentrations seems to involve all amino acids. In that context, the only point of importance to this discussion is that if one wants to standardize studies, one might think in terms of standardizing on the basis of the times of day the plasma is drawn rather than on the basis of protein intake.

E. AIRAKSINEN: I do not definitely know how many hours are needed after a meal for the blood levels of amino acids to return to fasting levels; but according to the studies of Stein and Frame (*Amino acid pools, distribution, formation, and function, proceedings.* Symposium on Free Amino Acids, City of Hope Medical Center, 1961, ed. J. T. Holden, Amer. Elsevier.) they stay high many hours (even more than eight hours). For practical reasons we took all our control specimens at 8 A.M. before breakfast, and we like to do the same with patients.

H. LEVY: I think it would be interesting for you to take a plasma at 8 A.M. and then take another one at 4 P.M. on the same patient.

E. AIRAKSINEN: We have some experiments on the effect of different diets: six children were placed on a low-protein diet, then changed to a high-protein diet. Blood specimens were taken always at the fasting state (8 A.M.) Each complex was higher when they were taking a high-protein diet a day before the specimen was drawn. We also have studies underway in which we give hydrolyzed casein to patients and then follow their plasma amino acid values. Preliminary results show that plasma amino acids clearly increase after ingestion of this amino acid mixture.

P. TOCCI: We inadvertently did a study like this on people who were using pesticides to analyze the effects of pesticides on a given amino acid. It was much easier for the public health people to get a sample in the morning. For a month or two we were finding abnormalities with people using pesticides as compared to the controls. Finally, we had our first meeting, and I discovered they were not telling these people to fast. We went back and got samples from the same men at the same time of day but while they were fasting; there were two-fold differences in lysine, valine, leucine, and isoleucine.

H. LEVY: Was it really the same time of day?

P. TOCCI: It was 8 A.M.

H. LEVY: In other words, if you got fasting samples, you could get them in the morning about 7 A.M.

P. TOCCI: No, we got them all at 8 A.M. They had to be at work at that time. We just forgot to tell them to fast from the night before.

H. LEVY: The reported studies in animals vary, but it seems to me that most of the studies would suggest that animals and humans raise their plasma amino acids little if at all following a normal meal.

H. BERRY: There are many studies on both humans and animals relating to the rise in plasma amino acids after a protein meal. An interesting nutritional study was carried out back in 1961 by Longenecker and House (1961, *Am. J. Clin. Nutr.* 9:356). They demonstrated that they could assess the nutritional quality of the protein by determining the rise in plasma amino acids from fasting and at one, two, three, four, and five hours after ingestion of standard protein meals. In dogs they found that the amino acids that were limited in a given protein rose to a lesser degree than those which were present in larger amounts. They later demonstrated the same relations in humans. As Dr. Airaksinen says, most people agree that plasma amino acids respond to protein meals. I really do not think there is much question about it.

H. LEVY: Well, I think there is a great deal of question about it. An analysis of several of the more recent studies published in the *Journal of Clinical Nutrition* would suggest strongly that the question is far from settled.

H. BERRY: I recently reviewed the literature on plasma amino acids, and I must have missed important references.

R. AN: I just want to comment on Dr. Levy's comment. The so-called circadian rhythms of plasma amino acids may be true to a certain extent, but I still believe that these rhythms might be related to the human eating habits like mealtime. It would be more relevant if we could prove this experimentally by altering the mealtime to see if this is still true.

H. LEVY: Well, I do not want to discuss Dr. Feigin's work in too much detail before its publication, but his was quite an interesting study. The study was very well done and utilized normal individuals under very close supervision. These individuals were fasted throughout a twenty-four–hour period so there was absolutely no question of protein intake. He showed that plasma amino acids rose continuously throughout the day from 8 A.M. to 8 P.M. with the upper limits arriving around 8 P.M. Since the postprandial blood samples in nutritional studies are usually taken at times when the plasma amino acids would be expected to rise on the basis of a normal circadian pattern, I do not think small rises can be attributed to the effects of protein intake.

D. KEELE: Mrs. Berry, what is the most appropriate time in relation to the meal at which the blood amino acids should be screened for hyperaminoacidemia?

H. BERRY: It depends on whether you are looking for large differences. We have never felt that it really made any difference if you are looking for gross abnormalities like phenylketonuria or maple syrup urine disease, but if you are attempting to use the amino acids as an index of protein nutrition, then you should standardize your values. Airaksinen, Farrell, and Johnson were very wise in their normal studies to bring all their children in and put them on a standard diet. Some of the amino acids will respond more to dietary changes than others. Much of what you find depends on what you are looking for. Phenylalaninemia, for example, is one of the changes found in malnutrition. Serum phenylalanine values are elevated in children with malnutrition, sometimes just from underfeeding. These are not necessarily children in underdeveloped countries. There are children in our own cities with malnutrition. Tyrosine is used preferentially for hormone production. The phenylalanine hydroxylase seems to be quite sensitive to protein malnutrition so phenylalanine accumulates. The nutritional state of the subject is reflected in the plasma amino acid levels. If you go through an institution and test everybody you would probably find that phenylalanine levels of phenylketonurics in institutions are relatively low. We assume that these low levels occur because the patients have a low-protein diet. By low, I mean phenylalanine levels in the 10 to 20 mg. per cent range with phenylpyruvic acid excretion. Dr. Airaksinen's purpose is to find distinct abnormalities that are grossly different from the normal so that fasting might not be critical, but I certainly would not see any objection to having a standard time for collecting a sample.

# REFERENCES

Berry, H. K., Sutherland, B. S., and Umbarger, B. 1966. Detection of phenylketonuria in newborn infants. *J.A.M.A.* 198(10):1114.

Bull, H. B., Hahn, J. W., and Baptist, V. H. 1949. Filter paper chromatography. *J. Am. Chem. Soc.* 71:550.

## Semiquantitative Analysis of Plasma Amino Acids

Carson, N. A. J., Cusworth, D. C., Dent, C. E., Field, C. M. B., Neill, D. W., and Westall, R. G. 1963. Homocystinuria: A new inborn error of metabolism associated with mental deficiency. *Arch. Dis. Child.* 38:425.

Childs, B., Nyhan, W. L., Borden, M., Bard, L., and Cooke, R. E. 1961. Idiopathic hyperglycinemia and hyperglycinuria: A new disorder of amino acid metabolism I. *Pediatrics* 27:522.

Dancis, J., Levitz, M., and Westall, R. G. 1960. Maple syrup urine disease: Branched-chain keto-aciduria. *Pediatrics* 25:72.

Efron, M. L.

1966a. Diseases of the urea cycle. In *The metabolic basis of inherited disease,* eds. J. B. Stanbury, J. B. Wyngaarden, and D. S. Fredrickson, p. 393. New York: McGraw-Hill.

1966b. Disorders of proline and hydroxyproline metabolism. In *The metabolic basis of inherited disease,* eds. J. B. Stanbury, G. B. Wyngaarden, and D. S. Fredrickson, p. 376. New York: McGraw-Hill.

Efron, M. L., Young, D., Moser, H. W., and MacCready, R. 1964. A simple chromatographic screening test for the detection of disorders of amino acid metabolism: A technique using whole blood or urine collected on filter paper. *New Eng. J. Med.* 270:1378.

Gerritsen, T., and Waisman, H. A.

1964. Homocystinuria, an error in the metabolism of methionine. *Pediatrics* 33:413.

1966. Hypersarcosinemia. *New Eng. J. Med.* 275:66.

Ghadimi, H., Binnington, V. I., and Pecora, P. 1965. Hyperlysinemia associated with retardation. *New Eng. J. Med.* 273:723.

Hirsch, W., Mex., A., and Vogel, F.

1961. Besonderheiten im Aminosaure-Stoffwechsel bei geistig abnormen Kindern in Vergleich zu Normalpopulation. *Mschr. Kinderheilk.* 109:445.

1963. Quantitative Abweichungen am Rande der Norm in den freien Aminosäuren von Serum und Urin bei schwachsinnigen Kindern. *Mschr. Kinderheilk.* 111:344.

Kay, R. E., Harris, D. C., and Entenman, C. 1956. Quantification of the ninhydrin color reaction as applied to paper chromatography. *Arch. Biochem. Biophys.* 63:14.

Knox, W. E. 1966. Phenylketonuria. In *The metabolic basis of inherited disease,* eds. J. B. Stanbury, J. B. Wyngaarden, and D. S. Fredrickson, p. 258. New York: McGraw-Hill.

La Du, B. N. 1966. Histidinemia. In *The metabolic basis of inherited disease,* eds. J. B. Stanbury, J. B. Wyngaarden, and D. S. Fredrickson, p. 366. New York: McGraw-Hill.

La Du, B. N., Howell, R. R., Jacoby, G. A., Seegmiller, J. E., Sober, E. K., Zannoni, V. G., Canby, J. P., and Ziegler, L. K. 1963. Clinical and biochemical studies on two cases of histidinemia. *Pediatrics* 32:216.

Schreier, K., and Müller, W. 1964. Idiopathic hyperglycinaemia ("glycinosis"). *Ger. Med. Monthly* 9:437.

Scriver, C. R., Davies, E., and Cullen, A. M. 1964. Application of a simple micromethod to the screening of plasma for a variety of aminoacidopathies. *Lancet* 2:230.

Shaw, N. F. K., Boder, E., Gutenstein, M., and Jacobs, E. E. 1963. Histidinemia (abstract). *J. Pediat.* 63:720.

Wada, Y. 1965. Idiopathic hypervalinemia: Valine and alpha keto-acids in blood following an oral dose of valine. *Tohoku J. Exp. Med.* 87:322.

Westall, R. G. 1963. Dietary treatment of a child with maple syrup urine disease (Branched chain keto-aciduria). *Arch. Dis. Child.* 38:485.

# Genetic Malformation Syndromes Associated with Mental Retardation[1]

JOHN M. OPITZ, M.D.

*Departments of Pediatrics and Medical Genetics, University
of Wisconsin Medical School, Madison, Wisconsin*

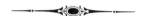

For prognostic and counseling purposes it is desirable, indeed vitally important, to make the diagnosis of congenital mental retardation as early in a given patient's life as possible. At the time of birth it is usually impossible to determine with any degree of certainty what the final, adult intelligence of an individual will be. What type of information is of value in assessing an infant's potential of normal or impaired intellectual functioning?

1. The *family history*. Only 0.5 per cent of children of normal parents who have normal siblings are mentally retarded. If it is true that approximately 3 per cent of all newborn infants will at some time of their lives be mentally retarded, then 2.5 per cent or some five-sixths of all the

[1] Research aided by a grant from The National Foundation–March of Dimes and by PHS/NIH Grants GM 08217 and GM 15422. Paper No. 1205 from the Genetics Laboratory.

This paper is based in part on:
1. Opitz, J. M. 1968. Genetics counseling in pediatric practice. In *Current pediatric therapy*, eds. S. S. Gellis and B. M. Kagan, pp. 974–983. Philadelphia: W. B. Saunders.
2. Opitz, J. M. 1968. Genetische Ursachen d. Schwachsinn's. In *Enzyklop. Hdb. d. Sonderpädagogik*. Part 16/17: 3055–3066. Berlin–Charlottenburg: Carl Marhold Verlagsbuchhandlung.

mentally retarded have a positive family history of mental retardation. E. W. Reed and S. C. Reed (1965) concluded that 2.5 per cent of the mentally retarded have at least one defective parent or a retarded aunt or uncle. This, the most important conclusion of the monumental and remarkable study by the Reeds, emphasizes the great value of a family history in assessing the likelihood of normal or abnormal intellectual functioning of a newborn child. Their book contains other empiric risk figures useful for genetic counseling in mental retardation.

2. Routine *biochemical screening tests* in the neonatal period may uncover inborn errors of metabolism which may lead to mental retardation. More extensive metabolic screening should be performed in any infant with idiopathic psychomotor retardation with or without seizures, hypotonia, and signs of CNS or visual and auditory impairment.

3. *Buccal smear screening* in the neonatal period may uncover a sex chromosomal abnormality in approximately one of every four hundred live-born children. Without doubt, such gonosomally aneuploid infants are at times predisposed to mental retardation. Lenz (1964) estimates that 1 per cent of all males with an I.Q. of 90 or less have Klinefelter's syndrome.

4. *Chromosome analysis* is presently not performed as a screening test in the neonatal period. If such tests were performed they would lead to the detection of all (nonmosaic) XYY cases that are not detectable by the buccal smear technique and of all (nonmosaic) autosomal aneuploidies that may account for another one in four hundred live-born infants. In the latter category there exists an almost absolute risk of *severe* mental retardation. It is estimated that altogether one in every two hundred live-born infants has a chromosome abnormality likely to lead to some degree of intellectual impairment.

5. A careful assessment of the *pregnancy history* may reveal factors frequently associated with a risk of mental retardation.

6. Finally one of the most useful means of detecting the potentially retarded child is the *physical examination*. It is becoming increasingly evident that many patients with "physiological, aclinical" mental retardation who were traditionally thought *not* to have congenital malformations do indeed, on closer scrutiny, reveal detectable abnormalities of morphogenesis which must have been present at the time of birth.

The following remarks are restricted to mental retardation associated with multiple, primary, discrete developmental anomalies. The presence of multiple anomalies in a retarded child suggests that the probability of chance concurrence of these defects and the retardation is less likely than a developmental relationship due to a single etiology. It is operationally useful to assume that the etiology is *genetic* until proven otherwise. In this paper I shall briefly and in general terms discuss the genetically determined malformation/retardation syndromes but shall exclude a consideration of the specific chromosomal aneuploidy syndromes that were presented by Drs. Trujillo and Sinha, and their co-workers.

Most of the anomalies that will be mentioned may be considered the result of incomplete, rarely abnormal morphogenesis. They are conventionally classified into *major* and *minor* anomalies of differentiation. The former are defects of surgical, medical and/or cosmetic importance to the patient and frequently lead to secondary functional aberrations; the latter are not of surgical or medical significance to the patient, although at times they cause cosmetic concern. Minor anomalies rarely, if ever, lead to secondary physiologic impairments. Although of little consequence to the patient, it is nevertheless of paramount importance to search for minor anomalies during the physical examination. Why is this so?

1. Minor anomalies may indicate the presence of a major anomaly. The study by P. M. Marden, D. W. Smith, and J. J. McDonald (1964) of several thousand newborn infants showed that some 15 per cent of them had one minor anomaly, 0.76 per cent had two, and roughly one in two thousand had three or more. Of the latter group over 90 per cent also had a major anomaly.

2. More important, several minor anomalies are frequently found in individuals with "idiopathic mental retardation." The study by D. W. Smith and E. Bostian (1964) showed that some 42 per cent of children with "idiopathic mental retardation" had three or more anomalies, 80 per cent of which were minor. At the present time it is impossible to state which individual and particular combinations of minor anomalies observed in the neonatal period are most frequently associated with later mental retardation. However, it is probably a truism to say that the risk of mental retardation increases directly with the number and severity of the anomalies in the patient. Many well-known, complex dysmorphogenetic syndromes accompanied by a high risk of mental retardation (for example, mongolism) are easy to recognize on a physical examination in the neonatal period.

3. The presence of three or more minor and/or major anomalies in an individual with mental retardation may indicate not just a developmental relationship between the retardation and the dysmorphogenetic

syndrome, but a common cause for the entire malformation/retardation syndrome. This conclusion is illustrated in a particularly striking manner by ongoing studies performed by Professor Klaus Patau at the University of Wisconsin Genetics Laboratory on individuals with idiopathic malformation/retardation syndromes—patients with an I.Q. of 70 or less and three or more minor and/or major anomalies. Patau estimates that in about 20 per cent of these patients the malformation/retardation syndrome was caused by a chromosomal abnormality, which, however, is microscopically detectable in only about half of such cases.

4. Finally it must be kept in mind that most of the abnormalities found in autosomal syndromes and almost all defects observed in sex chromosomal aneuploidy syndromes are *minor* anomalies. Dermatoglyphic changes alone form the basis of the mongolism-index methods devised by N. F. Walker (1957) and by L. Beckman, K. H. Gustavson, and A. Norring (1965).

There exists an extraordinary number of minor variations of normal morphogenesis. Most of the anomalies with which we are concerned are detectable on a "surface examination" of the patient; rarely do we perform extensive studies on the anomalies of the viscera, musculo-skeletal, nervous, and vascular systems.

At the present time it is probably impossible to prepare a comprehensive list of all minor anomalies detectable on a surface examination of infants and children. Instead of memorizing all possible minor abnormalities, it is probably far more important to be aware of the *normal* structure of a particular organ or region (that is, of the form occurring most commonly in the "normal" population) and then to be alert and to note any obvious variation from this "normal" pattern during the examination of a particular patient. The practical assessment of minor anomalies is further complicated by the fact that most of them have not yet been quantitated, at least not in infancy and early childhood, at which time evaluation of such defects is particularly difficult and yet of greatest importance. It is frequently very difficult to evaluate the validity of published claims that a particular patient had certain minor anomalies (hypertelorism, lowset ears, micrognathia, a highly arched palate) especially if these observations are not documented (if not by actual measurements then at least photographically). It is, therefore, urgently necessary for concerned physicians and competent anthropologists to begin collaborative studies now in order to find objective anthropometric criteria that can be used to describe all minor variations of normal development in quantitative terms.

If such collaborative work should succeed in producing a method of quantitative assessment of a given structure, then a survey of the (normal) population must be made to determine the distribution of values of the trait. If the trait is multifactorially determined, a "normal" distribution of values may be found in the population which will make it possible to determine relatively arbitrary cut-off points for a minor deviation ($>1\sigma<2\sigma$) from the normal population ($\pm1\sigma$), for "obvious abnormality" ($>2\sigma<3\sigma$), and for "highly abnormal" ($>3\sigma$) values of the trait. These distributions might differ in the two sexes and may change with age. Appropriate longitudinal studies in both sexes will, therefore, probably be required.

There exist very few traits of the present-absent type (preauricular, cervical, and commissural labial fistulae); however, even for these abnormalities population surveys are required to determine the relative frequency of the trait. For both types of abnormalities (continuously distributed and present-absent type), it will then be possible to determine if the distribution of values or incidence of the anomaly in a given syndrome is significantly different from the distribution or incidence in the normal population. It is presumed that both types of minor abnormalities are multifactorially determined in most cases, but that in the present-absent type a developmental threshold prevents the appearance of the anomaly in many of the cases. With the exception of a few, ever diminishing, relatively small groups of ethnically or racially "pure" people, the majority of the United States population is ethnically heterogeneous. This presents great problems in defining the "normal control population" for any given region or city in the United States.

Some traits of course can already be studied in a quantitative manner (head length and width, intercanthal distance, hand and finger length, palate height, width, and length). Some of the most useful traits of this type are the dermatoglyphic patterns of the digits, palms, and soles which have yielded much information of use in the diagnosis of chromosomal disorders and of some of the developmental defects of the extremities. Some of the pertinent implications of the evaluation of minor anomalies can be summarized as follows:

1. One minor anomaly per se does not necessarily indicate that the individual is abnormal or will be mentally retarded. Many persons become quite alarmed if they discover in themselves a simian crease, Brushfield spots, or several digital low-arch dermatoglyphic patterns. All of the minor anomalies observed to date in dysmorphogenetic syndromes are

also known to occur with variable frequencies in the normal population.

2. Some anomalies may change with *age*; moderate degrees of micrognathia or epicanthic folds observed at birth may disappear in the older child; other abnormalities may not become evident till later (for example, dental anomalies until the teeth erupt, abnormal skeletal growth rates resulting in distortions or hypoplasias where previously the structure had appeared relatively normal).

3. Some traits may differ in incidence and/or severity in one or the other *sex*.

4. There probably exist no morphologic traits *pathognomonic* for any one syndrome. Ten low arches may occur in arthrogryposis and brachydactyly as well as in the 18 trisomy syndrome, and it is, therefore, incorrect to say that the presence of ten low arches always identifies the patient as having the 18 trisomy syndrome.

5. There probably exist no *obligatory* anomalies (morphologic defects that occur in all cases of a given syndrome). Probably all anomalies are "facultative," and it is incorrect to say that a given patient cannot have the 18 trisomy syndrome because he does not have ten low arches.

6. *Severity* of given anomalies—if they can be assessed quantitatively—is likely to vary from patient to patient in a given syndrome; the distribution of values of the trait observed in the abnormal condition may overlap to a variable extent with that of the normal population.

7. Not all anomalies have the same frequency (*penetrance*) in a given syndrome. Some traits occur in many patients, others occur in very few patients. Regardless of how rare in the syndrome, the trait properly belongs to it if it occurs in the syndrome with a frequency significantly greater than in the normal control population.

The total number of anomalies in human dysmorphogenetic syndromes is almost impossible to assess, since we rarely scrutinize internal organs as carefully as we do the surface of the individual. Even many surface features of malformation syndromes remain completely unstudied.

It may also be found that the occurrence of two or more anomalies in a given syndrome is highly correlated. Such a correlation may reveal at times the presence of a "developmental field" (anomalies that occur as secondary manifestations of an underlying developmental defect of a certain anatomic region). For example, the correlation between clinodactyly, shortness, and the disappearance of one flexion crease of the fifth finger in mongolism seems to represent a developmental field.

8. If two or more different syndromes share one or more similar or

identical minor anomalies, then it is not necessarily true that these same anomalies occur with the same frequency and severity in the several syndromes.

In summary, it can be stated that the greater the total number of anomalies identified in a given syndrome and the greater the mean penetrance of the component anomalies, the greater will be the mean number of anomalies per patient and the greater is the chance that a reliable diagnosis can be made.

The process of defining a new malformation/retardation syndrome as a discrete nosologic and genetic entity generally passes through three stages.

1. The *physical examination syndrome* represents nothing more than the initial observation of *two or more anomalies in one patient.* These anomalies could have concurred in the patient by chance alone as the result of different etiologies acting in a developmentally unrelated manner. The probability of chance concurrence diminishes as the number of anomalies in the patient increases and as the frequency of a particular anomaly's appearance in the normal population decreases.

2. The *formal genesis syndrome* is defined as the presence of *n similar or identical sets of anomalies in n patients.* Such individuals may also be considered a group of patients with similar or identical physical examination syndromes. The assumption that these individuals are similarly deformed because of a similar developmental pathogenesis (formal genesis) unfortunately does not prove that the etiology of the syndrome is identical in all cases. Different mutations, chromosomal abnormalities, and environmental teratogens may produce syndromes of such nosologic similarity that they are frequently confused and considered a single pathogenetic entity. The converse is also true, namely that the same genetic cause may produce phenotypes that show striking clinical differences. The Lawrence-Moon-Biedl syndrome and the Fanconi anemia syndrome both provide frequent illustrations of striking variability. It should also be remembered that probably no two patients (including identical twins) with a given syndrome ever have exactly the same number and severity of anomalies. The validity of a defined formal genesis syndrome is directly proportional to the number, the rarity of the component anomalies, and the frequency of the syndromes in the population.

For most formal genesis syndromes it is difficult if not impossible to determine the true frequency in the population of patients with the condition, especially if there exist no diagnostic physiologic or biochemical tests for them. Theoretically the frequency could be determined by studying a population sample of predetermined size to see if the incidence of the syndrome in this sample significantly exceeds the incidence expected on the basis of random concurrence of *n* anomalies each with a known population frequency. The greater the number and the rarer the component anomalies the larger will be the population sample required, until it becomes so great that such a study is clearly impossible. The validity of the final results will be open to question, since such a study almost always involves a truncated sample of the patient population studied at a time when the complete phenotypic spectrum (frequency distribution of number of anomalies per patient) and the etiology are still unknown. The probability of discovering the syndrome in the first place is directly proportional to the severity of the disorder in the initial propositi. Lacking etiologic criteria or specific biochemical tests, the only reasonable assurance we have of defining an etiologically "homogeneous" formal genesis syndrome is to stick to patients who resemble the original cases as closely as possible. Such efforts almost invariably create an artificial homogeneity of the published patient material and tend to truncate the phenotypic spectrum of the disease ever more narrowly by focusing on the most extreme degrees of severity. Other investigators may possibly classify the milder cases of the disease as a different entity altogether (false splitting of syndromes). Ascertainment of patients with a given syndrome from specialty clinics may suggest the presence of obligatory anomalies and may lead to false inclusion of patients with the same anomaly (false lumping; for instance, Marfan's syndrome and homocystinuria).

If the disorder is due to multifactorial inheritance, a Mendelian mutation, or an inherited chromosome abnormality, then a fair idea of the complete phenotypic spectrum may be obtained by examining the sibs born after the ascertainment of the proband and by excluding the probands from the collected data.

3. The highest stage of syndrome definition is achieved in the *causal genesis syndrome*, which may be defined as *concurrence of causally related anomalies*. If the causal genesis (a chromosomal abnormality) or one of its primary effects (an inborn error of metabolism) can be determined at birth independently of clinical manifestations, then the total incidence, complete phenotypic spectrum, and entire natural history of the disorder can be established.

The genetic causal genesis of a syndrome is frequently very difficult to determine. The two greatest impediments to making a correct genetic diagnosis are etiologic heterogeneity and sporadic occurrence.

## Genetic Malformation Syndromes

1. *Etiologic heterogeneity* is at the present time the major methodologic handicap in human genetics. Many genetically distinct mutations express themselves in similar and sometimes identical pictures (Waardenburg 1964) so that as a good general rule it must be assumed until proven otherwise that all collected data from unrelated families on certain common and even some rare malformation/retardation syndromes are etiologically heterogeneous. Inspection of a catalogue of human mutations (McKusick 1968) still shows a preponderance of autosomal dominant mutations; this probably implies that hundreds, if not thousands, of recessively inherited conditions remain unrecognized and are at the present time frequently confused with known mutations.

2. *Sporadic occurrence* may refer either to the single case of an "idiopathic" condition in a family or to a greater than expected number of isolated cases in lists of cases of a given (genetic) disease entity. In the latter instance the excess of sporadic cases may be ascribed to new mutations or illegitimacies; nonpenetrance of the disease in heterozygous parents (in cases of dominant mutations) or in homozygous siblings (in cases of a recessively inherited condition); occasional penetrance in a heterozygote for a recessive mutation (possibly by deletion of the locus for the dominant allele); phenocopies and genocopies (chromosomal, multifactorial, other autosomal, and X-linked mutations). In case of a recessive mutation fatality may be so great that only an occasional case survives to postnatal life. With respect to autosomal recessive mutations it must be remembered that in over 65 per cent of marriages between two carriers producing two and three children and ascertained through an affected child, homozygotes appear not as familial but as chance isolated cases. It should, therefore, be evident that sporadicity does not speak against a genetic etiology or a high recurrence risk and that familial incidence is not a *sine qua non* of hereditary disease.

Many geneticists have reviewed evidence for the genetic etiology of a disease. A direct demonstration of causal genesis is possible only in chromosome abnormalities and clearcut cases of autosomal and X-linked inborn errors of metabolism. The only rigorous methods establishing genetic etiology from pedigree data are segregation and linkage analyses that have been reviewed extensively by N. E. Morton (1962) and by J. F. Crow (1965). Further evidence bearing on genetic etiology of a given malformation/retardation syndrome is obtained by more epidemiological investigations, including a study of the incidence of the disease in the general population, its incidence in special populations such as ethnic or religious isolates or in identical or fraternal twins; the study of mutation rates, selection coefficients, heritability estimates, and empiric risk estimates is also included. All these methods have been thoroughly reviewed in the volumes edited by W. J. Burdette and by J. V. Neel, M. S. Shaw, and W. J. Schull. In this discussion I shall review only a few of the most pertinent characteristics of the various genetic etiologies.

1. *Autosomal recessive inheritance.* This form of inheritance of human disease is probably the most common and numerous recessively inherited malformation/retardation syndromes are known. These syndromes frequently include extremely deleterious mutations, often leading to death, disability and/or infertility in a homozygous state. Evidence for recessive inheritance includes:

a. A segregation ratio of 25 per cent obtained with the appropriate methods. Parents and collateral relatives are usually normal if the trait is rare. With the exception of rare examples of sex limitation, both sexes are affected with equal frequency. If the recessive mutations are alleles, all offspring from two affected parents should be affected.

b. Discovery of an inborn error of metabolism with detection of the heterozygous carrier state in both parents and in two-thirds of the normal siblings of the homozygous patient; "dominant" inheritance of the carrier state and incidence of the carrier state in the population in accordance with the Hardy-Weinberg law.

c. A relatively high degree of parental consanguinity compared to the general population for rare recessive traits. Formal aspects of consanguinity analysis are reviewed by N. E. Morton (1961) and A. G. Steinberg (1962).

d. A probability of affected first cousins (from matings of unrelated individuals) approximately equal to $p/4$ (Crow) where $p = $ frequency of the gene in the population.

e. An incidence of the disease in 6.25 per cent of the double first cousins of the homozygous patient.

f. In inbred isolates affected homozygotes may marry heterozygotes and produce, on the average, 50 per cent affected offspring. If this occurs over several generations then an appearance of dominant inheritance may be produced.

2. *Autosomal dominant inheritance.* Observations are on record that the presumed homozygous state of some dominantly inherited mutations is much worse than the heterozygous state; most "dominant" mutations are probably incompletely dominant. Consanguineous matings between

two individuals with identical, relatively benign, dominantly inherited conditions may, therefore, be hazardous. Few dominantly inherited malformation/retardation syndromes are known. Evidence for dominant inheritance includes:

a. 50 per cent segregation ratio and recurrence risk if one of the parents is affected, with regular transmission from generation to generation.

b. Both sexes are affected with equal frequency and are equally able to transmit the disease to 50 per cent of their offspring unless there is limitation of expression of the trait to one sex.

The 50 per cent segregation ratio is not observed in sibships in which a patient's disease is due to a new mutation. The appearance of the latter may be associated with older paternal reproductive age. The 50 per cent segregation ratio may also not apply in traits with reduced penetrance.

3. *X-linked inheritance.* The majority of X-linked mutations studied to date are recessive and limited in full expression to the hemizygous male. There exist few well-documented X-linked malformation/retardation syndromes; one of the most striking is the Lenz-microphthalmia syndrome.

a. If the trait is rare and there are no consanguineous matings in the family, then the parents of the male with the X-linked trait will be normal; brothers of the mother or other male relatives in the female line may be affected. With the exception of mutations, every affected male comes from a carrier mother.

b. All daughters of a hemizygote will be carriers, all sons will be normal. One affected son from an affected father constitutes evidence against a hypothesis of X-linked inheritance of the trait. The probability of observing $n$ normal sons from an affected father under the hypothesis of autosomal dominant inheritance is $(\frac{1}{2})^n$ (that is, the more normal sons one observes among the progeny of an affected man the stronger is the case for X-linked inheritance and the less likely is autosomal dominant inheritance with male sex limitation). Close linkage with another X-linked trait constitutes further evidence for the hypothesis of X-linkage.

c. Heterozygous mothers transmit the mutant gene to half of their sons and half of their daughters.

d. Excluding an XO constitution or the feminizing testes syndrome, affected women usually arise only from the mating of a carrier mother and an affected father; their frequency in the population is somewhat less than the square of the frequency of affected males.

e. In a sporadic case it is frequently difficult to decide whether the patient's disease represents a new mutation. In hemophilia A, an unremarkable thromboplastin generation test does not constitute evidence against a carrier state of the mother; in Duchenne's progressive pseudohypertrophic muscular dystrophy serial determination of serum creatine phosphokinase, aldolase, and other muscle enzymes, evaluation of calf size and one or, if necessary, several muscle biopsies frequently allow for the detection of the carrier state. In Fabry's disease and Hunter's disease, specific cytochemical determinations on biopsy specimens permit an almost certain detection of all carriers and counseling of a negligibly small recurrence risk if the mothers, on careful investigation, are found to be normal. Counseling under such circumstances is discussed by E. A. Murphy (1968).

f. If it is impossible to differentiate X-linked from male-limited autosomal dominant inheritance, even by linkage studies, then large bodies of data might be examined to determine the ratio of familial to sporadic cases. For a lethal condition frequency of sporadic cases significantly less than one-half is evidence for X-linkage.

g. In X-linked dominant inheritance the heterozygous mothers, who are affected to a variable degree, transmit the trait with a segregation frequency of one-half to both sexes; if the trait is rare, the frequency of affected females is approximately twice as great as of males.

h. It is conceivable that in man also some dominant X-linked mutations (*incontinentia pigmenti*, the OFD syndrome) are lethal in hemizygotes, thus producing a two to one ratio of females to males amongst the progeny of affected women and inheritance solely in the female line.

Occasionally it is impossible to determine from pedigree data whether the disorder affecting several siblings is due to X-linked or recessive autosomal inheritance; this is particularly true if the parents are normal and not consanguineous, if no other cases have been observed in the family, and if the affected individuals are all males. Germinal mosaicism for an autosomal dominant mutation is admittedly difficult to exclude in such cases but is probably an extremely rare cause of such familial occurrence. Under such circumstances it is not possible to exclude the healthy sisters of the affected males as carriers of an X-linked mutation. If all attempts to detect carriers for the particular trait have failed, then provisional counseling advice may be offered to the sisters in question based on the likelihood of obtaining the observed distribution of healthy and affected brothers and sisters on the basis of autosomal recessive or X-linked inheritance (Frota-Pessôa *et al.*). Such "derived" risks are manifestly unsatisfactory and point again toward the urgent need of pursuing the phenogenetic problems as quickly as possible.

4. *Multifactorial inheritance.* Basic genetic aspects have been reviewed by J. A. Roberts (1964) and, recently, in a particularly brilliant exposition by F. Vogel (1966), who again pointed out how easy it is to confuse multifactorial inheritance and recessive or dominant inheritance with reduced penetrance. Empiric recurrence risks for the most important and common multifactorially determined congenital malformations are given by C. O. Carter (1965).

a. Multifactorially determined conditions are relatively common in the population; the more common they are the greater is the likelihood they will mimic autosomal dominant and recessive inheritance with reduced penetrance.

b. If the normal trait can be studied (serum uric acid levels, I.Q., height), it is frequently found to be normally distributed within a population, and the two extremes of the trait do not represent discontinuous phenotypic classes completely different from normal but are part of a continuum.

c. Multifactorially determined disorders have a relatively high concordance in monozygous twins (20 to 50 per cent) which, however, is usually lower than the concordance in monozygous twins with chromosomal abnormalities and Mendelian traits. The concordance in dizygous twins is relatively low and may not exceed the incidence of the disorder observed in siblings of the propositus.

d. Such traits have a low incidence in first-degree relatives; if both parents of a child are affected, then the recurrence risk is greater than if only one, or none, of the parents is affected. The greater the number of previously affected children the greater becomes the recurrence risk. The likelihood of being affected diminishes with decreasing degrees of relatedness from the proband; for a trait with the population incidence one in one thousand Grüneberg concludes that the proportion of first-, second-, and third-degree relatives affected would be approximately thirty-five, seven, and three times the population incidence; and Edwards, on the basis of $\rho^{2}\!/_{5}$, $\rho^{2}\!/_{3}$, and $\rho^{4}\!/_{5}$ for the first-, second-, and third-degree relatives (where $\rho$ is the population incidence—1/1000), computed an incidence sixty-three, ten, and four times the population incidence (Carter).

· e. Multifactorially determined traits may occur with a variable frequency in different races and geographic regions.

f. Environmental factors such as season and social class may influence the occurrence of the trait.

g. Parity and parental age may influence the occurrence of the trait.

h. Sex may influence the occurrence of the trait. If sex is a striking influence (pyloric stenosis) then the incidence of affected offspring from the less commonly affected sex will be greater than from the more commonly affected sex.

If the trait can be graded according to severity (degrees of cleft lip or palate deformity) then children from more severely affected parents have a greater likelihood of being affected than offspring from mildly affected parents. If only one parent is affected, the severity of the defect in the offspring is rarely greater than that of his parent and is usually less.

I suspect that some of the common malformation/retardation syndromes including Noonan's syndrome, the Williams hypercalcemia-supravalvular aortic stenosis syndrome, and the Prader-Willi, Rubinstein-Taybi, and Hallermann-Streiff syndromes may be multifactorially determined.

5. *Chromosomal abnormalities* are responsible for many cases of mental retardation (usually associated with minor and/or major malformations), infertility, some abnormalities of genital development, and many cases of spontaneous abortion. In general, *autosomal* anomaly syndromes represent some of the most complex of all malformation/retardation syndromes. Most cases represent sporadic instances in a family. Such abnormalities frequently cause death in infancy or early childhood. If survival to adult age is possible (as in mongolism), most patients are sterile. All gross unbalanced autosomal anomalies seem to be associated with mental retardation and growth impairment. Such patients frequently appear strikingly different from any of the patients' first-degree relatives (parents, sibs), and if they have an identical chromosome abnormality (trisomy G or mongolism) then two unrelated patients will resemble

each other far more than they will resemble their own parents and siblings. Autosomal aneuploidy, the XXX constitution and the $X^MX^MY$ type of Klinefelter's syndrome are associated with an increased maternal reproductive age ranging around a mean of approximately thirty-six years.

The overwhelming majority of patients with *gonosomal* abnormalities is represented by the XXY, XXX, and XYY syndromes. These cases are on the whole far less severely affected than is any patient with an unbalanced autosomal abnormality, and some of the individuals with an XXX and XYY constitution may, indeed, pass as normal in height, intelligence, and reproductive capacity. Most patients with the XO syndrome or evident deletions of the short arm of one X chromosome are more severely affected than the patients with forty-seven chromosome gonosomal aneuploidies (XXX, XXY, XYY) but less severely so than most autosomal aneuploidy syndromes. The gonosomal aneuploidies with forty-eight (XXXX, XXYY, XXXY) and forty-nine chromosomes (5X, 4XY, 3XYY) lead to rather severe impairment and may produce retardation and malformations comparable in severity to the autosomal aneuploidies.

If a cytologic analysis in a given malformation/retardation syndrome reveals no obvious chromosomal abnormality, then an examination of the patient's parents should be performed in an attempt to detect an obvious unbalanced translocation. Mosaicism should also be considered in such cases. The finding of apparently normal chromosomes does not by any means preclude the possibility that the patient's disorder may in fact be caused by a chromosome abnormality. It is quite easy to imagine that there exist many minor chromosomal abnormalities, undetectable by ordinary cytologic methods, which lead to malformation/retardation syndromes. Many of these cases will be sporadic; however, some of them may represent structural rearrangements in one of the parents with a relatively high recurrence risk.

## Summary

1. A complete family history and a thorough physical examination are the most effective means available to detect patients with a high risk of developing later mental retardation.

2. In describing and assessing minor anomalies, the physical examination as practiced at the present time is a very inexact and subjective method in need of urgent refinement.

3. At the present time most malformation/retardation syndromes represent formal genesis syndromes and are probably etiologically heterogeneous. Published descriptions do not yet represent the complete phenotypic spectrum of any malformation/retardation syndrome.

4. Most hereditary mutations leading to retardation in man have not yet been described.

5. "Apparently normal" chromosomes may be seen in patients whose malformation/retardation syndrome is in fact due to a chromosomal abnormality.

REFERENCES

Beckman, L., Gustavson, K. H., and Norring, A. 1965. Dermal configurations in the diagnosis of the Down syndrome. *Acta Genet. Basel* 15:3.

Carter, C. O. 1965. The inheritance of common congenital malformations. *Prog. Med. Genet.* 4:59.

Crow, J. F. 1965. Problems of ascertainment in the analysis of family data. In *Genetics and the epidemiology of chronic disease*, eds. J. V. Neel, M. S. Shaw, and W. J. Schull, pp. 23–44. Washington, D. C.: U. S. Department of Health, Education and Welfare.

Frota-Pessôa, O., Opitz, J. M., Leroy, J. G., and Patau, K. 1968. Counseling in diseases produced either by autosomal or X-linked recessive mutations. *Acta Genet. Statist. Med.* 18:521–533.

Lenz, W. 1964. Echtes, chromatin positives Klinefelter-syndrom (XXY Zustand). In *Hdb. d. Humangenetik*, ed. P. E. Becker, 3(1):333–347. Stuttgart: Thieme Verlag.

McKusick, V. A. 1968. *Mendelian inheritance in man. Catalogs of autosomal dominant, autosomal recessive and X-linked phenotypes.* 2nd ed. Baltimore: Johns Hopkins Press.

Marden, P. M., Smith, D. W., and McDonald, J. J. 1964. Congenital anomalies in the newborn infant, including minor variations. *J. Pediat.* 64:357.

Morton, N. E.

1961. Morbidity of children from consanguineous marriages. *Prog. Med. Genet.* 1:261.

1962. Analysis of human heredity: Segregation and linkage. In *Methodology in human genetics*, ed. W. J. Burdette, pp. 17–52. San Francisco: Holden-Day.

Murphy, E. A. 1968. The rationale of genetic counseling. *J. Pediat.* 72:121.

Patau, K. Personal communication.

Reed, E. W., and Reed, S. C. 1965. *Mental retardation: A family study.* Philadelphia: W. B. Saunders, Co.

Roberts, J. A. 1964. Multifactorial inheritance and human disease. *Prog. Med. Genet.* 3:178.

Smith, D. W., and Bostian, E. 1964. The frequency of associated congenital anomalies in children with idiopathic mental retardation. *J. Pediat.* 65:189.

Steinberg, A. G. 1962. Population genetics: Special cases. In *Methodology in human genetics*, ed. W. J. Burdette, pp. 76–91. San Francisco: Holden-Day.

Vogel, F. 1967. *Multifactorial determination of genetic affections.* Proc. III International Congress Human Genetics, pp. 437–445. Baltimore: Johns Hopkins Press.

Walker, N. F. 1957. The use of dermal configurations in the diagnosis of mongolism. *J. Pediat.* 50:19.

Waardenburg, P. J. 1964. Problems der Heterogenie phänisch gleicher Abweichungen. *Z. menschl. Vererb. -und Konstitutionslehre* 37:269.

# Transplacental Psychotropic Agents and Mental Retardation

JOSEPH CLAYTON SCHOOLAR, Ph.D., M.D.

*Drug Abuse Research Section, Texas Research Institute of Mental Sciences, Houston, Texas*

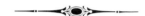

## Introduction

The influence of prenatal environment on offspring is a long-recognized factor, the importance of which has already been mentioned by several members of this symposium. Many references may be found to such influences throughout classical antiquity and mythology; in our own era, folklore claims that pregnant women should beware of certain actions, lest they unwittingly visit harm on the unborn child. Sir James Frazer (1959, p. 18) reports that "—among the Ainos . . . a pregnant woman may not spin or twist ropes for two months before her delivery, lest the child's guts might be entangled like a thread." And again (p. 176), "among [certain] tribes of New Guinea [an expectant mother] should not use sharp instruments, lest she . . . 'stab' [or 'harm'] the child in her womb."

In our own Southern states there are popular accounts of mothers rocking during pregnancy, for example, to impart in utero a sense of rhythm to the unborn child; and of the somewhat fanciful relationship of childhood behavioral difficulties to the fact that the mother suffered fear, panic, or the like during pregnancy. These beliefs were at one time common concerning the genesis of nevi in children.

## Transplacental Psychotropic Agents

The ideas to which Dr. Desmond and I will address ourselves are not new; we hope, however, that we are becoming more precise in separating fact from fantasy.

### Methodology

This task of separating scientific fact from fantasy is not easy, even in these days of increasing methodological sophistication. In reviewing the literature concerning the infrahuman animal (and I shall confine my remarks to animal work, leaving the human studies to Dr. Desmond), several problems inherent in methodology are pointed out by the various authors, and others occur to the reader. In the study of any drug, utilization of several species—rodents, nonrodents, primates—is of course mandatory. Likewise, comparison of results obtained from the *study of different species* must be made knowledgeably. Sometimes species selection is made merely on the basis of the investigator's familiarity with that species. In our own laboratory, for example, I have been guilty of turning to the cat, not necessarily because it is the best animal to prove a given point, but because it is the species with whose neuroanatomy I am most familiar.

*Maternal placental differences* may be important. From membrane studies we now are virtually certain that almost any agent incorporated by the mother will ultimately reach the fetus (Werboff and Gottlieb 1963). But the importance to transplacental kinetics of such factors as total placental surface area and blood supply is obvious.

*Biotransformation* may vary for different species, illustrating differences in critical enzymatic complement. For example, if one is to relate experimental animal studies on Vitamin C to humans, it would be well to remember that only the guinea pig is, like humans, totally dependent on exogeneous sources for its ascorbic acid supply, other species being able to synthesize their own supplies.

What for one drug may be a *critical period of gestation* may not be true for another agent, or there may be differences for the same agent in different species. The *blood supply to the brain* varies from species to species. Looking again at the cat, for example, we know that there is in that species virtually no vertebral artery supply. Yet we blithely dismiss this fact—I suspect, because we are not really certain of its significance.

There are *structural differences* in the central nervous system in the fetus and in the very young animal that are not reflected in the adult. *Rates of myelinization* are known to differ, and the rate of entry of certain drugs into brain tissue has been clearly shown to vary with brain fat content (Dobbing 1961). Likewise, *the water content* of the brain varies with area and with age (Schoolar 1957). Thus, Domek and Barlow have shown quite definitely that phenobarbital distribution is ubiquitous in the neonatal kitten, quite a different situation from that seen in the adult, in which there is sharp anatomical delimitation of phenobarbital distribution (Schoolar, Barlow, Roth 1960).

Here again, for the developing neonate there may be *enzymatic differences*, as mentioned in the case of the adult. Too often, as J. Werboff and J. S. Gottlieb (1963) point out, the assumption is made that the fetus and neonate possess the same facility for metabolism of a drug that the mother does. Yet sharp contrasts have been reported for such divergent agents as amidopyrine, phenacetin, hexobarbital (Jondorf, Maickel, Brodie 1958) and certain antibiotics (Michael and Sutherland 1961).

*Factors in research design* that may constitute uncontrolled variables are obvious, and one need not spend much time on them. As regards the current topic, however, there are noted variations of telling significance in reading over the reports. Some of these variations are discussed below. The *volume of injection* sometimes varied widely, and in one case by a factor of 1,200 (Hoffeld and Webster 1965). To a small animal, this is significant. The *mode of injection* is likewise important. J. Werboff and R. Kesner (1963) noted in rats that maternal injection with distilled water significantly decreased maze learning in offspring if the mother was injected intraperitoneally, but not if injected subcutaneously. That *animal handling* is a significant variable is well known. Edelman has reported that control rats may show a decrease in white blood cells of 70 to 80 per cent, due to experimental conditions alone (Jones 1952). How much more might excitation influence such an elusive variable as performance! *Dosages* are often high, much higher on a weight basis or even on a surface area basis, than one would encounter clinically. Finally, most of the experiments are *acute studies* without a dosage schedule approximating human therapeutic usage. At least in the same generation, we need more chronic studies.

Variables in measurement and in interspecific comparison also occur. J. L. McGaugh and L. F. Petrinovich (1965) have called attention to the importance of distinguishing properly among *learning, behavior*, and *performance*. The inadvertency here is that what actually measures one factor may be interpreted as representing another. H. C. Blodgett (1929), studying rats, found that they were quite capable of learning under his research design, yet they performed only when rewarded. He calls this an example of "latent learning."

Lastly, one must of course keep in view *differential responses to social situations*, when relating data to humans. I often say, only partially in jest, when one of my colleagues points out one or another effect of an antipsychotic drug in monkeys, "Fine. The next time a psychotic monkey wanders into my office, I'll try it."

## Data

Yet, the very simplicity of the laboratory animal is often advantageous. Obviously, it is because there are fewer parameters to hold constant that the experimental animal is a less encumbered research tool. Keeping these considerations in mind, let us turn to representative animal data concerning psychotropic agents. In all subsequent data, we are considering the effects on offspring of agents given to the mother. Table 30 represents the effects of some of these agents.

TABLE 30

Deficiencies in Offspring of Treated Rats

| Author | Agent | Effect | |
|--------|-------|--------|--|
| Harned *et al.* 1940 | NaBr | Decreased: | Maze learning |
| | | | Problem solving |
| | | Increased: | Seizure threshold |
| Vincent 1958 | Alcohol | Decreased: | Maze learning |
| Armitage 1952 | Pentobarbital | Decreased: | Maze learning |
| | Barbital | | |
| Murai 1966 | Phenobarbital | Decreased: | Maze learning |
| | | | (early) |

Perhaps the oldest sedative in medical usage (except alcohol) is the *bromide ion.* Bromides are not used in psychiatry anymore, and bromide-containing patent medicines are not as popular as they once were, but the bromide ion is still significant. B. K. Harned, H. C. Hamilton, and J. C. Borrus (1940) have found that the bromide ion when used in rats decreases maze learning as well as the reasoning ability necessary to solve simple problems. It also increases audiogenic seizure threshold. Some authors have correlated this latter finding with decreased intelligence, although it may be more inferential.

As regards ethanol itself, N. M. Vincent (1958) published data indicating that ethanol given to gravid rats was capable of decreasing intelligence to a significant degree.

The barbiturates barbital, pentobarbital (Armitage 1952), and phenobarbital (Murai 1966) have likewise been shown to lengthen the time required for rats to learn a maze. Murai's findings were true only if the gravid animals were treated early in pregnancy.

Werboff and his co-workers (1961), again examining rats, have studied a variety of drugs important in psychotropic activity, such as reserpine, meprobamate, iproniazid, serotonin, and a benzyl serotonin derivative. Interestingly, all these agents affected neonatal activity and emotionality, and all acted in the same manner, despite their structural disparity. Only meprobamate decreased learning ability. In further studies comparing the two antidepressants, iproniazid and isocarboxazid, Werboff and his associates found both drugs to be toxic to offspring survival; for isocarboxazid toxicity occurred only if the drug were administered in the first trimester of pregnancy; in contrast, there was no difference in iproniazid effect, regardless of gestational stage at injection.

TABLE 31

Effect of Maternal Chlorpromazine on Offspring (Rat)

| Author | Learning | Activity Level | Seizure Threshold | Remarks |
|--------|----------|----------------|-------------------|---------|
| Werboff & Kesner 1963 | 0 | — | — | No stage difference (5–8, 11–14, 17–20 days) |
| Jewett & Norton 1966 | — | Decreased | Decreased | 4–7 days |
| Hoffeld & Webster 1965 | Decreased | — | — | Early only |
| Murai 1966 | Decreased | 0 | Increased | Differences diminished late in pregnancy |

In Table 31 the importance of the stage of gestation at treatment time is raised. Using chlorpromazine alone to focus on this point, and compiling data from different authors, Werboff and Kesner (1963) found no learning deficit at any stage. On the other hand both D. R. Hoffeld and R. L. Webster (1965) and N. Murai (1966) found learning to be decreased if the mothers were injected at about the sixth day of pregnancy. Hoffeld and Webster found no effect if injection was in late pregnancy; and Murai found that the deficit, although present, was less for the late-injection group.

Different findings are also reported for activity level and for audiogenic seizure threshold. Thus R. E. Jewett and S. Norton (1966), studying only early animals, found both activity and seizure threshold decreased, whereas Murai reports no discernible effect on activity level and an *increase* in seizure threshold. As previously mentioned, some workers equate brain electrical activity with intelligence and think it is correlated with motor activity level.

TABLE 32

Effects of Maternal Injection on Offspring (Rats)

| | Early (5–8 days) | | | Late (17–20 days) | | |
|---|---|---|---|---|---|---|
| | No Change | Decreased | Increased | No Change | Decreased | Increased |
| Learning | Res | CPZ Mep Pb | | CPZ Pb Res | Mep | |
| Motor activity | Res CPZ Pb | Mep | | Res CPZ Pb | Mep | |
| Electroshock seizure threshold | Res | | CPZ Mep Pb | Res Pb | | CPZ Mep |

| Res = reserpine | Pb = phenobarbital | (Murai, 1966) |
|---|---|---|
| CPZ = chlorpromazine | Mep = meprobamate | |

Table 32 is compiled from Murai's work (1966) with rats, comparing the effects of four agents of timely significance on three parameters—learning, motor activity, and electroshock seizure threshold. He further compared results of the early- with the late-injection group. The results are most intriguing. He found that injection at five to eight days, with chlorpromazine, meprobamate, and phenobarbital, resulted in a learning deficit whereas in late pregnancy only meprobamate decreased learning. Reserpine was ineffective in either case. In motor activity, only meprobamate gave a significant decrease and did so at both stages of gestation. Murai concludes, therefore, that activity (a performance) and intelligence are not correlated. He reports a stage difference again as regards electroshock seizure threshold: chlorpromazine, meprobamate, and phenobarbital are all significant in the early-treated animals, with phenobarbital becoming insignificant in the late-injected group. Reserpine again showed no difference. Murai concludes that the earlier stage of gestation is more vulnerable than the late stages; his findings agree generally with findings for congenital malformations.

TABLE 33

Effect of Gestation Stage on Offspring Learning
(Hoffeld & Webster)

| Early | Middle | Late |
|---|---|---|
| a. CPZ slower than Mep or Controls | Controls & Res slower than CPZ | No difference |
| b. Mid-pregnancy treated took significantly longer than early or late, for all agents. | | |

Hoffeld and Webster (1965) likewise studied the effect of gestation stage at injection on offspring learning. In Table 33 are reported slightly different results. In the early stage chlorpromazine animals are slower learners than meprobamate animals; there is no difference in the late group. Perhaps of greatest interest is the middle-gestation group, in which both reserpine-treated and control rats were slower than chlorpromazine animals. Also, the midpregnancy group took significantly longer than either the early or late groups for all agents. The authors attribute this difference to possible handling effect or to anxiety—one of the "social" factors mentioned earlier.

These findings are in sharp contrast to those of Werboff and Kesner (1963), who reported that among reserpine, meprobamate, and chlorpromazine, only meprobamate produced a learning deficit, and that there was no stage difference. Not directly applicable here, but interesting, is the finding of R. D. Young (1964) that chlorpromazine decreases maze learning ability in the two-day-old neonate.

The situation concerning antidepressant medications is perhaps less confusing, but only because there is less data available. A. Pletcher and K. F. Gey (1962) have reported species variation in the effect of monoamine oxidase inhibitors on cerebral catecholamine level, but beyond this we know very little.

Of current interest and unique relevance are the effects of these agents when taken as a result of psychic aberration rather than for therapeutic benefit. N. M. Vincent's studies showing deleterious effects of alcohol have been mentioned. G. J. Alexander and his co-workers (1967) have reported a remarkably high incidence of abortions, stillbirths, and offspring-stunting in rats given LSD early in pregnancy, and many workers have warned of possible mental retardation in humans. Studies ·in the area of the psychedelics have barely begun.

## Conclusions

What conclusions can we draw from these rather conflicting data? They mean that caution is needed and that further work is mandatory. I do not intend, on the basis of these reports, categorically to condemn any agent, or even to recommend its proscription during pregnancy. Rather, I have attempted briefly to emphasize the many-faceted nature of the problem and to increase the index of inquiry in both researcher and clinician.

## REFERENCES

Alexander, G. J., Miles, B. E., Gold, G. M., and Alexander, R. B. 1967. LSD: Injection early in pregnancy produces abnormalities in offspring of rats. *Science* 157:459.

Armitage, S. G. 1952. The effect of barbiturates on the behavior of rat offspring as measured on learning and reasoning situations. *J. Comp. Physiol. Psychol.* 45:146.

Blodgett, H. C. 1929. *Univ. Calif. Publ. Psychol.* 4:113.

Dobbing, J. 1961. The blood-brain barrier. *Physiol. Rev.* 41:131.

Frazer, Sir James G. 1959. *The New Golden Bough*, pp. 18, 176. New York: Criterion.

Harned, B. K., Hamilton, H. C., and Borrus, J. C. 1940. The effect of bromide administration to pregnant rats on the learning ability of offspring. *Am. J. Med. Sci.* 20:846.

Hoffeld, D. R., and Webster, R. L. 1965. Effect of injection of tranquilizing drugs during pregnancy on offspring. *Nature* 205:1070.

Jewett, R. E., and Norton, S. 1966. Effect of tranquilizing drugs on postnatal behavior. *Exp. Neurol.* 14:33.

Jondorf, W. R., Maickel, R. P., and Brodie, B. B. 1958. Inability of newborn mice and guinea pigs to metabolize drugs. *Biochem. Pharmacol.* 1:352.

Jones, H. B. 1952. Some physiological factors related to the effects of radiation in mammals. In *Symposium on radiobiology. The basic aspects of radiation: effects on living systems*, ed. J. J. Nickson. New York: J. W. Wiley & Sons.

McGaugh, J. L., and Petrinovich, L. F. 1965. Effects of drugs on learning and memory. *Int. Rev. Neurobiol.* 8:139.

Michael, A. F., and Sutherland, J. M. 1961. Antibiotic toxicity in newborn and adult rats. *Am. J. Dis. Child.* 10:442.

Murai, N. 1966. Effect of maternal medication during pregnancy upon behavioral development of offspring. *Tohoku J. Exp. Med.* 89:265.

Pletcher, A., and Gey, K. F. 1962. Pharmacodynamics of monoamine oxidase inhibitors of the hydrazine type. In *Psychosomatic medicine*, eds. J. H. Nodine and J. H. Moyer, p. 595. Philadelphia: Lea & Febiger.

Schoolar, J. C. 1957. Studies on the localization of urea-$C^{14}$, acetazolamide-$S^{35}$, and isonicotinic acid hydraziade-$C^{14}$ in specific areas of the cat brain. Ph.D. dissertation, University of Chicago.

Schoolar, J. C., Barlow, C. F., and Roth, L. J. 1960. The penetration of carbon-14 urea into cerebrospinal fluid and various areas of the cat brain. *J. Neuropath. Exp. Neurol.* 19:216.

Vincent, N. M. 1958. The effects of prenatal alcoholism upon motivation, emotionality, and learning in the rat. *Am. Psychol.* 17:401.

Werboff, J., and Gottlieb, J. S. 1963. Drugs in pregnancy: Behavioral teratology. *Obstet. Gynec. Survey* 18:420.

Werboff, J., Gottlieb, J. S., Havlena, J., and Word, T. J. 1961. Behavioral effects of prenatal drug administration in the white rat. *Pediatrics* 27:318.

Werboff, J., and Kesner, R. 1963. Learning deficits of offspring after administration of tranquilizing drugs to the mothers. *Nature* 197:106.

Young, R. D. 1964. Drug administration to neonatal rats: Effects on later emotionality and learning. *Science* 143:1055.

# Behavioral Alterations in Infants Born to Mothers on Psychoactive Medication during Pregnancy[1]

MURDINA M. DESMOND, M.D., ARNOLD J. RUDOLPH, M.D.,
REBA M. HILL, M.D., JAMES L. CLAGHORN, M.D.,
PHILIP R. DREESEN, M.D., and IMOGENE BURGDORFF, R.N.

*Department of Pediatrics, Baylor University College of Medicine, the Harris County Hospital District, the Texas Research Institute of Mental Sciences, and the Public Health Nursing Division, Department of Health, Houston, Texas*

The subject, the effects of antenatally administered psychoactive agents on the clinical behavior of the young infant, concerns an area in which our knowledge is meager and fragmentary. It is also an area in which the need for knowledge is urgent.

It has been known for many years that pharmacologic agents given to or taken by the maternal organism may cross the placenta and reach the fetus (Moya and Thorndike 1962). A few compounds that act during embryogenesis are teratogenic—thalidomide, aminopterin, certain pro-

[1] This research was supported by The John A. Hartford Foundation, Inc., the Maternal and Infant Care Project #535, Children's Bureau, and the Maternal and Child Health Division, Texas Department of Public Health.

The authors are indebted to Benjamin Sher, M.D., Willie Verniaud, D. Ed., Robert R. Franklin, M.D., Elna White, Ph.D., Carl Smith, M.D., Mrs. Hope Sessions, P. H. N., Barbara Kidd, M. S. W., and Betty Barnard, R. N., for their assistance with these patients.

gestins—while others may alter the structure of specific tissues—tetracycline, antithyroid agents (Yaffe 1966).

## Opiates

Drug-induced behavioral effects on the human infant without the concurrent presence of malformations caused by morphine and its cogeners have been described since the late nineteenth century (Cobrinik *et al.* 1959; Hill and Desmond 1963; Claman and Strang 1962; Perlstein 1947). Pregnant women actively addicted to morphine or heroin have given birth to infants who are often small in size and not infrequently depressed at delivery (especially if the mother has received narcotics close to or during labor). A syndrome considered to represent withdrawal usually occurs within twenty-four hours in 80 to 90 per cent of these infants. The signs of withdrawal include restlessness, tremors, hyperactivity, excessive crying, swift vasomotor changes, hyperreflexia, diarrhea, and poor food intake. Less frequent manifestations include convulsions, twitching, yawning, sweating, and respiratory difficulties.

Of the ten infants we have observed, four were depressed at and following birth. The onset of withdrawal (excitation) ranged between forty minutes and twenty-four hours with a median time of onset of fourteen hours. Symptoms lasted for as short a period as forty-eight hours and as long as ten weeks. Sedation was required by nine of the ten.

None of these infants were cared for by the mother on discharge from the hospital. Since eight were placed for adoption, the follow-up period has been limited. The characteristic developmental pattern shows a delay in motor behavior and socialization during early months followed by a period of rapid development. All infants followed for nine months or longer appeared to be making adequate developmental progress. However, very little information is known to us or is reported in the literature concerning the later cognitive development of infants who have shown postnatal withdrawal phenomena.

Three of our ten infants weighed below 2500 gm. at birth and five appeared malnourished or undergrown. The factor of undernutrition alone should keep us from assuming that the learning process has been totally unaffected, since undernutrition at birth has been related to learning deficits (Warkany, Monroe, and Sutherland 1961).

## Rauwolfia

The Rauwolfia compounds, introduced in 1954 (Kline 1954), have been utilized in the care of women with essential hypertension and pregnancy toxemia. Side effects have been reported to occur in 15 per cent of infants (Desmond *et al.* 1957; Budnick *et al.* 1955). The early effects are nasal congestion, bradycardia, vasodilation, thermal instability, hypertonicity, and tremors lasting for twenty-four hours to five days. In rare patients the hypertonicity and tremors may persist into early infancy.

## Alcohol

Alcohol withdrawal has been described in the newborn (Schaefer 1962). This syndrome has long been suspected, but few precise descriptions have been available. A newborn patient with irritability, convulsions, and jaundice following maternal alcoholism was recently reported by Nichols (1967).

## Tranquilizers

The early experience with infants born to mothers on therapy with phenothiazines was favorable (Kris *et al.* 1957; Kris 1965; Sobel 1960).

Our interest in the possible effects on the infant of tranquilizers that were taken antenatally by the mother for therapeutic purposes was aroused by the clinical course of an infant who demonstrated signs of an extrapyramidal disorder (hypertonicity, a wide amplitude, tremor, and abnormal hand posturing) which persisted for at least five months. The mother of this child was a schizophrenic under treatment with phenothiazine derivatives during pregancy. The hypertonicity persisted to ten months. No abnormalities were noted at thirty-two months. The child subsequently did well and entered school at the age of six (Hill, Desmond, and Kay 1966).

Since that time we have seen abnormal patterns of clinical behavior in twenty-two additional patients during the period of neonatal adjustment and during early infancy. Eighteen of the twenty-two mothers received major or minor tranquilizers (usually mixtures) in large dosages throughout pregnancy or during late pregnancy. Four of the mothers received continuous therapy with barbiturates to allay anxiety or as anticonvulsants.

In this group birth weight varied widely—six were of low birth weight. The majority were well nourished. A few showed deep skin creases and persistence of intrauterine position—a finding perhaps suggestive of diminished movement *in utero*.

The syndrome shown by these infants has many similarities to the withdrawal syndrome encountered in infants following maternal opiate addiction. The syndrome may be present as postnatal depression followed by agitation, or agitation may begin within minutes of delivery.

Postnatal depression was seen in nineteen of the twenty-two infants. Nine had some difficulty in establishing respiration after birth and showed low one-minute Apgar scores (Apgar 1953). The remaining ten established respiration efficiently but became depressed after the initial onset of respiration. Depression was characterized by diminished spontaneous movement and cry, brief response to stimulation, vasomotor instability, thermolability, and difficulty with oral feeding. This phase of the syndrome lasted from twenty-four hours to five days.

The phase of agitation developed gradually or abruptly and became evident from birth to two weeks of age.

Findings of this phase were excessive motion (especially when supine), excessive crying, alerting behavior (head side-to-side, rooting, sucking, flinging of pelvis), hyperreflexia, hypertonicity with tremor, excessive sucking drive (increased intake), vasomotor instability, low-grade fever, and hyperacusis. Less frequent findings were abnormal hand posturing (hyperextension of fingers, pronation at wrist), prolonged tongue protrusion, uncoordinated suck and swallow mechanism, hyperperistalsis, and seizure-like movements.

The duration of the agitative phase was variable, from one to seven months. The intensity of this phase varied widely.

Many types of psychoactive agents were taken in large dosages during or late in pregnancy by the mothers of these infants. They were often taken in combination or in series and not infrequently in association with alcohol or barbiturates (see Table 34). In addition to the mental disorder, many of these mothers (60 per cent) had major complications of pregnancy or of labor and delivery. Prenatal care was often inconsistent or absent. No statement can be made concerning the incidence of the behavioral alterations in the infants of such mothers since information relating to maternal problems and therapies was often incomplete on pregnancy and delivery records. The mother was not uncommonly under the care of separate clinics or physicians, each working independently. (During the past two years, information has become more readily available, because of the active participation of the psychiatric clinic of the Harris County Hospital District, the Texas Research Institute for Mental Sciences, and public health nursing.)

The depression and agitation are nonspecific in relation to type of psychoactive agent taken by the mother. These effects are not seen in all

TABLE 34

Psychoactive Therapy during Pregnancy in Mothers of Twenty-two Infants Exhibiting
Abnormal Behavioral States Postnatally

| | |
|---|---|
| Phenothiazine derivatives | Antibiotics* |
| Rauwolfia compounds | Diuretics* |
| Chlordiazepoxide | Thyroid hormone* |
| Barbiturates | Antiasthmatic drugs* |
| Meprobamate* | Quinidine* |
| Hydroxyzine* | |
| Imipramine* | |
| Amitriptyline* | |
| Trimethylbenzamide* | |
| Dilantin* | |
| Alcohol* | |
| Electroshock treatment* | |

* In combination with other agents.

infants born to mothers on psychoactive therapy and they vary widely in intensity and duration. They have not been encountered when the mother's medication was infrequent or taken only during the first two trimesters.

In differential diagnosis of the agitative phase, other syndromes leading to agitation must be considered:

1. *During the immediate neonatal period*—septicemia, encephalitis, meningitis, cerebral hemorrhage, cerebral malformation, hypocalcemia, hypoglycemia, hypomagnesia, inborn errors of metabolism, pyridoxine dependence, and congenital hyperthyroidism.

2. *During early infancy*—colic, severe pain (otitic, abdominal), bilirubin encephalopathy, residua of encephalitis, and postanoxic CNS irritation.

## Management

In management the most important factors are reassurance of the parents or parent substitutes concerning the temporary nature of the agitation and establishment of communication with the physicians responsible for the care of the mother.

1. Diminishing the sensory input by providing a quiet environment, swaddling, and warmth.

2. Use of the pacifier between feedings.

3. Holding and walking with the infant in an upright position; plac-

ing of the infant in the prone position for sleeping. (Spontaneous Moro reflexes and startle responses are more frequent when the infant is supine.)

4. Frequent feedings. These infants often require a large caloric intake to compensate for the energy expended in activity.

5. Sedation—the minimum necessary.

6. Frequent consultations with mother during the agitated period.

## Conclusions

The biochemical mechanism underlying the symptomatology is obscure. *In utero* the infant has adapted to the continued presence of a potent pharmacologic agent in his tissues. After birth the drug supply is discontinued, and the infant must readapt to its absence. The symptoms may represent drug effects or drug withdrawal effects. The agitation may also be related to a prior drug-induced intrauterine sensory deprivation. Investigation of drug concentrations in the tissues, its duration in the body, its mode of excretion, and its relationship to enzymatic processes must be clarified before the pathophysiology can be outlined.

Are these behavioral alterations significant in regard to the cognitive process? We do not know at this time that they are, but, more important, we do not know that they are not.

The effects described above occur during the early cognitive period of infancy. Motor development after three to six months is not appreciably affected. Socialization and learning are delayed early. Can the infant catch up at a later age?

These effects are extremely disruptive to maternal-infant interaction and communication. Many of the mothers relapse under the twofold pressure of their disorder and the agitation of the infant.

Patients with psychiatric problems maintained on psychoactive therapy are not, in this time of community-centered mental health centers, unusual patients in an obstetrical population. In Jefferson Davis Hospital obstetrical patients with psychiatric problems occur in a proportion of twelve in every one thousand deliveries. These patients tend, as shown by Sobel (1961), to have many complications of pregnancy and delivery, a finding consistent with our experience. Since complicated pregnancy is now considered to be one of the many factors contributing to mental retardation, unusual effort may be required to provide comprehensive and team care for the psychiatric patient and her infant (Lilienfeld, Pasamanick, and Rogers 1955).

## Summary

Alterations of postnatal clinical behavior have been described in some infants born to mothers on intensive psychoactive drug therapy during late pregnancy. These effects appear during the neonatal period and during early infancy and last for a period of months. Their significance in regard to later cognitive development is not known.

# DISCUSSION

M. Airaksinen: I want to call attention to the effects of general anesthesia during the pregnancy and delivery and the choice of anesthetics. I have been interested in the toxic effects of halothane—and of halothane metabolites—because in Finland Dr. Tammisto and I found myoglobinuria and other signs of muscular damage in several cases after repeated doses of succinylcholine and other depolarizing agents. These signs appeared only if the doses were given during halothane anesthesia—not during ether, barbiturate, $N_2O$ (nitrous oxide), or methoxyflurane anesthesia. Muscles of children seemed to be more seriously and more often affected than those of adults; in particular, women seemed to be less affected.

Because liver toxicity of halothane has also been suspected but not conclusively demonstrated, despite the discovery of several cases of liver necrosis, we decided to study its metabolites, trifluoroethanol and trifluoroacetic acid. The latter seemed to be rather nontoxic to mice, $LD_{50}$ over 2 gm. per kg. intraperitoneally and nearly 2 gm. per kg. intravenously, but the former, trifluoroethanol, had a considerable toxicity, $LD_{50}$ about 160 mg. per kg. i. p. This toxicity was late; the mean living time with 250 mg. per kg. dose was about twenty-four hours. Young, vigorous mice seemed to die faster and with lower doses than did the old ones. This result suggested a metabolic toxicity, and we found a drop of pyruvate and lactate in liver and muscle, often to zero values after trifluoroethanol administration. This finding means that the trifluoroethanol blocks the glycolysis as does iodoacetate. This blocking was well demonstrated by giving neostigmine and causing fibrillation that normally increases the lactate level. In mice and guinea pigs receiving trifluoroethanol, however, the lactate level decreased as happens in iodoacetate poisoning and McArdles disease. Both trifluoroethanol and trifluoroacetate also slightly increased citrate values in the kidney, brain, and heart. This increase was not as high as the increase monofluoroacetate causes by blocking the Krebs cycle. This slight citrate increase may not be important; perhaps, however, it really can block the tricarboxylic acid cycle, too, but the decreased amount of available pyruvate prevents the increase of citrate. According to some authors trifluoroethanol is enzymatically formed when debromination and dechlorination of halothane occur, and 18 to 20 per cent of the halothane absorbed is metabolized in the human body in this way.

Although the fate of trifluoroethanol is not known, one can suppose that it affects the fetus in the same way ethanol affects the fetus. So far, the susceptibility of the fetus to this compound is not known—as I mentioned, young mice seemed to die at lower doses than adults. Neither is it known how long the enzyme inhibition lasts. If the trifluoroethanol or aldehyde derived from this are only competitive inhibitors of some enzymes and remain a short time in the body, the effect might be rather harmless—but if they cause a permanent block of the enzymes (in the way that iproniazid inactivates monoamine oxidase), the effect lasts until enough new enzymes are synthesized.

J. SCHOOLAR: We have no such clear-cut data on the effects of the agents under consideration. There has been some preliminary work showing diminished activity *in utero* in rats receiving barbiturates.

# REFERENCES

Apgar, C. 1953. Proposal for new method of evaluation of newborn infant. *Anesth. & Analg.* 32:260.

Budnick, I. S., Leikin, S., and Hoeck, L. E. 1955. Effect in the newborn infant of reserpine administered antepartum. *Am. J. Dis. Child.* 90:286.

Claman, A. D., and Strang, R. I. 1962. Obstetric and gynecologic aspects of heroin addiction. *Am. J. Obst. & Gynec.* 83:252.

Cobrinik, R. W., Hood, T. R., and Chusid, E. 1959. The effect of maternal narcotic addiction on the newborn infant. Review of the literature and report of 22 cases. *Pediatrics* 24:288.

Desmond, M. M., Rogers, S. F., Lindley, J. E., and Moya, J. H. 1957. Management of toxemia of pregnancy with reserpine. II: The newborn infant. *Obst. & Gynec.* 10:140.

Hill, R. M., and Desmond, M. M. 1963. Management of the narcotic withdrawal syndrome in the neonate. *Pediat. Clin. N. Am.* 10:67.

Hill, R. M., Desmond, M. M., and Kay, J. L. 1966. Extrapyramidal dysfunction in an infant of a schizophrenic mother. *J. Pediat.* 69:589.

Kline, N. S. 1954. Use of rauwolfia serpentina in neuropsychiatric conditions. *Ann. N.Y. Acad. Sci.* 59:107.

Kris, E. B. 1965. Children of mothers maintained on pharmacotherapy during pregnancy and postpartum. *Curr. Therap. Res.* 7:785

Kris, E. B., and Carmichael, D. M. Oct. 1957. Chlorpromazine maintenance therapy during pregnancy and confinement. *Psychiat. Quart.* 31:1.

Lilienfeld, A. M., Pasamanick, B., and Rogers, M. 1955. Relationship between pregnancy experience and the development of certain neuropsychiatric disorders in childhood. *Am. J. Pub. Health* 45:637.

Moya, F., and Thorndike, V. 1962. Passage of drugs across the placenta. *Am. J. Obst. & Gynec.* 84:1778.

Nichols, N. M. 1967. Acute alcohol withdrawal syndrome in a newborn. *Am. J. Dis. Child.* 113:714.

Perlstein, M. A. 1947. Congenital morphism—a rare cause of convulsions in the newborn. *J.A.M.A.* 135:633.

Schaefer, O. 1962. Alcohol withdrawal syndrome in a newborn infant of a Yukon Indian mother. *Canad. Med. Ass. J.* 87:1333.

Sobel, D. E.

1960. Fetal damage due to ECT, insulin coma, chlorpromazine, or reserpine. *Arch. Gen. Psychiat.* 2:606.

1961. Infant mortality and malformations in children of schizophrenic females. *Psychoanal. Quart.* 35:60.

Warkany, J., Monroe, B. B., and Sutherland, B. S. 1961. Intrauterine growth retardation. *Am. J. Dis. Child.* 102:249.

Yaffe, S. J. 1966. Some aspects of perinatal pharmacology. *Ann. Rev. Med.* 17:213.

# The Role of Early Mother/Child Relations in the Etiology of Some Cases of Mental Retardation[1]

DAVID A. FREEDMAN, M.D.

*Department of Psychiatry, Baylor University College of Medicine, Houston, Texas*

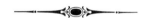

L. S. Penrose (1963) proposes that the distribution of I.Q. does not follow the normal curve. Rather, he suggests a skewing on the low side (Fig. 56) which is the result of the superposition of a relatively small group of cases designated as "organic" on what would otherwise be the low end of the normal curve. When these organic cases are removed, the remaining individuals with I.Q. up to 70 are considered to be instances of "familial mental deficiency."

Controversy concerning the etiology of familial cases has polarized around two points of view. One group of workers feels that specific genetic factors must be operative whereas the other opts for the multi-factorial solution. For the latter group, individuals with familial mental deficiency are seen as coming from the same genetic pool as the general population and should be distinguished from their more fortunate brethren only in terms of the quantity of their intelligence. As E. Zigler (1967) points out, this assumption generates the proposition that such individuals should function at the same cognitive level as do normal

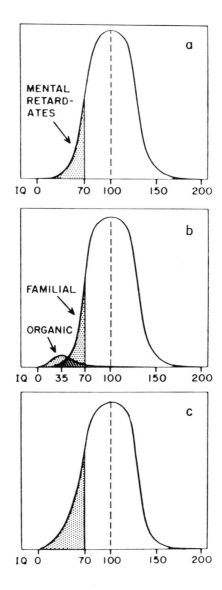

FIGURE 56. (a) Conventional representation of the distribution of intelligence. (b) Distribution of intelligence as represented in the two-group approach. (c) Actual distribution of intelligence. (After Penrose 1963.)

people of the same mental age (that is, in terms of their cognitive functioning a six-year-old with an I.Q. of 100 and a twelve-year-old with an I.Q. of 50 should be identical). The fact that this proposition is contravened by the repeated observation of marked differences in the performance of normals and retardates has been taken to support the specific gene-determined hypothesis.

The cases that will now be reported confirm the observation that retardates show significant cognitive differences when compared to normals. They are being presented, however, because the available data point to a nongenetic etiology—one related to the subjects' very early postpartal experience rather than to intrinsic gene determined disabilities.

Tables 35 and 36 demonstrate the level of intellectual functioning of the subjects. Their I.Q.'s have remained in the neighborhood of 40 during the twenty-month period of observation. By contrast performance on the Vineland Scale has shown striking changes (Table 37).

These youngsters are the middle children of a sibship of four. Their parents are intellectually within the normal range; both are high school

TABLE 35

Summary of Psychologic Tests

| Ann | ♀ D. O. B. 4/27/58 | | | |
|---|---|---|---|---|
| Date | 6/1/65 | 1/10/66 | 5/3/66 | 9/7/66 |
| Test | Stanford-Binet | Stanford-Binet | Stanford-Binet | Stanford-Binet |
| Score | C. A. 7–2 | C. A. 7–8 | C. A. 8–0 | C. A. 8–4 |
| | M. A. 2–5 | M. A. 3–3 | M. A. 3–11 | M. A. 3–7 |
| | I.Q. "Minimal" < 67 | I.Q. 39 | I.Q. 46 | I.Q. 40 |

TABLE 36

Summary of Psychologic Tests

| Albert | ♂ D. O. B. 3/14/60 | | |
|---|---|---|---|
| Date | 1/24/66 | 5/3/66 | 9/8/66 |
| Test | Stanford-Binet | Stanford-Binet | Stanford-Binet |
| Score | C. A. 5–10 | C. A. 6–2 | C. A. 6–6 |
| | M. A. 2–6 | M. A. 2–10 | M. A. 2–10 |
| | I.Q. Est. 36 | I. Q. Est. 42 | I. Q. Est. 38 |

TABLE 37

Summary of Psychologic Tests

| Albert | ♂   D. O. B. 3/14/60 | | | |
| --- | --- | --- | --- | --- |
| Date | 6/1/65<br>C. A. 5/3 | 5/18/65 | 7/23/65 | 1/24/66 |
| Test | Cattell Infant<br>Intelligence<br>Score | Vineland Social<br>Maturity Scale | Vineland | Vineland |
| Score | Inconsistent<br>Avg.—M.A.<br>6 mos. | S. A. 0–10<br>S. Q. 17 | S. A. 2–4<br>S. Q. 37 | 5–6<br>94 |

graduates. There is no known history of mental deficiency in either of their very large and extended families. The older sibling has been able to maintain himself at expected grade level in a regular school setting. Of the younger child, born since our observations began, we know nothing. It seems that during her second and third pregnancies the mother developed the conviction that her offspring would be born defective. In the light of this foreordained conclusion, she elected both to keep them isolated from birth on and to devote a minimum of her time to them. For reasons known only to herself, she also elected to treat the children somewhat differently.

The little girl was confined to a room she shared with her older brother. He had a bed, but she slept on a straw pallet on the floor. He came and went as he pleased, but she remained totally confined to the room. The little boy, by contrast, was confined by himself to a room eight by ten feet in size. Aside from a crib and a potty, this room was bare of furniture. There was a single electric light bulb in the ceiling. The only window was covered by burlap sacking.

The following is a description of their behavior when they were found and of its evolution over the next thirty months.

Ann, at age 6, was unable to feed herself or to talk meaningfully although she did repeat some words and sentences in echolalic fashion. She displayed no affective reaction either to her mother or to the strangers who came to investigate. Subsequently when she was removed from the home she showed no response either to the leaving or to the new environment and handling. The social worker commented that when Ann was picked up she offered no resistance. Her body, however, remained unresponsive (that is, she did not mold in response to the worker's handling).

On admission to the John Sealy Hospital her height was noted to be 42.5 inches and her weight 30 pounds. By both criteria she ranked below the third percentile in physical development. She was incontinent of urine and feces and indifferent to the overtures of the staff. Much of her time she spent sitting up in bed rocking. She was, however, able to stand and walk without assistance. During the relatively brief hospitalization (8 weeks) she is said to have become continent, learned to feed herself, learned to call some objects by name and at times seemed to display affectional responses to members of the staff. She was returned to her family for another nine months before the slowly moving legal process eventuated in placement in a foster home.

The description from the foster mother indicates that the gains made during her hospitalization were short-lived. Although she was able to pass objects from hand-to-hand and to her mouth, this nearly seven-year-old child could neither handle eating utensils nor feed herself by hand. (At home her only food is said to have been moderately thick gruel served in a nursing bottle.) She was described as extremely obedient, and it was noted that when told to she would sit for hours in one position. She exhibited no interest either in her environment or in her body. At no time was she observed to engage in masturbatory activity. On the Vineland Social Maturity scale, she scored at the ten-month-level.

After her placement in the foster home, she very quickly learned such basic skills as eating and toileting. Unlike her younger brother she has consistently shown evidence of awareness of and concern for the reaction of adults in her immediate environment. Her foster parents described her as timid because she neither took food or water nor played with objects without obtaining permission. We assume that this characteristic must reflect her long experience of confinement with another child whose spontaneous coming and going she could watch but was not permitted to emulate.

She now responds more or less in kind to the affectionate overtures of adults. The quality of her response is, however, distinctive. She continues unable to mold her body to another person. To the casual observer she appears to be a friendly affectionate little girl. On closer inspection, however, her outgoing qualities prove more apparent than real. She makes no discrimination among people and goes willingly to anyone, friend or stranger, who makes an overture to her. Five months after she came to foster care she and her brother were presented to a large conference. There were well over one hundred people present. The examiner, who up to that time had only seen them through a one-way screen, picked them up and carried them into the room. During the demonstration, which lasted nearly three-quarters of an hour, they showed absolutely no concern. Not only were they unaffected by the examiner's handling, but also they went willingly to various members of the audience. Their response to their teachers who were present was not noticeably different from their response to the total strangers.

At present both children continue to show this lack of concern with people whom they encounter. They will go without question or hesitation to and with anyone who wishes to take them. They show nothing to suggest that their awareness of, or attachment to, any one person, place, or object is sufficient to lead them to be concerned with the strange as opposed to the familiar or the dangerous as opposed to the safe and secure.

Their lack of capacity to make attachments was most dramatically illustrated when they were adopted. After some sixteen months in a warm and loving environment, they moved to their new homes without displaying any evidence of a sense of grief or loss. They have never even mentioned, let alone inquired for, their foster parents. When the adoptive parents elected to change their given names, they accepted the new ones as though they had never had any others.

When they are engaged in play these characteristics persist. The examiners as people seem to be of little interest to them. Their concern is with part objects—pieces of anatomy like the nose, mouth, or ear, or with articles of dress. It is not possible to involve either child in games that require spontaneity and mutual interchange.

Ann has progressed from an echolalic repetitious and meaningless use of a few words to a considerable vocabulary. She now uses some abstract concepts. However, she continues to articulate poorly. She was in foster care a year before she began to use the first person pronoun. Six months later, differentiation of herself from the environment was still incomplete. The following episode is illustrative. She was holding a doll as she sat on the examiner's lap and was asked to show the doll's ear. At once she reached for her own ear, hesitated, and then touched the doll's. The question, "Where is the other ear?" evoked reaching again for the same ear. Further questions made it clear that the concept of "other" as well as of two, like the image of the ear as something both she and the doll possess, remained extremely tenuous in this eight-year-old girl. A psychological report from roughly the same time noted it was frequently difficult to determine whether she was referring to the examiner or to herself.

During a visit shortly after they were adopted, their new mother wished to show off Ann's accomplishments. She asked her, "What do we say at the table?" Ann replied in a high-pitched sing-song voice, "Don't talk with your mouth full." When the foster mother repeated the question and emphasized sitting down at the table, Ann crossed herself and rattled off grace. In both instances it was as though a switch had been turned and a preprogrammed performance had been run off. One had the feeling that what she said was as meaningful to the child as the music on a tape is to the tape deck.

The younger sibling, Albert, was isolated *in toto*. Like Ann, he was fed exclusively by bottle. His diet also consisted of a gruel that would pass through an enlarged nipple hole. We have reason to believe that his mother only entered the room to feed and diaper him. In his later years we know that it was her wont to place him on the potty where he would, on command, sit for long hours. However, he never learned the intended connection between the potty and excretion.

When he was hospitalized at age four he was thirty-seven inches in height and weighed twenty-three pounds. Like his sister he was well below the third percentile in both weight and height. He walked with a peculiar waddling gait, and he was incapable of even the most elementary use of his hands. Neither the manipulation of objects nor hand-to-mouth activity were present; he was unable to masticate, was incontinent of urine and feces and totally devoid of articulate speech. The only vocalizations recorded were grunting sounds and at times screams.

During the hospitalization locomotion improved, and he became able to hold his cup and clutch toys. He was never observed to play with objects or people.

Nine months later, when he came to foster care, he too had lost most of his paltry advances. Like his sister, he would sit for long hours, almost immobile. He was unable to handle objects or to feed himself. Head banging and rocking were chronic. He was unable to walk. Subsequently his gait became similar to that described at the time of his earlier hospitalization.

In addition to their intellectual and behavioral pecularities these children displayed certain other traits that seem worthy of mention. Albert, for instance, showed no evidence of pain sensibility during the first months

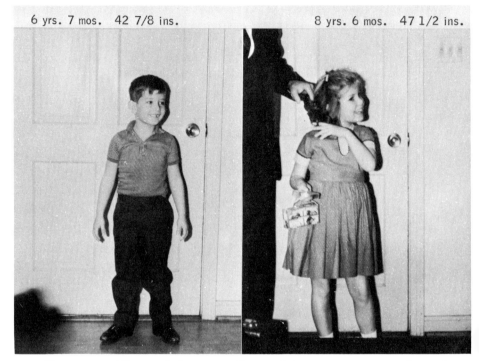

6 yrs. 7 mos.   42 7/8 ins.                    8 yrs. 6 mos.   47 1/2 ins.

FIGURE 57. Albert and Ann, mentally retarded as a consequence of experiential factors.

of the observation period. His foster mother reported that he would repeatedly fall and bruise or cut himself, sometimes quite severely, without ever a whimper. It was only when he had begun to have some interest in her that he would come crying—or make any complaint—after such an injury. While many of us have had the experience of not noticing a cut or bruise during a period of excitement, such behavior as a matter of routine in a five-year-old is certainly atypical. Yet in the past both J. M. G. Itard (1932) and R. M. Zingg (1940) reported similar behavior in youngsters who had spent long periods of time in isolation.

Both children, when they were taken into foster care, also showed evidence of defective visceral sensation. This defect persisted in Albert much longer than it did in his sister. For nearly a year, he would eat anything and everything placed in front of him. It was only possible to stop his eating by forcibly removing him from the supply of food.

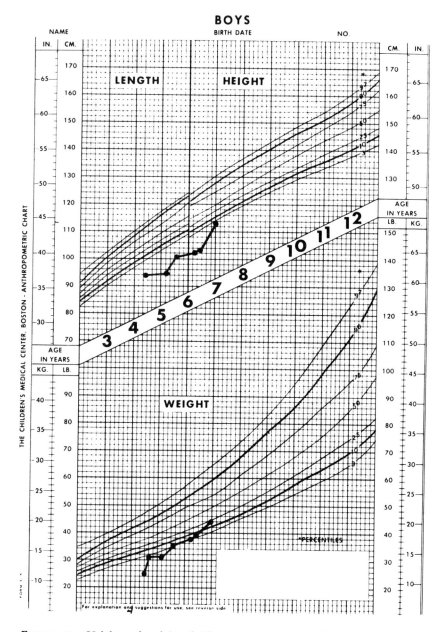

FIGURE 58. Height and weight of Albert (•——•) compared to those of normal boys.

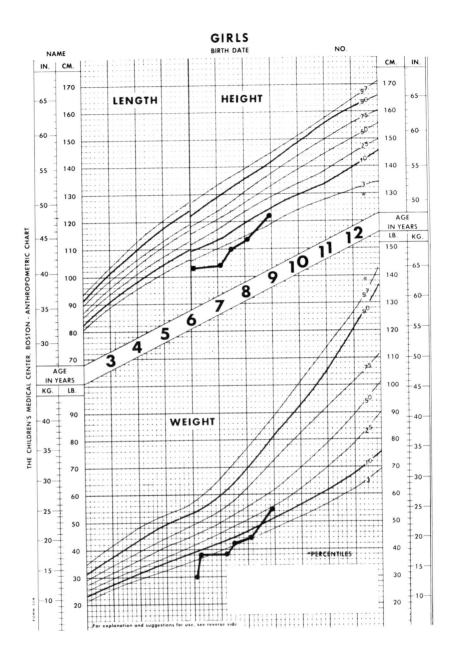

FIGURE 59. Height and weight of Ann (●——●) compared to those of normal girls.

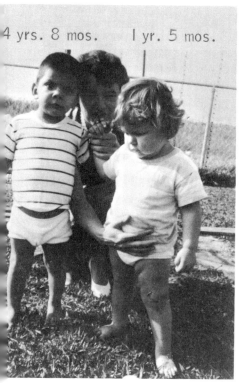

4 yrs. 8 mos.    I yr. 5 mos.

FIGURE 60. Growth retardation due to maternal deprivation. The boy was deprived; the girl was not.

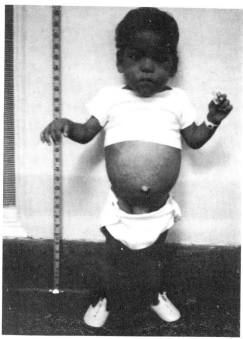

3 y 10 m 13 d

Wt: 20 1/2 lb.    Ht: 29 1/2 in.

FIGURE 61. Growth retardation due to maternal deprivation.

The children's diminutive stature has already been mentioned. Figure 57 shows Albert at six years, seven months and Ann at eight years, six months, nearly two years after they came into foster care. Their parents, it should be noted, are of average stature. Figures 58 and 59 illustrate that the height and weight of both children remained below normal over the period of study, despite adequate nutrition.

The degree of physical retardation, as well as its persistence, is so striking that we have found ourselves looking for evidence of similar delays in other children. In the last year we have found several such cases. Figures 60 and 61 illustrate two of them. The children came to attention because of failure to thrive, and there was evidence of significant maternal deprivation.

F. M. Blodgett (1963) has already described the phenomenon of growth retardation in an emotionally deprived child, and G. F. Powell (1967) has reported thirteen such cases, which were brought to him as instances of suspected primary hypopituitarism. In each he came to the conclusion that the problem was of psychologic origin. Powell seems to have excluded malnutrition as the explanation for growth retardation because with no endocrine therapy his subjects responded very quickly to placement in a secure and psychologically benign environment. Ann and Albert (Fig. 57), however, did not show a significant acceleration of growth rate despite ample diets over a period of nearly twenty months. More recently under a regime of almost forced high caloric feedings they have gained in weight. Their heights, however, continue to lag (Figs. 58 and 59). In another case that we have followed, the child seems to have eaten sporadically. At times he would gorge himself, whereas on other occasions he would go on what his foster parents called a hunger strike. These strikes, which were accompanied by diarrhea, were closely related temporally to events that he found upsetting. Apparently he was doing well until age two when the birth of a baby to his foster mother led him to feel set aside. His present, and we hope permanent, foster mother has noted a recurrence of symptoms of watery diarrhea and anorexia each time she accepts a new baby for care as well as each time she herself is upset.

This latter observation seems to us to have considerable prognostic significance. This child, unlike Albert and Ann, gives evidence of much concern for those in his environment who provide care. It is, we suspect, of more than passing significance that he seems to have made rapid strides in learning during the past five or six months.

An implication to be derived from this case is the possibility that the factors underlying growth retardation are different from those accounting for intellectual and emotional deficiencies. This is a possibility that remains to be explored.

For the present, it is sufficient to say that our observations suggest that maternal deprivation and isolation during infancy and childhood result in a devastating syndrome even when the child is not cruelly treated in any active sense. This syndrome includes, in addition to its behavioral elements, at least one very dramatic biochemical defect—failure of either production or utilization of growth hormone. What other alterations in intimate metabolism may occur has to date not been investigated.

If one entertains the hypothesis that neither the intellectual nor the physical retardation is of genetic origin in these cases, the question must be raised whether it is possible to determine more precisely what factors in the patient's experience may have had the retarding effect. There are several lines of clinical evidence as well as at least one series of experiments which have relevance to the question. Because numbers tend to be more convincing than isolated case studies, I will cite the problem of the congenitally and neonatally blind. At least two series of cases (Norris, Spalding, and Brodie 1958 in Chicago, and Fraiberg and Freedman 1964 in New Orleans) make it clear that 25 per cent of congenitally blind youngsters develop a striking and uniform syndrome.

Whether the child is two, five, nine, or even thirteen years old, the picture is almost unvarying. Typically he spends hours in bed or in a chair or lying on the floor absently mouthing an object. There is no interest in anything that is not in itself pleasurably stimulating to the mouth. Contact with human objects is often initiated by biting and even more often by a primitive clutching and clawing with the hands. For all these children, the mouth remains the primary organ of perception. New objects are at once brought to the mouth and are rarely explored manually.

The behavior of the hand is striking. While many can use it for self-feeding and can even use spoons and forks, the hand appears to have no autonomy of its own. It can serve the mouth, it can bring objects to the mouth, but it is not employed for examination or manipulation. Among these children objects seem never to be of interest as such; they are important not for their own characteristics, but for their qualities in stimulating the mouth.

In addition, deviant blind children display behavior such as body rocking, head banging, arm and hand waving, and bizarre posturing, which is strikingly similar to posturing observed in the sighted autistic child. Language is rarely employed for communication or expression of need. It consists mainly of echolalia and the repetitive use of apparently meaningless words and phrases. Discrimination of "I" and "you" is not made, and self-reference is in the third person.

The very early developmental histories of these deviant blind children are not significantly different from the histories of those who, though blind, achieve a good level of ego formation. Both groups are characterized as quiet babies, content to lie for long hours in their cribs. Gross motor development follows parallel courses for the first nine months of life. Holding the head up, turning over, and sitting independently, are achieved at roughly the same age. However, deviant children either never learn to creep or do so at a very delayed age. Some do not achieve independent walking until four or five years of age.

The picture of developmental arrest is most striking. The thirteen-year-old is not different in any significant way from the two- or three-year-old. In one case, it was possible to compare a ten-year-old boy in the deviant group with home movies of him taken at age 3. Some progress in independent locomotion aside, there was no difference in the behavioral achievements.

To reiterate, only 25 per cent of congenitally blind children show this picture. The other 75 per cent fade off in the direction of less and less evidence of psychological disturbance. Many children with blindness of the same etiology are able to attend sighted school, college, and even graduate school. The English pianist Alec Templeton is a case in point. It should be emphasized that the 25 per cent figure holds, whatever the etiology of the blindness.

When the living circumstances of deviant and nondeviant blind youngsters are investigated, very definite differences can be defined. The youngster whose plight first brought our attention to this problem is a poor little rich boy. His mother reacted to his birth and blindness with a frenzy of activity which kept her so occupied with the problems of the blind in general that she had no contact with her blind son in particular. Confined to an upstairs back room in a very large house, he offered no complaint and was, therefore, left alone. A succession of nursemaids provided perfunctory care. It was only as the mother discovered in the course of her activities that not all blind children were like her child that she sought an explanation for his difficulties.

Inadequate and temporally inappropriate stimulation during early life seems to be crucial in the evolution of the deviant syndrome in blind children just as it does in the cases already reported.

Additional support for this view comes from the case reports of Marie Mason (1942) and Kingsley Davis (1940, 1947). Mason reported her experience with a girl born illegitimately to an aphasic mother. The mother was totally uneducated, could neither read nor write, and communicated with her family only by gesture. From the time the pregnancy was discovered, she, and subsequently her child, were kept in a locked room behind drawn shades. Six and one-half years later, carrying her child, the mother made her escape, and the child came to the attention of public authorities. Mason saw the latter when she was admitted to the

Children's Hospital in Columbus, Ohio. The first two days the child spent in tears. Mason's overtures were greeted by a gesture of repulsion from, to quote her, "the wan-looking child whose face bore marks of grief and fear."

Sensing that no direct approach was possible, Mason attempted to involve her by playing dolls with another little girl while ostensibly ignoring her. By this method, which would have been entirely inapplicable to the apathetic children described above, she was able to engage the child's interest and establish a mutual relation with her. Within a year and a half she had acquired a vocabulary of between 1500 and 2000 words, could count to a hundred, identify coins, and perform arithmetic computations to ten. Mason describes her at $8\frac{1}{2}$ as having an excellent sense of humor, being an inveterate tease and an imaginative, affectionate, and loving child. In less than two years she made the transition from a world of silence, fear, and isolation to an excellent adjustment in the average expectable social world of childhood.

In contrast to Albert and Ann, this child was isolated with her mother. Despite the paucity of all other modes of stimulation, she had ample opportunity for body contact. Undoubtedly, too, she was held, cuddled, played with, and was able to engage in a variety of other forms of non-verbal communication. Support for the assumption of the mother's crucial role is also found in the case reported by Davis. He describes a youngster born illegitimately to a woman who confined the child to a room by herself. Eight years later, when the little girl was found, she was totally uneducable.

Two additional sources of evidence support the view that the quality of early postpartal experience plays a crucial role in later mental development. The story of Helen Keller (Dahl 1965) is one. She was a normal healthy eighteen-month-old when she was struck deaf and blind by meningitis. Despite many years of markedly disturbed behavior during which, by the definition of the intelligence tests she was retarded, Miss Sullivan was ultimately able to make contact with her. The results are familiar to us all.

Finally, the observations of H. F. and M. K. Harlow (1962) and William A. Mason (1967) on the role of mothering in the primate require mentioning. The Harlows have demonstrated that in the absence of adequate mothering infant monkeys develop very dramatic behavioral syndromes. Not only are these animals defective as infants, but they persist in being markedly deviant as adults. When on rare occasions a female monkey of this sort becomes pregnant, she proves to be totally incapable of rearing her youngster. Thus, she passes on the malignant effects of her own rearing to the next generation. It is not difficult to understand how, in the comparable human situation, an investigator seeing a mentally defective child of a mentally deficient parent might invoke genetic factors as an explanation.

William Mason has attempted to learn what in the experience of the infant monkey determines whether or not it will develop a deprivation syndrome. He found that when he modified Harlow's experimental situation so that the surrogate mother moved freely and, from the standpoint of the infant, unpredictably in three dimensional space the entire syndrome was averted. Such a moving surrogate seems to add two elements to the experience of the developing infant which are absent in the presence of Harlow's fixed surrogate. In the first place when the infant is on the "mother" its labyrinths are being stimulated. Secondly, since "mother" approaches and withdraws unpredictably the infant must be constantly aware of her whereabouts both in order to reach her when he feels the need and to avoid being bumped by her as he goes about his own activities.

In summary, it has been the purpose of this report to present data from a variety of sources, all of which point to the importance of both the amount and quality of early postpartal stimulation in physical and mental development. These data seem relevant to the present symposium on two scores. In the first place, they emphasize the importance of not assuming that biochemical abnormalities are prima-facie evidence for an inborn error of metabolism. Even in very young children so drastic a disturbance as failure either to elaborate or to utilize growth hormone can be environmentally determined. Secondly, the data lend support to that school of thought which attributes familial mental deficiency to experiential as opposed to genetic factors.

# REFERENCES

Blodgett, F. M. 1963. Growth retardation related to maternal deprivation. In *Modern perspectives in child development*, eds. A. Solnit and S. Provence, p. 83. New York: International University Press.

Dahl, H. 1965. Observations on a natural experiment: Helen Keller. *J. Am. Psychoanal. Assn.* 13:533.

Davis, K.
    1940. Extreme social isolation of a child. *Am. J. Soc.* 45:454.
    1947. Final note on a case of extreme isolation. *Am. J. Soc.* 52:432.

Fraiberg, S., and Freedman, D. A. 1964. Observations on the development of a congenitally blind child. *Psychoanal. Study of the Child* 19:113.

Harlow, H. F., and Harlow, M. K. 1962. The effects of rearing conditions on behavior. *Bull. Menninger Foundation* 26:213.

Itard, J. M. G. 1932. *The wild boy of Aveyron.* Translated by George and Muriel Humphrey. New York: Century Co.

Mason, M. K. 1942. Learning to speak after 6½ years of silence. *J. Speech & Hearing Disorders* 7:295.

Mason, W. A. April 1967. The primate deprivation syndrome: The search for sources. Manuscript presented at Society for Research in Child Development, New York.

Norris, M., Spalding, P. J., and Brodie, F. H. 1958. *Blindness in children.* Chicago: University of Chicago Press.

Penrose, L. S. 1963. *The biology of mental defect.* London: Sidgwick and Jackson.

Powell, G. F., Brasel, J. A., and Blizzard, R. M. 1967. Emotional deprivation and growth retardation simulating idiopathic hypopituitarism. *New Eng. J. Med.* 276:1271.

Zigler, E. 1967. Familial retardation: A continuing dilemma. *Science* 155:292.

Zingg, R. M. 1940. Feral man and extreme cases of isolation. *Am. J. Psychol.* 53:487.

# The Effect of Malnutrition on the Physical and Mental Development of Children

ROBERTO RENDON, M.D.,* JUAN JOSE HURTADO, M.D.,
and MARIA CHRISTINA ARATHOON

*Department of Neurology, Roosevelt Hospital, Guatemala City, Guatemala*

Translated by Vicente Estevez

*Texas Research Institute of Mental Sciences*

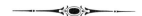

## Introduction

It is estimated that more than half the world's population suffers some form or degree of malnutrition. The protein and caloric deficiency in infancy and childhood is the most generalized nutritional problem and at the same time one of the most important factors in the development of pre-industrialized countries. It is the indirect or direct cause of the high infantile mortality, and since more children survive than die of malnutrition, it is a cause of poor productivity in the adults.

In Latin America at present there are not adequate statistical figures for the incidence of malnutrition or for the mortality related to it because the system by which the causes of death are recorded in most Latin

*Present address: Jefferson Medical College, 11th and Chestnut, Philadelphia, Pennsylvania 19107.

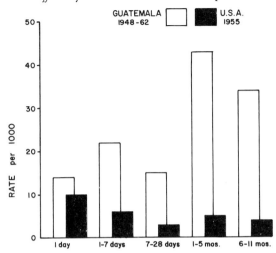

*Effect of Malnutrition on Development*

FIGURE 62. Evaluations of mortality by specific age during the first year of life in rural area of Guatemala (1948–1962) and in the United States of America (1955). (From J. Cravioto 1966.)

American countries, especially in Guatemala where accurate analysis is not allowed, is inadequate. R. Calder (1966) has mentioned that 70 per cent of the preschool children in underdeveloped countries suffer protein and caloric malnutrition, and in the cases of surviving children their growth and development is altered, sometimes in an irreparable form.

Investigations of every death that occurred during a two-year period in four rural towns in Guatemala reported that of 109 deaths in children of less than five years, 38 were cases of grave protein and caloric malnutrition; this finding means that 33 per cent of those deaths were related to malnutrition (Behar *et al.* 1963). In a previous study it was estimated that in about 50 per cent of the deaths among preschool children malnutrition was a very important factor (Behar, Ascoli, and Scrimshaw 1958). The evaluation of specific mortalities by age among preschool North American and Guatemalan children from rural areas is quite similar the first day of life, but later respiratory and gastrointestinal infection factors are considered primary causes of death, and it seems obvious that malnutrition is a contributing factor of great importance. This conclusion can be better seen in Figure 62 (Behar *et al.* 1963).

263

In recent years there has been a growing interest in the effects of the nutritional deficiencies on the central nervous system. Although there is some evidence of this effect (Cavak and Najdanvic 1965; Cordano *et al.* 1963; Craviato 1966; Acheson 1960), there is still a lack of thorough studies on preschool children. Other factors that could possibly affect the psychobiological development of the child in a permanent way and that are frequently associated with malnutrition have not been adequately evaluated: for example, the sociocultural aspect by which parents are functioning at a subnormal level because they themselves have grown and developed with marked multisensory limitations. Since we do not know the vulnerability age of the child, it may be possible that the nutritional state of the mother is one of the most important factors in the development of the central nervous system of her child because the myelinization occurs during pregnancy. Once the myelin constituents are deposited, they have an apparent metabolic stability. Although adverse factors may decrease the speed of the myelin formation, it is less probable that they could reduce the amount of the metabolic stable material already there (Davidson and Dobbing 1965). This time factor could, in a way, explain the previous concept that malnutrition did not affect the human brain. However, the vulnerability of myelin to adverse external factors seems to be confined to the periods of active myelinization, and the mechanisms and reactions observed during recuperation are related to the time in which the myelinization is still active (Eayrs and Levine 1963). Myelin does not determine the intellectual or emotional development; neither is it necessarily related to the voluntary or sensory motor functions, but it does constitute quantitatively the greatest part of weight at the early stages of development (Tanner 1961).

It has been mentioned that the period of vulnerability in the human being is from the seventh month of intrauterine to the first months of postnatal life (Davidson and Dobbing 1965). Malnutrition during acute myelinization could retard this process and produce a permanent deficit. There is evidence that the synthesis of one specific component of myelin, the sulfatide 3 sulfate-ester of galactocerebroside, is notably decreased in nutritionally deficient rats (Chase, Dorsey, and McKhann 1967).

Frequently the motor or intellectual defects of a child are attributed to factors such as prematurity, asphyxia, and neonatal anoxia when these same findings could be explained on the basis of a pre-existent pathology. It is known that the incidence of prematurity in a Negro population in

Baltimore was 11 per cent compared to 5 per cent in the white population of the same city, where the socioeconomic conditions were the main factor of difference (Pasamanick 1959; Pasamanick and Lilienfeld 1955). The same figures could be compared with an urban and suburban population in Guatemala, where the incidence of nutritional factors lacking in the mother are high and where prematurity has been shown to occur in 16 to 17 per cent of reported cases (Publicación 1962; Rendón 1965; Montiel 1960). There seems to exist a correlation of prematurity with the nutritional state and the socioeconomic conditions of the mother (Council of Foods 1958; Jeans, Smith, and Stearns 1955). A correlation with the socioeconomic conditions of the parents of the mother has also been reported because of the possible influence of the nutritional habits of the mother during her childhood which may be continued in her future home (Wolf and Drillien 1958). If the period of vulnerability does lie between the seventh month of intrauterine and the first months of postnatal life, then the full-term newborn child and, especially, the premature child would be exposed to a great risk when additional factors of malnutrition exist (Wigglesworth 1966).

There are three groups of women particularly vulnerable to malnutrition: adolescents, who are not prepared for the extra load of pregnancy, chronically undernourished women, and older women with poor feeding habits who develop more deficiency with several pregnancies in rapid succession (Council of Foods 1958).

With respect to the neonatal asphyxia or extended periods of apnoea, one could speculate in a similar way. Recently H. Knoblock and B. Pasamanich (1962) suggested that in many circumstances a pre-existent factor may exist in the child which determines the child's inability to initiate the respirations; although no studies have been carried out to relate this problem to the malnutrition of the mother, this possibility is something to keep in mind.

In anthropometric studies of newborn Guatemalan babies from rural areas and from middle and upper classes in urban areas, a significant difference among the diameters, especially in the cranial circumferences (Departmento de Estadística), is apparent (Herrera Chávez 1944; Montiel 1958; see Table 38).

Some nutritional diseases affecting the central nervous system are known among adults, but little is known about their progress and pathology (Victor and Dreyfus 1961). More has been learned about biochemical changes in the child (Edozien 1965), about the child's

TABLE 38

Comparison of Measurements of Weight, Height, and
Cranial and Thoraxic Diameters in Guatemalan Newborn Babies*

| Groups Studied | Weight (in gm.) | Height (in cm.) | Cranial Diameter (in cm.) | Thoraxic Diameter (in cm.) |
|---|---|---|---|---|
| General Hospital | 2600 | 47.30 | 31.30 | 30.20 |
| Roosevelt Hospital | 2934 | 49.14 | 33.75 | 32.22 |
| Santa Maria Cauqué | 2220 | 48.00 | — | — |
| Newborns Studied | 3261 | 49.90 | 34.29 | 33.42 |

*The children of the General Hospital represent a socioeconomic class lower than those of the Roosevelt Hospital, and those described as newborn belong to a higher socioeconomic class.

metabolisms, and about his physical recovery, but little is known about the child's intellectual recovery (Dreyfus 1966).

## Purposes

This paper has the following purposes:

1. To determine at what degree malnutrition affects the psychobiological development of the child.

2. To determine age of vulnerability.

3. To evaluate the interpolation of environmental factors not related to malnutrition.

The research was begun in April 1966, and the study of eighteen children with the same number of controls has been processed. The study will be continued in a longitudinal way until the children reach school age, and at the same time additional cases will be analyzed, according to the number of admissions to this hospital. Hence, the present work is but the beginning of this investigation and should be considered a preliminary report.

## Material and Methods

Children were chosen from the Roosevelt Hospital admissions (Pediatric Department) in Guatemala City, from April 13, 1966, to October 5, 1967, because they had the following characteristics:

1. Obstetric care (delivery assistance) at this hospital and acknowl-

edgment that such delivery was considered normal by the obstetrician and the pediatrician.

2. No history of infections, traumatisms, or toxicity that could affect the central nervous system of the child.

3. No previous chronic neurological disease.

4. Age of less than twelve months at the date of readmission to the hospital.

5. A protein and caloric malnutrition state of II and III degrees (II equals 25 to 40 per cent; III equals +40 per cent deficit in weight at the time of readmission).

6. For practical reasons (availability for home visits, control regulations at the hospital clinics, homogeneity of the groups) residency in Guatemala City.

A group of eighteen patients and eighteen controls was studied (normal children were examined at the Clinica del Niño Sano in the hospital). Records of the prenatal, delivery, growing, and developmental history of the children were gathered in detailed form. Past family history, feeding habits, and socioeconomic situation were included in the evaluation of each case. Once the infectious problems, dehydration, and electrolytic imbalance shown at the time of admission, were corrected, each child was submitted to pediatric, neurological, psychological, and ophthalmological evaluation and was observed daily during the time of hospitalization. The following complementary investigations were carried out: hematometry (hemoglobin, red cell count, differential, hematocrit), serum calcium, phosphorus, alkaline phosphatase, cholesterol, total proteins, and albumin globulin ratio; also radiological evaluation to determine osseous maturity, and electroencephalography.

Whenever the cultural and socioeconomic conditions were studied it was for the purpose of determining which cases existed with collateral or contributing factors such as culture, the child as a member of the family, the family as part of a social group, the type of social group, the attitude of the mother, and the level of sensory deprivation.

## Evaluation of Results

*Pediatric evaluation*

In those cases in which any respiratory and/or gastrointestinal infection problem existed, correction was made immediately after admission to the hospital.

According to the standards suggested by the National Board of Re-

DEFICIENCY IN BODY WEIGHT ON ADMISSION

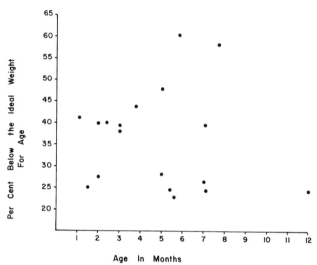

FIGURE 63. Deficiency in body weight in the group of children in Guatemala; the diet supplied at home was of poor nutritional quality.

search of the United States (Brozek 1956; Keys 1956), the following measurements were taken in each case:

1. Height, length of the trunk, and weight.
2. Circumference of the head, thorax, and abdomen.
3. Bicrestal and biocromial diameters.
4. Size of the adipose tissue in triceps, subscapular region, and abdomen, using a caliber gauge according to Franzen, with a pressure in its branches of 10 gm. per cm.

To determine the physical growth of the children, the combined auxometric method was used; recordings were made on the Wetzel chart to determine the weight and height deviation with respect to the average values for age and size, the physical configuration, the line of expected growth compared to the percentile curves of the group, actual growth curve of the child, and his growth situation. Radiological studies of hands and wrists were made, including the terminal phalanges and the distal aspect of the ulna and radius. It could be observed that the children were, at their admission, on an auxodromic curve corresponding to small premature children. Analyzing the Wetzel chart, on which the average

DEFICIENCY IN HEIGHT ON ADMISSION

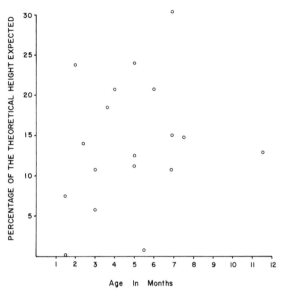

FIGURE 64. Deficiency in body height in the group of Guatemalan children.

results of five hundred Guatemalan children of a high socioeconomic class have been plotted (Hurtado 1967), we can see that the eighteen children under study are well below the average values for well-nourished children and that they fall on the auxodromic curves of prematures. The same figure shows the low cranial circumference in these children when compared to the resulting curve of the average values of 300 control children.

The deficiency in body weight is represented in Figure 63. This deficiency is expressed as a percentage of the theoretically ideal weight expected for each child. Sixteen of the children show a weight deficiency of 25 to 48 per cent of their ideal weight; two of the cases show 59 to 60 per cent, and one shows 22 per cent deficiency.

Figure 64 shows the height deficiency expressed as a percentage of the theoretical height expected for each child, plotted against its age at the date of the admission to the hospital. Only four children showed deficiencies smaller than 10 per cent, while the remaining fourteen had between 10 and 30 per cent deficiency.

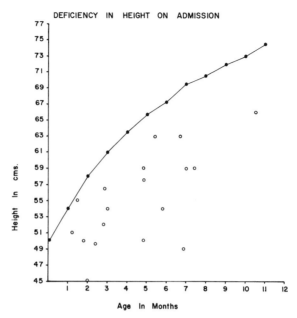

FIGURE 65. Comparison of the height of the undernourished children (o) with that of well-nourished children from the same city ( •——• ).

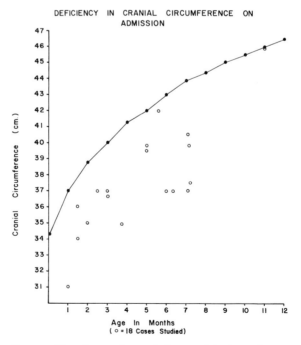

FIGURE 66. Comparison of the cranial circumference of the undernourished children (o) with that of well-nourished children from the same city ( •——• ).

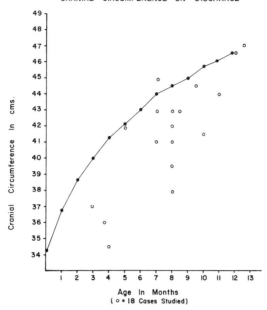

CRANIAL CIRCUMFERENCE ON DISCHARGE

Cranial Circumference In cms.

Age In Months
( o = 18 Cases Studied)

FIGURE 67. The cranial circumference of the undernourished children on discharge from the hospital, following a
period of good nutrition (o), as compared to cranial circumference of well-nourished children (●——●).

In Figure 65 the height of these children is compared to a local standard for well-nourished children (Hurtado 1967). The low values of the
children under study are evident.

The plotted weight values of these children were compared to the
figures recommended by the Institute of Nutrition of Central America
and Panama (INCAP) for the control of growth in male and female
children. The children of both sexes were below the inferior limiting
values of the chart and fell inside the group of the undernourished children: the girls were below the boys.

In Figure 66, when the values for cranial circumference of the children
under study are given in relation to a local standard (Hurtado 1967) for
children of similar age and under ideal nutritional conditions, the small
cranial circumference is noticeable. Although the cranial circumference
shows an increase at the date of discharge from the hospital, it does not
reach the normal curve, as seen in Figure 67.

As soon as the children started to receive an adequate diet, they showed
an initial period of fast nutritional recovery, their growth rate being

faster than the growth rate observed for normal children of similar chronological age. However, their auxodromic curves show a deceleration in growth rate and do not reach the values of the corresponding normal curves. These findings agree with previous reported results (Barrera-Moncada 1963; Dean 1960; Rueda-Williamson 1966). Work on weight and body measurements of rehabilitated cases shows that after children have recovered, their heights remain below their chronological levels and their skeletal development is retarded when compared to development of normal children of similar age and ethnic group (Dean 1960). Similar results were obtained on children studied until ten years of age (Barrera-Moncada 1963).

*Case Presentation*

Case No. 1:VAH: This case describes a girl, seven months old, whose measurements at birth were below the 50 percentile on the Wetzel chart. From birth to seven months her nutritional history was very deficient, and at seven months her dimensions were below the corresponding auxodromic curve for small premature children. She was hospitalized for a period of three months. After the first week on an adequate diet, her growth rate was twice as fast as normal. During the first four weeks there was no change of the adipose tissue, but since then a progressive increase has been observed. The measurements of the adipose tissue at the time of admission were 5.0 mm., 3.5 mm., and 3.3 mm. for the triceps, subscapular area, and abdomen respectively; at her discharge from the hospital they were 6.8 mm., 8.5 mm., and 5.4 mm. However, at the time of discharge, and by following evaluations, the measurements and growth rate were well below the expected theoretical curve calculated for this girl's age.

Case No. 2:MRG: This case describes a boy, seven months old, with severe malnutrition (edematous). At birth his measurements were slightly below the 50 percentile on the Wetzel chart; his nutritional history was deficient; he reached seven months of age with a deceleration process in his growth and development; and his dimensions placed him on an auxodromic curve of a premature child in spite of his being edematous. During the first four weeks of hospitalization the boy lost weight; according to the Wetzel chart this phenomenon represents a change to the lower growth curve of a small premature child. This loss of weight coincided with a decrease in the thickness of the adipose tissue; from 16 mm., 6 mm., and 7 mm., for the right arm, dorsum, and abdomen to 7.0 mm.,

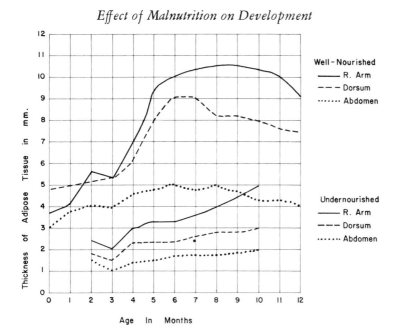

FIGURE 68. Failure of a malnourished premature infant to deposit normal amounts of subcutaneous fat even when placed on an adequate diet in the hospital at the age of two months.

3.0 mm., and 2.5 mm., respectively. After the fourth week the rate of growth was normal and after the tenth month this rate was even greater. This rate coincided with an increase of the adipose tissue thickness, which after eight weeks reached normal values. However, when he was discharged and afterward, the measurements of the boy and his rate of growth remained below the expected theoretical curve for this child (see Fig. 68).

Since it is known that protein and caloric malnutrition produces a delay in ossification and thus alters the linear and transversal growth of bones,[1] X-ray radiographs of hands and wrists were taken, including the terminal phalanges and the distal extremes of the ulna and radius. In all cases a decrease in cortical thickness and in the volume of the compact bone was found, with no difference at the date of the discharge.

[1] Garn 1966; Garn and Rohmann 1960; Garn *et al.* 1964; Garn, Silverman, and Rohmann 1964; Jones and Dean 1956.

*Neurological Evaluation*

To correlate the neurological status of the children with different degrees of malnutrition, a detailed developmental history was taken, and psychological tests and electroencephalographic studies were done in each case. These tests were run at the time of admission to the hospital and were repeated during hospitalization, just before discharge, and at succeeding evaluations at the outpatients clinic.

The neuromuscular development of infants and children depends on the potential inherent in their neurological maturity. A child of more than three years of age may be neurologically evaluated in a manner similar to the way in which an adult would be measured. However, with children below this age, especially from birth to twelve months, the evaluation requires special attention.

Maturation is associated with the process of myelinization, and with neurochemical and electrophysiological changes (Illingworth 1960).

The common neurological test performed on an adult is not adequate to determine the neuromuscular development in infancy. Spontaneous reflexes elicited in this period are the products of a mechanism that is not entirely known. Frequently, the modification of the response to the same stimulus tends to complicate the problem rather than to simplify it (Jabbour 1964).

The neurological evaluation is more complete and reliable if psychological factors are also incorporated, especially if these are evaluated and compared to local standards.

The neuromuscular development of the infant and child depends on the cerebral maturation, on the functional maturation and integration of tracts, and on other cerebral structures. The concept of maturation has been correlated to a great extent with the myelinization process, and it is known that maturation takes place at different periods depending on the area of the nervous system which is involved.

The aspect of the malnourished child, as well as his attitudes and behavior, constitutes the most dramatic area of the neurological test. These children may show apathy of different degrees or well-marked irritability. In the child older than twelve months of age apathy has been divided into different categories (Wilson 1964): physiological, communal, and cultural. The children under study did not seem to fit into any of the categories mentioned above; rather, the emotional alteration was that of a sick child, who looked miserable and unhappy and who behaved similiarly in

274

the presence of the mother, whether in the hospital environment or in the home.

The degree of apathy or irritability began to decrease between the second and fourth weeks in the hospital, coinciding with some improvement in other aspects of their adaptive behavior and also with better neuro-muscular responses.

In general the child improved so much that the examiners were satisfied with the results. Especially when compared with his condition at the date of admission to the hospital, the child showed an extraordinary recovery. When compared with local standards, however, the child was well below the behavior level of the expected theoretical curve for a given age. With respect to the psychobiological development, shortcomings were observed in different areas. The crying was of a poor quality with high pitch; it was intermittent and could be present with little or no stimulus. Moro and tonic neck reflexes were not found in any of the children of less than four months of age, and during the periods of nutritional recovery, while the patients were within the four-month period, these reflexes were not observed.

The sucking reflex was, during the critical period of the disease, weak and the activation by stimulation of the lips or cheeks did not produce the common response. After the third week of nutritional recovery the sucking reflex began to appear and after the fifth week was already effective. This activity coincided with the general improvement of the child, who already showed more interest in the environment and was less irritable and apathetic.

The grasp reflex was weak or absent during the critical period even when the predominant position of the limbs was of flexion or semiflexion with clenched hands. The grasp reflex at the toes was also very weak or absent.

The spontaneous and assumed postural attitudes of the child when suspended by the legs, by the abdomen (prone), or by the dorsum (supine), were evaluated. Through these observations it was possible to learn more about the tone, muscular strength, and posture attitudes of the child. Active and passive movements as responses to stimuli are slow in the child during the critical period.

The muscular hypotonicity was predominant; when the limbs were in flexion it was easy to get them stretched by passive movements. The stretch reflex was weak if present at the lower extremities. A delay in the psycho-motor development of the child was found at all classical reference points.

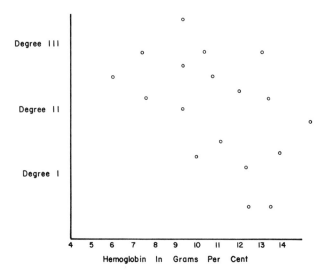

FIGURE 69. Hemoglobin values among the malnourished infants in this study revealed that many of them were anemic; the degree of anemia was correlated with pallor of the optic disk. Degree I—light pallor; II—moderate pallor; III—marked pallor.

Among the significant findings related to the cranial nerves were the extreme pallor of the optic disk and the decreased corneal reflex.

The eye grounds were examined at different stages of the disease by several investigators including an ophthalmologist. During the critical period almost invariably (15 of the 18 cases) an extreme pallor of the disks was found. We attempted to determine whether the observed paleness, which decreased progressively during the recovery period, was related to the degree of anemia in the child. Figure 69 shows the relation of the pallor of the optic disk to the degree of anemia expressed in grams of hemoglobin.

It is interesting to note that the pallor of the optic disk persisted in spite of the fact that the level of recovery seemed clinically satisfactory. Examination of the eye grounds of other children whose hemoglobin was 9 gm. per cent did not reveal the marked paleness of the optic disk found in the undernourished children.

During the critical period the child did not focus his eyes toward the appropriate stimulus, although in twenty-week-old children it is already possible to determine if there is any gross defect of the optical field or lack of interest (apathy). The winking response in front of the stimulus of an intense light was obtained faster during the critical period of the first four months of age; later, the response was similar to the one obtained from well-nourished children.

Responses to a voice, to the snap of the fingers, or to a tuning fork of 128 v.p.s. were recorded as movements of the eyes or head toward the source of sound and as change in attitude or rate of respiration. During the critical period and during convalescence, the responses were always negative, but during recovery a regular response was already observed. Negativity was interpreted as indifference to the stimuli during apathy period, since in the recovery stage the response was normal.

The phasic myotatic reflexes were universally decreased or absent during the critical period in all the patients investigated. The abdominal reflexes were absent in eight cases and decreased in the others.

The circumference of the head of these children at birth coincided with the dimensions or diameters obtained for normal children born at the Roosevelt Hospital in Guatemala (Montiel 1958), and the growth was progressive. At the time of discharge, however, growth did not reach the expected curve according to the age.

*Electroencephalographic studies*

Electroencephalographic studies were carried out on these children using a Grass machine of eight channels with eighteen electrodes on the scalp and two electrodes on the ear lobes. Recordings were taken while the patient was awake and asleep.

By the use of the criterion of the postnatal development described by Lindsley (1936; 1939) the electroencephalographic characteristics found in the children under study at their admission as well as at their discharge agreed with the norms for their ages; that is Delta activity as a dominant rhythm appeared in a diffuse and generally symmetric form.

In children of less than four months of age, potential changes were observed to be irregular and slow in the occipital regions with a rhythmic activity of three to four seconds. A slight increase between six months and one year of age with from five to seven cycles per second was noted.

In studies made while the patients slept, activity of seven cycles per second at the central areas could be observed in some cases. Only on one occasion was a paroxysmal activity with the presence of nongeneralized

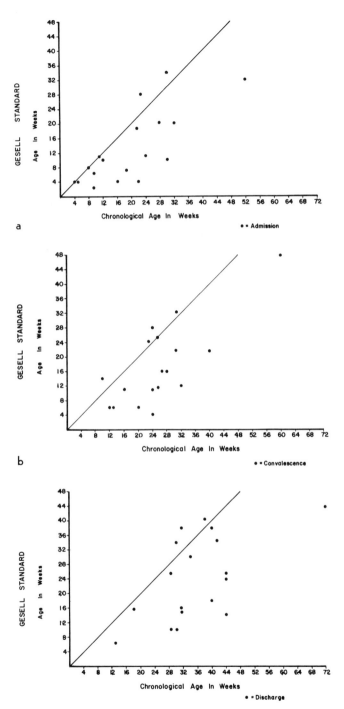

FIGURE 70. Evaluation of motor development of undernourished children by the Gesell method. The straight line indicates normal development. The dots ( • ) indicate values for the undernourished children, a) on admission to the hospital, b) during convalescence between the second and fourth week of hospitalization, and c) àt the time of discharge from the hospital.

spike waves obtained. The focal changes previously described in the temporal areas (Nelson and Dean 1959) were not found. The only difference observed between the admission and discharge time was that in the sleeping studies fast activity induced by the chloral hydrate was not observed at admission but was positive at discharge.

*Psychobiological Evaluations*

All children under study were evaluated psychologically, using the Gesell test. The test was repeated several times during hospitalization, upon discharge, and on further evaluations at the outpatients clinic. Patients were also submitted to an observation program including activity, attitudes, emotionality, communications, sociability, feeding, playing, nature of the sleep, and quality of crying.

E. Wug de León previously demonstrated that the responses of the Guatemalan children born in the rural areas and in the Roosevelt Hospital did not show any difference during the first twelve months of life when compared to standards given by Gesell—a standard considered satisfactory in order to evaluate the psychomotor development of the children under study. To evaluate results, these responses were analyzed in three stages: upon admission, at which stage the child is characterized by his apathy and irritability; the second stage of convalescence, characterized by a passive receptivity (Barrera-Moncada 1963); and the third stage upon discharge when the patient was considered nutritionally recovered.

*Motor Area.* Thirteen children showed defects in this area when admitted to the hospital, three were functioning at the expected level and two were functioning above normal. During the convalescence period, between the second and fourth week of hospitalization, there was some improvement among the children with defects, but they did not reach the expected level; two improved in this area, becoming slightly above normal. On discharge, when considered nutritionally recovered, only three were slightly above normal, and the remainder were below the expected curve. This finding suggests there is not a parallel between the motor development and the chronological age (see Fig. 70).

*Adaptive Area.* On admission fourteen children were functioning below normal, two on the expected curve and two above. During the convalescence period, one of the children who originally functioned above normal improved his level even more, but the remainder did not show any change. On discharge, when they were nutritionally recovered, the two children originally on the expected curve were above it, but all those who

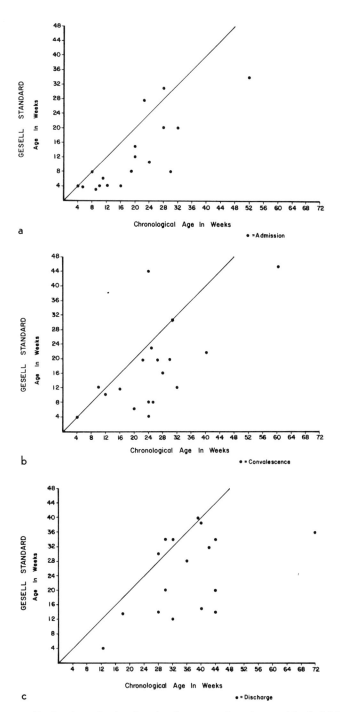

FIGURE 71. Evaluation of adaptive development of undernourished children by the Gesell method. The straight line indicates normal development. The dots ( • ) indicate values for the undernourished children, a) on admission to the hospital, b) during convalescence between the second and fourth week of hospitalization, and c) at the time of discharge from the hospital.

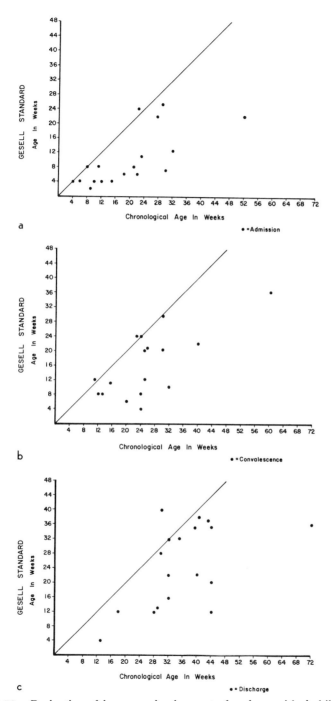

FIGURE 72.   Evaluation of language development of undernourished children by the Gesell method. The straight line indicates normal development. The dots ( • ) indicate values for the undernourished children, a) on admission to the hospital, b) during convalescence between the second and fourth week of hospitalization, and c) at the time of discharge from the hospital.

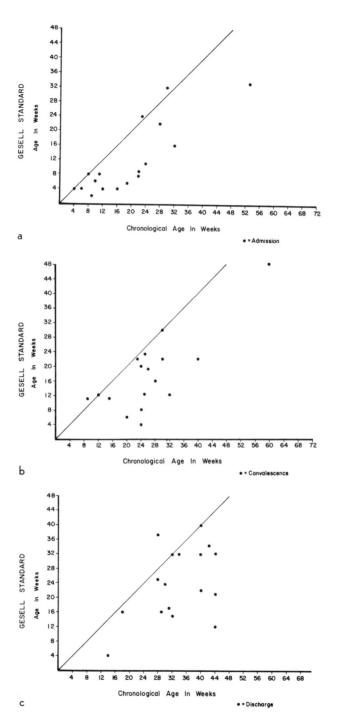

FIGURE 73. Evaluation of social-personal development of undernourished children by the Gesell method. The straight line indicates normal development. The dots ( • ) indicate values for the undernourished children, a) on admission to the hospital, b) during convalescence between the second and fourth week of hospitalization, and c) at the time of discharge from the hospital.

were functioning below the curve, although they showed slight improvements, did not reach the normal values (see Fig. 71).

*Language Area.* There were fifteen children on admission who functioned below normal, two on the expected curve, and one slightly above. During the convalescence period of the children on the expected curve, one dropped to the deficiency area and the other remained the same. No change was observed in the child who was above normal. Of the fifteen children functioning below normal, eight dropped even lower and none of the others showed any improvement (see Fig. 72). The information obtained upon discharge was similar to information obtained during the convalescence period.

*The Social-Personal Area.* On admission, fourteen children functioned below normal, two children were on the expected level, and two above. During the convalescence period one of the children above normal dropped to the expected curve and one normal child dropped to the deficiency area. Among the fourteen who were below normal, a slight improvement was observed although the patients did not reach the expected curve of normality. On discharge only one child continued functioning above normal, two were on the expected curve, and the rest below that curve (see Fig. 73).

During the observation program to which these children were submitted, it was noticed that on their admission they showed marked irritability or apathy, muscular hypotonicity, poor socialization and communication, with irregular and poor sleeping patterns, and with intermittent crying of high pitch. Between the second and third week an improvement in all areas was observed, although it was more noticeable and faster in the motor and adaptive areas. In the language and social-personal areas, however, the recovery was slower and smaller. It was interesting to notice that on discharge only six children functioned at a normal level, while the rest were below the expected level for their chronological age. This deficiency was more noticeable in the language and social-personal areas.

### Socioeconomic and Cultural Evaluations

All the cases were studied through a socioeconomic cultural evaluation carried out by a social worker. From the beginning we tried to limit this investigation to those cases in which the mothers agreed to have their children studied for a period of seven years. All the cases were residents of Guatemala City and their socioeconomic situations were considered bad or very bad, with an average income of $50.00 to $75.00 per month. All the children came from broken homes and were mainly dependent on their mothers. The factor of poor protein and caloric intake existed concurrently with other factors (poor environmental stimulation, poor education of the parents, some of whom had subnormal intelligence, and deficient hygienic conditions).

## Conclusions and Comments

Findings are described for eighteen undernourished children below one year of age under multidisciplinary studies made with the same number of controls.

Children with perinatal antecedents controlled at the same hospital and residing in urban areas later developed different degrees of malnutrition. The results obtained were compared to local standards. Findings from the pediatric, neurologic, and psychobiological point of view are in accord: on discharge the children seemed to be nutritionally recovered and to present a generally satisfactory state, but when their anthropometric measurements, development, and functioning levels were graphically compared with local standards, an evident and noticeable deficiency was noted.

It is interesting to observe that the diameters of the cranial circumference and the height were significantly low. Although there was an improvement on discharge with respect to the admission date, the children never attained the expected curves for their ages. The marked pallor of the optic disk noted on admission seemed not to be related to the degree of anemia or hemoglobin level. Psychological tests, using the Gesell scale for mental development in infants, showed deficiencies in all areas but especially in the development of language and social-personal attitude. These deficiencies persist even after a satisfactory nutritional recovery.

Since there are multiple interrelated factors (the lack of environmental stimulation, parents functioning at a lower than average intellectual level, extreme poverty), the deficiencies of the child cannot be attributed only to the low protein and caloric intake.

No definite conclusions can be drawn by the present investigations because they are only the beginning of a longitudinal study, and the results must be considered preliminary.

# DISCUSSION

R. HILL: We have found similar results in infants who are dysmature or malnournished at birth. I have studied these infants biochemically and developmentally from birth to three years of age. The infants are patients of private physicians in Houston and come from high and middle socio-economic background. You would anticipate then that they would have a good developmental potential, home environment, and prompt care of medical disease. We found that the physical stature continued to be small, between the 10 and 25 percentile, even at three years of age. Clinically, they remained slender until four to six months of age. Gesell Development ment Schedule Testing has shown persistent delay in language development.

D. BUENO: I will take just a minute to comment. I have worked for many years with rural teachers in Mexico. I organized a mental hygiene service for a big state; it is the state around the Federal District in my country, and all the country teachers have a special way of selecting the children they want to teach. They take the height of the children. They clump all the children together and the smartest teachers get the tallest and the new teachers get the shortest. And so, the new teachers have no trouble with the little ones. All we know is that there is a correlation between height and mental evolution.

B. KOLENDA: May I ask please, how much and how varied is the stimulation these youngsters receive in the hospital? You have mentioned that the psychologist sits by the crib and observes rather than interacts. Are these children essentially isolated in their cribs or is there frequent contact with, and, therefore, stimulation from, others?

R. RENDON: We have been quite interested in having the psychologist develop a close relationship with these children. Besides the routine type of observation, which includes time while the children are awake, sleeping, and during the feeding periods, the psychologist plays with them, and soon the relationship is a close one. The mother is encouraged to develop a similar relationship.

# REFERENCES

Acheson, R. M. 1960. *Effects of nutrition and disease on human growth.* Symposium *Soc. Hum. Biol.* 31:73.

Arroyave, G. August 1962. Biochemical signs of mild moderate forms of protein-caloric malnutrition. Symposium of the Swedish Nutrition Foundation.

Barrera-Moncada, G. 1963. *Estudios sombre alteraciones del crecimiento y del desarrollo psicológico del síndrome pluricarencial (Kwashiorkor).* Caracas: Ed. Grafos.

Behar, M., Ascoli, W., and Scrimshaw, N. S. 1958. Children's malnutrition. *Boletín de la Organizacion Mundial de la Salud.* 19:1093.

Behar, M. *et al.* 1963. *Death and diseases in the rural area.* 14. Guatemala: Congreso Nacional de Medicina de Guatemala.

Brozek, K. 1956. Recommendations concerning body measurements. *Hum. Biol.* 28:2.

Calder, R. 1966. Food supplementation for prevention of malnutrition in the pre-school child. International Conference on Prevention of Malnutrition in the Pre-school Child. *Proc. Natl. Acad. Sci.* (U.S.A.) 251.

Cavak, V., and Najdanvic, R. 1965. Effect of under-nutrition in early life on physical and mental development. *Arch. Dis. Child.* 40:532.

Chase, H. P., Dorsey, J., and McKhann, G. M. 1967. Effect of malnutrition on synthesis of a myelin lipid. *Pediatrics* 40:551.

Council of Foods and Nutrition. 1958. Nutrition in Pregnancy. Symposium IV. *J.A.M.A.*

Cordano, A., Baertl, J. M., and Graham, G. G. 1962. Growth sequences during recovery from infantile malnutrition. Paper presented at Am. Soc. Pediat. Res.

Cravioto, J. 1966. La desnutrición protéico-calórica y el desarrollo psico-biológico del niño. *Bol. Sanit. Panam.* 4:285.

Cravioto, J., and Robles, B. August 1962. The influence of protein-caloric malnutrition on psychological test behavior. p. 115. Proceedings of the Swedish Nutrition Foundation. A Symposium on Mild-moderate Forms of Protein-caloric Malnutrition, Bastad and Gothenburg.

Davidson, A. N., and Dobbing, J. 1965. Myelination as a vulnerable period of brain development. *Br. Med. Bull.* 22:40.

Dean, R. F. A. 1960. The effects of malnutrition on the growth of young children. *Mod. Prob. Pediat.* 5:111.

Dekaban, R., 1959. *Neurology in infancy.* Baltimore: Williams and Wilkins.

Departamento Estadística, INCAP. Personal communication.

Dreyfus, P. M. 1966. Nutritional disorders of obscure etiology. *Med. Sci.* 17(4): 44.

Eayrs, J. T., and Levine, S. 1963. Influence of thyroidectomy and subsequent replacement therapy upon conditioned avoidance learning in the rat. *J. Endocr.* 25:505.

Edozien, J. C. 1965. Protein and aminoacid metabolism in malnourished children. *Israel J. Med. Sci.* 6:1384.

Garn, S. M., Rohmann, C. G., Behar, M., Viteri, F., and Guzmán, M. A. 1964. *Proc. Natl. Acad. Sci.* (U.S.A.) 43.

Garn, S. M., and Rohmann, C. G. 1960. Variability in the order of ossification of the bony centers of the hand and wrist. *Am. J. Phys. Anthropol.* 18:219.

Garn, S. M., Rohmann, C. G., Behar, M., Viteri, F., and Guzmán, M. A. 1964. Compact bone deficiency in protein-caloric malnutrition. *Science* 145:114.

Garn, S. M., Silverman, F. N., and Rohmann, C. G. 1964. A rational approach to the assessment of skeletal maturation. *Ann. Radiol.* 7:297.

Herrera Chávez, O. 1944. Contribución al estudio del recién nacido Guatemalteco. Graduate thesis, Faculty of Medical Sciences, Guatemala.

Hurtado, J. J. 1967. Estudio longitudinal del crecimiento en 500 niños Guatemaltecos bien nutridos durante el primer año de vida. Central American Congress of Pediatrics.

Illingworth, R. S. 1960. *Development of the infant and young child.* Baltimore: Williams and Wilkins.

Jabbour, J. T. 1964. Developmental neurological examination of the infant. *South West Med.* 45:1.

Jeans, P. C., Smith, M., and Stearns, G. 1955. Dietary habits of pregnant women of low income in Iowa. *J. Am. Diet. Assn.* 31:576.

Jones, P. R. M., and Dean, R. F. A. 1956. The effects of kwashiorkor on the development of the bones and the hand. *J. Trop. Pediat.* 2:51.

Keys, A. 1956. Recommendations concerning body measurements for the characterization of nutritional status. *Hum. Biol.* 28:111.

Knobloch, H., and Pasamanich, B. 1962. Environmental factors affecting human development before and after birth. *Pediatrics* 26:210.

Lindsley, D. B.
1936. Brain potentials in children and adults. *Science* 84:354.
1939. Longitudinal study of the occipital alpha rhythm in normal children. *J. Genet. Psychol.* 55:197.

Montiel, R.
1958. Datos antropométricos en 1,000 niños nacidos en Guatemala. *Revista de la Juventud Médica* Epoca IV, 14(81).
1960. Consideraciones sobre algunos aspectos de recién nacidos prematuros. *Rev. Colegio Medico de Guatemala* 11(3):163.

Nelson, M. A., and Dean, F. A. 1959. The electroencephalogram in African children: Effects of kwashiorkor and a note on the newborn. *WHO* 21:779.

Pasamanick, B. 1959. Influence of socio-cultural variables upon organic factors in mental retardation. *Am. J. Ment. Defic.* 63:316.

Pasamanick, B., and Lilienfeld, A. 1955. Association of maternal and fetal factors with development of mental deficiency. *J.A.M.A.* 159:155.

Publicación, Dirección General de Estadística. 1962. Datos para Hospital Roosevelt, Guatemala.

Rendón, R. October 1965. Informe sobre la incidencia de retraso mental en la República de Guatemala. Inter-American Seminar on Mental Retardation. Puerto Rico.

Rueda-Williamson, R. 1966. The measurement of physical growth in the pre-school child. Pre-school Child Malnutrition. *Proc. Natl. Acad. Sci.* (U.S.A.).

Tanner, J. B. 1961. *Education and physical growth*. London: University of London Press.

Victor, M., and Dreyfus, P. M. 1961. Nutritional diseases of the nervous system. A statement of some current problems and suggestions for further investigation. *World Neurol.* 2:862.

Waterlow, J. C. August 1962. Metabolic disturbances in protein-caloric malnutrition. Symposium of the Swedish Nutrition Foundation.

Wigglesworth, J. W. 1966. Foetal growth retardation. *Br. Med. Bull.* 22:13.

Wilson, A. T. M. 1964. *Fostering nutritional change. Some points from social research.* Proceedings of the 6th International Congress on Nutrition. Edinburgh and London: E. S. Livingston.

Wolf, A., and Drillien, C. M., mentioned by Masland, R. L. 1958. *The mental subnormality.* New York: Basic Books.

Wug de León, E. 1966. Patrón de desarrollo psicomotor y adaptativo en niños del medico rural en Guatemala. Graduate thesis, Guatemala.

# Drug Treatment of Mental Subnormality

JAMES L. CLAGHORN, M.D.

*Division of Professional Services, Texas Research
Institute of Mental Sciences, Houston, Texas*

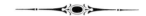

The introduction of tranquilizers has brought as much euphoria to clinicians as ataraxia to a multitude of patients. After early reservations about the effectiveness of this group of drugs, their widespread use has resulted in an annual decline in hospital beds used for psychiatric patients, reminiscent of the years following the introduction of isoniazid and para-aminosalicylic acid (PAS) into the treatment of pulmonary tuberculosis. It is hardly surprising that a group of drugs with such dramatic beneficial effects on behavioral disorders should also be studied in related conditions such as mental retardation. The large contribution of interpersonal and psychological factors in some kinds of retardation suggests a further benefit from the use of neuroleptic medications.

### Methods of Clinical Drug Evaluation

In evaluating drug effects, it is necessary first to establish some frame of reference against which drug actions will be measured. There are five postures from which a clinical investigator may set out to examine drug effects. The first and most obvious of these relates to standard diagnostic categories of disease. Many investigators in studying the effects of drugs on retarded children use as diagnostic categories mild, moderate, and severe grades of limitation in intellectual function. They are limited to statements relating treatment success to intelligence quotient. Another version of this method which is less commonly used is the examination of a drug effect in terms of benefit on children retarded as a result of cerebral agenesis or maternal deprivation or phenylketonuria. In fact, few papers indicate any attempt to differentiate on the basis of organic, psychological, or metabolic causes the etiology of retardation in the children treated.

The second technique for evaluating drug effect is popular in the field of drug evaluation in psychiatric patients. The concept of target symptom control is utilized here. Diagnostic categories are not central to the evaluation, and symptoms like aggression, anxiety, manifest psychotic thought processes, or social interest are assessed, pre- and posttreatment. Little emphasis is placed on the etiology of the primary psychiatric disorder. Many clinicians feel this method of viewing drug effects has been highly successful. Though many tranquilizing drugs function primarily in the control of symptoms, it must also be admitted that by controlling disabling symptoms over long periods of time the entire life history and life adjustment pattern of the patient may be changed. Secondarily, the drug can have long-term effects on the patient's psychological make-up. It is important in the measurement of symptoms to keep in mind the operation of the law of initial values. Where symptoms are most dramatic and acute, the measurable change will be large. Where symptoms are relatively less severe, the amount of change that can be expected is considerably less. Degree of change is, therefore, only in part a function of drug effect and in part a function of the acuteness and severity of symptoms.

Thirdly, drug effects can be viewed in terms of general patterns of relating to others. This is an extremely important aspect of drug action which is difficult to measure. The patient's general pattern of relating to other people will also be the pattern by which he relates to the evaluating physician and to the physician's prescribed treatment. Most patients who have been under long-term treatment are placed in a position of comparative helplessness and dependency. When approached with new treatment the opportunity is created for the patient to hang on and cling, and his wish to please and placate the therapist will result in a deceptive appearance of benefit from drug treatment—a particular disaster in the case of uncontrolled experimentation. In problems arising from basically defensive and suspicious people, particularly where psychotic disorders or paranoid modes of adaptation are noted, medication will be seen as an attempt to control. Another alternative is to fear the medication and resist its effects. An example of this resistance occurs in the patient who suffers insomnia when given a sedative or heightened anxiety when taking a mildly tranquilizing drug. Some people who protect themselves by maintaining an isolated independent status will tend to disrupt the treatment plan by passive means. Such comments as, "I got to the pharmacy too late to fill the prescription," "I keep forgetting to take my medication," are all indications of this kind of disruptive pattern of relating. The danger in all these instances is that events relating primarily to personality patterns will be seen as drug effects. The final consideration in evaluating psychoactive drugs is concern of third parties, such as parents, in cases dealing with children. A case in point concerns a young child who was referred for the treatment of hyperactivity. She was a quite limited youngster, who at age five had a vocabulary of only a few words and had been in special schools from early in life. She was, however, bright, cheerful, and active. Her play was enthusiastic, but not destructive. Initially, she was treated with dextroamphetamine at doses up to 5 mg. of the elixir by mouth four times daily. At first, reports at home and school were favorable. As time passed complaints that she was no longer the cheerful, endearing youngster she had been earlier gave way to outright hostility about her moping, slow-moving, morbid behavior. Drug dose was then put on intermittent schedule at the option of teacher and mother. After a period of experimentation, it was agreed upon by all that they would much prefer having an active, delightful, though tiring youngster than a mute, quiet, nonparticipating child. Drug treatment is now used periodically to provide rest to those tired middle-aged people who cannot keep up with this active, cheerful child.

## Psychotropic Drugs Currently in Use

To give a review and to establish a vocabulary, I will go over the chemistry and pharmacology of the major classes of the psychotropic drugs currently used in psychiatric practice, many of which have been studied and are used in the treatment of mental retardation. The best-known class of compounds, those which started the tranquilizer era, are those of the phenothiazine class. The phenothiazine nucleus illustrated in Figure 74 is usually substituted in positions R1 and R2. Substitutions in the R2 position tend to effect potency and substitutions in the R1 position effect the quality of actions attributed to the drug. The usual system of classification divides them on the basis of substitution at the R1 position into aliphatic, piperazine, and piperidine groups. Examples of the aliphatic drugs are chlorpromazine (Thorazine), triflupromazine (Ves-

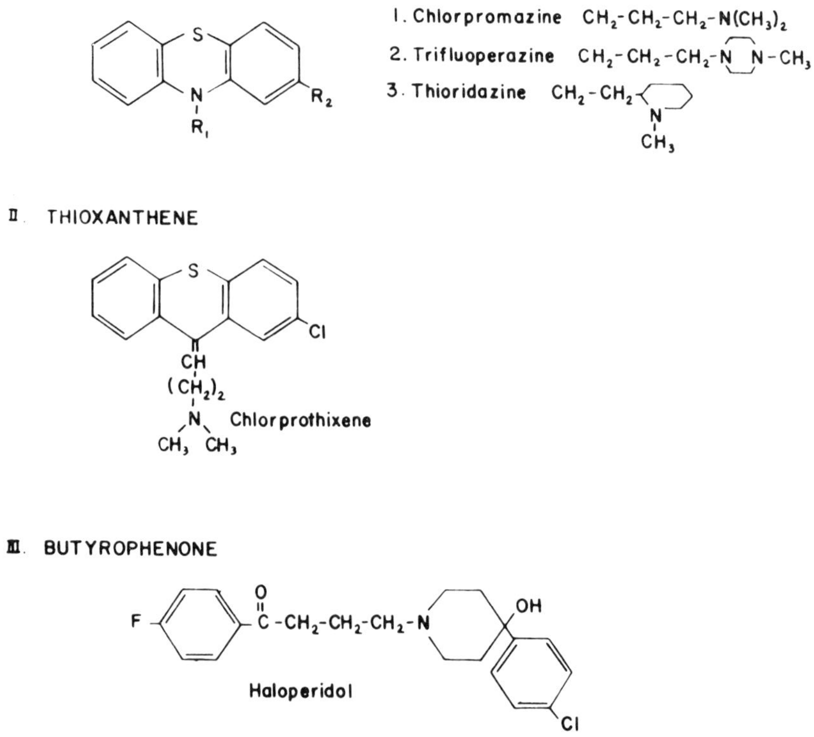

1. Chlorpromazine   $CH_2-CH_2-CH_2-N(CH_3)_2$

2. Trifluoperazine   $CH_2-CH_2-CH_2-N\phantom{N}N-CH_3$

3. Thioridazine   $CH_2-CH_2$ ...

    CH₃

II. THIOXANTHENE

Chlorprothixene

III. BUTYROPHENONE

Haloperidol

FIGURE 74.   Chemical structures of tranquilizers in common use.

prin), and promazine (Sparine). When the R1 substituent group has a six-member ring substituted with nitrogen in the para positions, then the class is called piperazine drugs, examples of which are trifluoperazine (Stelazine), and prochlorperazine (Compazine). When the six-membered ring has one nitrogen atom in the ortho or meta positions the drugs are known as piperidine drugs. The only current marketed drug of this class is thioridazine (Mellaril).

A variety of changes have been made in the chemistry of the central phenothiazine ring and have produced drugs of the thioxanthine and iminodibenzyl groups. A new and somewhat different class of compounds, known as butyrophenone compounds, has been introduced to the American market. The only currently marketed butyrophenone in this country is haloperidol (Haldol). This drug is substantially like the piperazine drugs in most of its actions. These drugs are often called "antipsychotic" or "major tranquilizers."

Drugs of this class would be most beneficial in the treatment of retarded children when psychotic disorders or symptoms such as aggressiveness or agitation are present. Where personality factors make drug administration a problem, there is now available an injectable form of fluphenazine (Prolixin). Surprisingly, some people who otherwise resist taking medication tend not to think of their every second week injection of a long-acting phenothiazine as being a drug administration. In their minds, anything they do not notice happening within thirty minutes or an hour of the injection, they do not associate with that event. I have had the experience of patients coming to me a month or six weeks after having made rather remarkable improvement on fluphenathiazine enanthate and asking me when they were going to begin taking the medication I had mentioned earlier.

Antianxiety drugs, or minor tranquilizers, are in common use. Meprobamate (Miltown, Equanil) is a drug of the propandiol class and is related to drugs that are muscle relaxants. A second group of commonly used antianxiety drugs includes chlordiazepoxide (Librium) and diazepam (Valium). Diazepam (Valium) is a sedative and muscle-relaxant drug that has proved to be quite effective in reducing anxiety. Hydroxazine (Vistaril, Atarax) and azacylonol (Frenquel) are used less often than the previously mentioned antianxiety drugs.

In children stimulant drugs are commonly used with good effect in the control of agitation. The drugs currently used are amphetamine, methamphetamine, and methylphenidate (Ritalin).

A few studies of retarded children that utilize drugs that are described as antidepressant in action have been reported (see Fig. 75). Few people would argue that there are any extremely potent antidepressant drugs currently available. There are two major classes of drugs in use. The first class includes drugs that inhibit the enzyme monoamine oxidase; iproniazid (Marsilid), phenelzine (Nardil), and tranylcypromine (Parnate) are commonly used examples. The second major class includes iminodibenzyl drugs, imipramine (Tofranil), and amitriptyline (Elavil); these drugs do not inhibit monoamine oxidase.

Just prior to the introduction of the drugs of the phenothiazine class reserpine came into use as a tranquilizing medication. Its use was somewhat shortlived because of the effectiveness of the phenothiazines and problems of parkinsonism, hypotension, and at times, severe gastro-

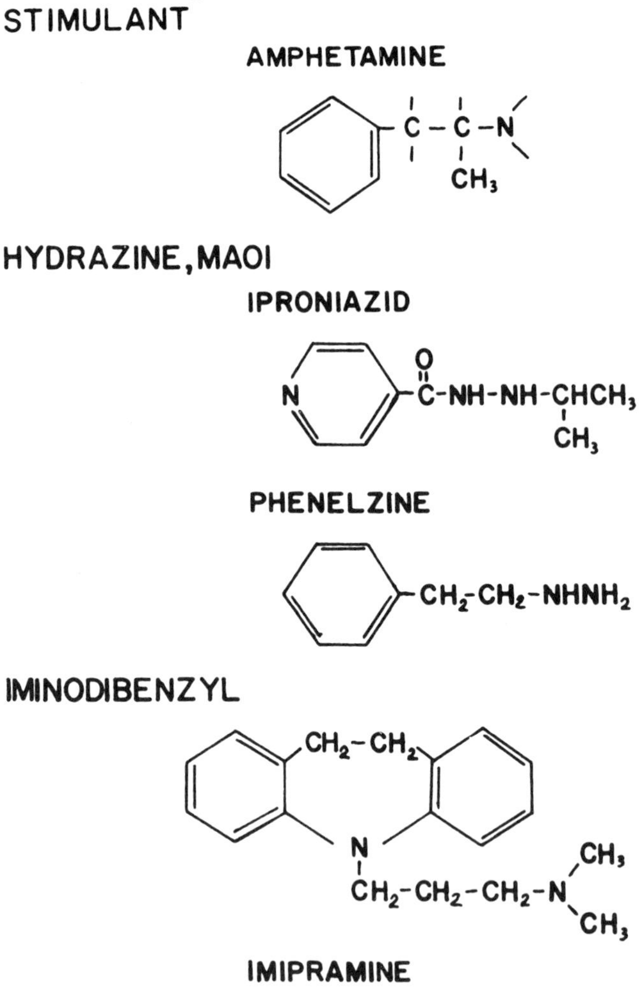

# STIMULANT

## AMPHETAMINE

# HYDRAZINE, MAOI

## IPRONIAZID

## PHENELZINE

# IMINODIBENZYL

## IMIPRAMINE

FIGURE 75. Chemical structures of antidepressant drugs in common use.

intestinal symptoms. Like reserpine, tetrabenazine (Nitoman) depletes central nervous system serotonin but lacks the side effects of reserpine. This drug is not generally used in clinical psychiatry but is used in screening drugs for potential antidepressant activity.

## Drug Treatment

### A Review of Recent Publications

Though our focus is on the use of tranquilizing medications, it is a matter of some interest to note the wide variety of areas in which at least small research probes have been undertaken. There has been little effort to pursue the work, but the variety indicates the uncertainty that exists about the etiology, pathogenesis, and treatment of mental retardation. Good results are reported with the use of subconvulsive electrical stimulation of the brain (Schutt 1960), the use of bovine brain extract (Tokizane and Schade 1966), the use of 1-glutamic acid monoamine (Beley, Caustier, and Olievenstein 1965) and the beneficial effect of large doses of α-tocopherol—vitamin E (Houze, Wilson, and Goodfellow 1964–1965). The lack of controls in these studies, as well as the absence of any follow-up by other groups, is indicative of the status of these experimental efforts.

Although most studies of the effects of psychotropic drugs deal with only one medication, the following studies compare several drugs. L. H. Rudy, working at the Galesburg State Research Hospital in Galesburg, Illinois (Rudy, Himwich, and Rinaldi 1958), reports the results of a study in a large state school where target symptoms of untidiness, failure to participate in programs, obstinacy, feeding problems, ineffective interpersonal relationships, destructiveness, and frequent quarrels with resulting physical injuries were chosen for treatment. The technique of study consisted of a four-week treatment period with active medication followed by a two-week placebo period for purposes of comparison. Reserpine and chlorpromazine were by far the most common medications used, causing improvement in target symptoms of seventeen and twenty-two of twenty-five patients respectively. Promazine and mepazine, drugs of the aliphatic and piperidine drug groups respectively, caused improvement in nine or ten of twenty-five patients. Two antianxiety drugs, azacyclonol (Frenquel) and meprobamate (Miltown, Equanil), showed poor performance with improvement in only three to four of twenty-five patients treated. These results are very compatible with the kinds of effects one would see in treating similar symptoms in psychiatric patients. Promazine (Sparine) and mepazine (Pacatal) are considerably less potent than reserpine or chlorpromazine (Thorazine), and azacyclonol (Frenquel) and meprobamate (Miltown, Equanil) have very minimal effects in the treatment of aggressive syndromes. Working at the Fountain Unit in Surrey, England, Brian H. Kirman (1964) surveyed prescribing practices in two large state schools. Drugs were used primarily for patients who showed overt emotional disturbances such as withdrawal from or disruption of group activities. Most commonly used were phenothiazine drugs with a somewhat uniform distribution among the potent drugs of all three chemical classes. Minor tranquilizers and barbiturates combined accounted for approximately 25 per cent of the drugs used, and anti-depressants and stimulants were hardly used at all. In an article published in *Review of Infantile Neuropsychiatry*, F. Brauner and G. Pringuet discussed the French literature and concluded that slightly and moderately deficient children are improved by tranquilizers but grossly deficient children are refractory. Where apathy, inhibition, and autistic behavior dominate the picture, stimulant and antidepressant drugs may be helpful. They note that amphetamines and monoamine oxidase inhibitor anti-depressant drugs may stabilize agitated children.

In general, however, reserpine, chlorpromazine (Thorazine), and pro-chlorperazine (Compazine) have proved in wide experience to be effective in controlling agitation, hyperactivity, and disorders of affect. Minor tranquilizers such as hydroxazine (Vistaril, Atarax), azacyclonol (Frenquel), and chlordiazepoxide (Librium) have proved to be of considerably less value. Chlorprothixene (Taractan), a thioxanthene derivative of less effectiveness than the phenothiazines, is similar in potency to the minor tranquilizers.

Specific drug studies dealing with individual medications can be readily separated in terms of reported effect largely on the basis of the degree of experimental control employed. As might be anticipated, controlled studies have generally been far less enthusiastic than have uncontrolled studies. Uncontrolled trials of triflupromazine (Vesprin), trifluoperazine (Stelazine), fluphenazine (Prolixin), and thioridazine (Mellaril) have in general reported a good effect in half to three-quarters of the patients treated.[1] Controlled studies on promazine (Sparine), chlorpromazine (Thorazine), trifluoperazine (Stelazine), prochlorperazine (Compazine), and fluphenazine (Prolixin) have shown no more effect on hyperactivity than was seen in placebo groups.[2] Most noteworthy was the report of

[1] Himwich *et al.* 1960; Mises and Beauchesne 1963; Badham *et al.* 1963; Waites and Keele 1963; Hunter and Stephenson 1963; Fine 1963–1964; Badham *et al.* 1963; Robb 1959.
[2] Sharpe 1962; LaVeck, Cruz, and Simundson 1960; Rosenblum and Buoniconto 1960; Schulman and Clarinda 1964; Robb 1960.

improvement on I.Q. scales which clearly reflects the value of motivation in improving the patient's capacity to attend to learning tasks.

No consideration of the use of these drugs is complete without an adequate discussion of the potential hazards. The physician's responsibility to balance his therapeutic ambitions against the known shortcomings of drugs is of paramount importance. The motor retardation, blunting, and dulling produced by these drugs can sharply impair certain necessary functions. Some poorly controlled individuals are able to remain calm and under control only by exercise of considerable psychological effort. Depriving them of their full capacity of self-discipline inevitably results in outbursts of temper and, at times, of violence. In addition to psychological difficulties, the effects of these drugs on the extrapyramidal system can produce Parkinson-like syndromes as well as a motor restlessness called akathisia. There are extremely small numbers of reported fatalities due to hepatic and bone-marrow difficulties as well as relatively rare reports of deaths of unknown etiology. It is unsettled whether these are spontaneous occurrences or whether they represent drug-related mortalities.

Use of stimulant and antidepressant drugs in treating the target symptoms of stuttering, hyperactivity, and withdrawal is based on a relatively small number of studies. In a controlled study of 106 retarded children with speech defect, half of the eleven stutterers treated with dextroamphetamine showed improvement as compared to only one of eleven stutterers treated with placebos. Two patients in the amphetamine group developed increased psychotic disturbance. Athetosis and excessive weight loss were noted in four other subjects (Fish 1962). Control of hyperactivity and increased attention span with rise in I.Q. have also been reported with stimulant drugs. One postulated mechanism for the calming effect of amphetamine is based on the raised threshold of neurones in the diencephalon in children. Although not definitely established as causally related, this postulated mechanism offers a highly appealing explanation of the action of this group of drugs. Insomnia and weight loss complicate treatment. Some children become more agitated. Each case must be given a therapeutic trial at low dose with rapid increments to therapeutic level after three to five days at minimal dose. J. Jacobs has shown that deanol, a mildly stimulating drug that is a derivative of choline and may be a precurser of acetylcholine, causes improvement in frequency of tantrums, nervousness, and attention span (Jacobs 1965).

An antidepressant drug, nialamide, which is an inhibitor of the enzyme monoamine oxidase, has been reported in a controlled study to cause maximum improvement in children suffering from primary amentia in the I.Q. range of 75 to 100. Improvement in memory and vocabulary were also noted though none of these changes could be described as large. No improvement was noted in the control group (Krupanidhi *et al.* 1964; Mackay *et al.* 1963). Iproniazid (Marsilid) was used by B. H. Kirman and C. M. B. Pare in 1961 in the treatment of phenylketonuria. They reasoned that others have reported that 5-hydroxytryptamine has been lowered in patients with PKU. Iproniazid (Marsilid) presumably would raise this level. In their carefully controlled study they found no effect from Iproniazid (Marsilid) or nialamide on mongols or on patients retarded due to the effects of PKU (Kirman and Pare 1961).

The most potent of the iminodibenzyl antidepressants, imipramine (Tofranil), has been used in only one study for the treatment of mental retardation. T. L. Pilkington (1961) treated thirty-nine mentally defective patients who were divided between those suffering affective disorders and those with symptoms primarily associated with schizophrenia. Over half of his sample of the nonschizophrenic, affective group responded favorably whereas the schizophrenic group showed a worsening of symptoms.

Barbara Fish in her careful review of drug therapy in children (1960) reports good experience with diphenhydramine hydrochloride (Benadryl). This safe, well-established drug, which is primarily used as an antihistamine, calms the anxieties and symptoms of agitated, hyperactive, retarded children under the age of ten years. Following the age of ten these children require phenothiazine medications for control of symptoms. Nowhere in the recent literature have I been able to find any reports of large-scale testing of this old, very safe, and reliable medication in the control of agitation, restlessness, and hyperactivity, in retarded children (Fish 1960).

Minimal brain damage and cerebral dysfunction of varied cause are found in hyperactive, impulsive children. Unfortunately EEG changes are unreliable diagnostic indicators. Many clinicians use diphenylhydantoin (Dilantin) alone or in combination with amphetamine. Reduction of protein-bound iodine (PBI) levels, gingival hypertrophy, hirsutism, and motor hyperactivity have been noted with treatment. Therapy is contraindicated in known liver disease. When used in cases of conduct disorder, hyperactivity, and in some psychotic disorders good results have been reported.

*Drug Treatment*

## Recommendations for Drug Use

Treatment is always individualized; this is no less true with psychotropic drugs than with any other class of compound. In general, however, a clear list of priorities can impose a rational order on treatment programs. In children under ten years of age the drugs of choice for controlling symptoms of hyperactivity and anxiety are diphenhydramine (Benadryl) and amphetamine. Diphenylhydantoin (Dilantin) singly and in combination with amphetamine may be the drug of choice in treatment of conduct disorders, school refusal, and hyperactive impulse disorders. Where age or failure to control symptoms requires the use of phenothiazine tranquilizer, then medication choice is determined by the degree of hypo- or hyperactivity noted in the child. Where hypoactivity is a problem, trifluoperazine (Stelazine), perphenazine (Trilafon), or related tranquilizers are suggested. Where hyperactivity is a severe management problem, chlorpromazine (Thorazine) or similar aliphatic phenothiazine should be used. The use of minor tranquilizers for symptoms of lesser intensity is less well established but well worth therapeutic trial. All available studies on the use of antidepressants are inconclusive.

## Conclusion

Systematic large-scale trials of medications in retarded children have not been done. There is a great need for carefully planned well-controlled studies that would give a reasonable comprehension of the relative effectiveness and special qualities of the major groups of psychoactive drugs. The very evident placebo effects of staff attention and study do result in an improvement in children and emphasize the need for rigid experimental control. Enthusiasm for the newer and very potent phenothiazine medications has drawn attention away from older and better-understood compounds, which are as beneficial to the younger child and less hazardous than the phenothiazines.

Drugs of the stimulant and antidepressant types have poorly understood actions in retarded children and need exploration. Amphetamine is widely used but experimental evidence for its usefulness is incomplete. Antidepressants of the monoamine oxidase-inhibiting or iminodibenzyl types are also inadequately studied in children.

# REFERENCES

Badham, J. N., Bardon, L. M., Reeves, P. O., and Young, A. M. 1963. A trial of thioridazine in mental deficiency. *Psychopharm. Absts.* 3(2):61. Also *Brit. J. Psych.* 109:408.

Beley, A., Caustier, M., and Olievenstein, A. 1965. Favorable action of 1-glutamic acid monoamine (levoglutamine) on qualitative efficiency of the mentally deficient pupil (tests relating to two groups, using pairing and placebo). *Psychopharm. Absts.* 4(9):735.

Brauner, F., and Pringuet, G. 1964. Drug treatment of mentally defective children. *Psychopharm. Absts.* 3(8):618.

Fine, R. H. 1963–1964. Clinical experience with trifluoperazine in the severely retarded. *J. Neuropsych.* 5:370.

Fish, B.
1960. Drug therapy in child psychiatry: Pharmacological aspects. *Comprehen. Psych.* 1:212.

1962. Editorial. Dexamphetamine administered to 106 mentally retarded patients with speech defects for 3 months. *Phychopharm. Absts.* 2(12):1132.

Himwich, H. E., Costa, E., Rinaldi, F., and Rudy, L. H. 1960. Triflupromazine and trifluoperazine in the treatment of disturbed mentally defective patients. *Am. J. Ment. Def.* 64:711.

Houze, M., Wilson, H. D., and Goodfellow, H. D. L. 1964–1965. Treatment of mental deficiency with alpha tocopherol. *Am. J. Ment. Def.* 69:328.

Hunter, H., and Stephenson, G. M. 1963. Chlorpromazine and trifluoperazine in the treatment of behavioral abnormalities in the severely subnormal child. *Brit. J. Psych.* 109:411.

Jacobs, J. 1965. A controlled trial of deanol and a placebo in mentally defective children. *Psychopharm. Absts.* 5:582.

Kirman, B. H. 1964. Drugs in the treatment of mental deficiency. International Copenhagen Congress on Scientific Study of Mental Retardation. *Proceedings* 1:241.

Kirman, B. H., and Pare, C. M. B. 1961. Amine-oxidase inhibitors as possible treatment for phenylketonuria. *Lancet* 1:117.

Krupanidhi, I., Gowda, K. A., and Nirmala, N. S. 1964. The use of nialamide in mental retardation in childhood. *Psychopharm. Absts.* 4(12):1021.

LaVeck, G. D., Cruz, F. de la, and Simundson, E. 1960. Fluphenazine in the treatment of mentally retarded children with behavior disorders. *Dis. Nerv. Syst.* 21:82.

Mackay, R. I., Wiseman, A. G. M., Harding, P., and Riley, M. A. 1963. Monoamine oxidase inhibitors and mental subnormality: Experiences with nialamide. *J. Ment. Def. Res.* 7(2):107.

# Drug Treatment

Mises, R., and Beauchesne, H. 1963. A test of perphenazine in infants and adolescents. *Psychopharm. Absts.* 3(5):330.

Pilkington, T. L. 1961–1962. A report on "Tofranil" in mental deficiency. *Am. J. Ment. Def.* 66:729.

Robb, H. P.

1959. The use of chlorpromazine in a mental deficiency institution. *J. Ment. Sci.* 105:1029.

1960. A comparison between prochlorperazine and chlorpromazine in mental deficiency. *J. Ment. Sci.* 106:1413.

Rosenblum, S., and Buoniconto, P. 1960. "Compazine" vs. placebo: A controlled study with educable, emotionally disturbed children. *Am. J. Ment. Def.* 64:713.

Rudy, L. H., Himwich, H. E., and Rinaldi, F. 1958. A clinical evaluation of psychopharmacological agents in the management of disturbed mentally defective patients. *Am. J. Ment. Def.* 62:855.

Schulman, J. L., and Sister Mary Clarinda. 1964. The effect of promazine on the activity level of retarded children. *Pediatrics* 33:271.

Schutt, C. C. 1960. The efficacy of sedac therapy with maladjusted mentally retarded girls. *Am. J. Ment. Def.* 64:978.

Sharpe, D. S. 1962. A controlled trial of trifluoperazine in the treatment of the mentally subnormal patient. *J. Ment. Sci.* 108:220.

Tokizane, T., and Schade, J. P., eds. 1966. Correlative neurosciences. *Prog. in Brain Res.* 21B:37.

Waites, L., and Keele, D. K. 1963. Fluphenazine in management of disturbed mentally retarded children. *Dis. Nerv. Syst.* 24(2):113.

# Preschool for the Mentally Retarded: A Training Program for Parents of Retarded Children[1]

SAM E. TOOMBS, Ph.D., SALLY O'NEILL, R.N., B.S.,
and BOBBYE M. ROUSE, M.D.

*Child Development Clinic, Department of Pediatrics, The
University of Texas Medical Branch, Galveston, Texas*

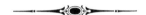

There seems to be little doubt that programs designed to combat mental retardation and promote mental health will be most effectively carried out only when they are based and implemented at the community level. In most communities there is a notable lack of personnel trained to work with the problems associated with mental retardation. The vocational school, junior college, and university programs have been unable to meet the demands for personnel.

Institutions that need personnel to work with the severely mentally retarded child in most instances must take the responsibility for instituting in-service training programs to qualify their own attendant personnel to carry out the service program of the institution. Professional persons should feel a similar responsibility for initiating action at the community level.

[1] This study was made possible through partial support from Children's Bureau Grants No. 409 and 240.

*Preschool for the Mentally Retarded*

In the 1967 report from the President's Committee on Mental Retardation, the problems of utilization of community facilities and mobilization of manpower resources to work in the area of retardation were considered to be two of the ten areas that most urgently needed the President's attention. The literature on programs for the mentally retarded reveals that considerable effort has been directed toward training of the mentally retarded child in institutional settings (Baer, Peterson, and Sherman 1965; Ellis 1963; Girardeau and Spradlin 1964; Hundziak *et al.* 1963; and Spradlin 1964). Other programs to help the mentally retarded have been directed primarily either at additional training for technical and professional personnel or at helping mothers gain insight into and understanding of the mentally retarded child (Chisholm, Haar, and McCarty 1966). L. Headley and H. Leler (1964) described a nursery school program for cerebral palsied children some of whom were reported to be mentally retarded. Although they involved mothers in the program, emphasis was upon the professional therapist, and the mothers played a relatively minor role. There have been, however, few reports of any systematic approach using parents to function as teacher-trainers of the mentally retarded child. Parents of the mentally retarded represent a logical source of manpower which has not been fully explored.

## Materials and Methods

In November 1966 the authors, members of the Child Development Clinic at The University of Texas Medical Branch, and the Island Council for Retarded Children (Galveston, Texas) established a training program for mothers of retarded children. Four mothers and their children were selected for this training program. During the operation of the program, four other mothers and their children became involved to a varying degree; however, the initial four mother-teachers continued throughout the program. The purpose of the training program was to prepare these mothers to work constructively with children to teach the skills that have adaptive value. The training for the mothers required approximately forty hours of teaching time spread over a two-month period. Each teaching session the authors held with the parents lasted from one to two hours. The frequency of the teaching sessions was determined by the daily schedule commitments of the parents and the authors. The group met from one to three times a week.

*Teaching the Mentally Retarded, a Handbook for Ward Personnel,* edited by Gerard J. Bensberg, was used as a text. This source gives additional introduction in the problems of mental retardation as well as very specific techniques for teaching the mentally retarded.

The study sessions consisted of lectures designed to clarify points brought up by the mothers, to give demonstrations of the principles of behavior-shaping, and to provide actual practice under supervision in using the principles set forth in the textbook. One of the final tasks each mother completed prior to beginning work with a child was to outline her own child's achievements and deficiencies. Each mother was further asked to put in writing the goals she wanted to see the child reach during the time he participated in the preschool program.

Each mother selected as her student a child other than her own and then began working with the child. There was a determination made of an effective reinforcer for the given child. Usually the determination was nothing more than asking the parent, "What does the child like?" For one child it was candy; for another child Cheerios; yet another effective reinforcer was pudding. The presentation of the reinforcer on the contingent basis confirmed the effectiveness of the reinforcer for a given child.

After the mother-teacher selected a student, she made an analysis of a probable hierarchy in the acquisition of goal behavior along lines the mother had set forth. There was further analysis of the specific behavioral components that seemed to make up the terminal or target behavior. With the help of the authors, the mother-teacher then arranged the component behaviors in what appeared to be a reasonably natural sequential order.

Each mother-teacher was encouraged to keep daily records of her work and of the child's behavior. In most instances the records were narrative comments. One mother-teacher kept more quantitative data: duration of temper tantrums, total time spent on a task, and number of instances of social interaction. The data from this mother-teacher's records will be presented in detail to illustrate the results of the program.

One of the authors met weekly with the parents to discuss problems for which no technique or solution had been set forth during the training period. The preschool program has been in operation from January 1967 until the present time. The classes are held for two hours, three times a week, in a regular kindergarten classroom at one of the local churches.[2]

[2] Moody Memorial First Methodist Church, Galveston, Texas.

Results

The results of the preschool program were most dramatically illustrated in the case of the mother-teacher working with Michael, a 7%12-year-old with Down's syndrome. Prior to the child's exposure to the preschool program an attempt had been made to evaluate psychologically. Excerpted from the psychological report is the following paragraph:

A hyperactive boy who must be constantly attended. He understands a few simple words but can speak no words at all. He was unable to respond to the most simple instructions. He can be controlled only by physical restraint. He was only able to do one test out of six which would be expected from one who is functioning at the two year level. This would place his mental age below two years and his estimated I.Q. below 25.

The child's measured intelligence level would place him within the severe if not the profoundly retarded range.

Michael appeared to have had very little control or limited-setting at home. His chief method of locomotion was crawling around the floor, although he could walk. He would resort to temper tantrums when he did not have what he wanted. His parents responded to these by soothing him or by rubbing his back, but the tantrums would last a considerable time. Michael's mother had determined these goals for Michael in this program:

1. Learn to pay attention.
2. Obey simple commands such as "sit" or "come here."
3. Independence in toileting and dressing.
4. Independence in eating.

These, then, were the areas in which Michael's mother-teacher worked with Michael. Gradually he learned these tasks; as he began to make progress, social reinforcement as well as consumables began to have some meaning. The verbal responses "good boy" or "that's very good" became as reinforcing as the food he was receiving earlier. Since his temper tantrums were ignored, they diminished in a relatively short time. The decline in duration of temper tantrums is shown in Figure 76a. There was a progressive decrease in the duration of time that temper tantrums continued during successive training periods. The mother-teacher's daily records indicated that with decreasing amounts of time expended in temper tantrums there was a concurrent improvement in performance

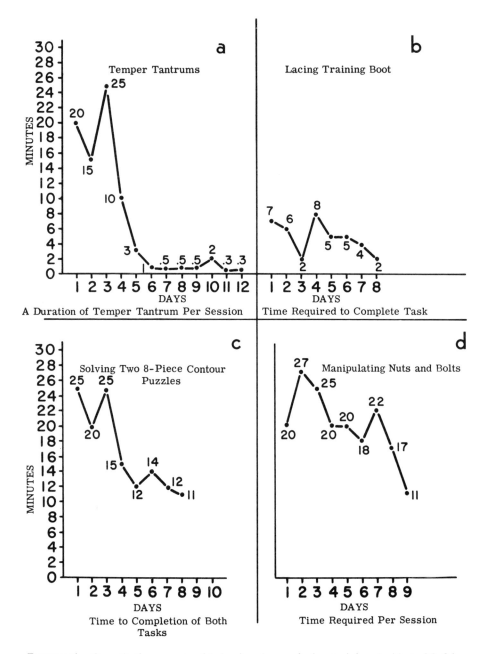

FIGURE 76. Quantitative aspects of behavior change during training (subject: M. S.).

of developmental tasks. These improvements are shown in Figures 76b, 76c, and 76d. The figures show increased efficiency in lacing a training boot, in solving two eight-piece contour puzzles, and in manipulating colored plastic nuts and bolts.

A five-minute film made after four months of training depicted Michael correctly matching all five color forms from the Gesell Development Scale, lacing a training boot with minimum assistance from his mother-teacher, and successfully completing other manipulative tasks requiring both color and form discrimination. The child walked with assistance on a balance board and gave no evidence of hyperactivity or temper tantrums. The film also depicted a rather lean schedule of consumable reinforcements.

The Denver Developmental Screening Test was administered to Michael prior to training and after nine months in the program. The results are shown in Figure 77 and indicate a gain of eighteen months' development. These results probably do not reflect development per se, but rather show a child who was much more amenable to assessment and consequently was able to demonstrate skills that were not demonstrated earlier. It was probably the training in attending and responding socially to other people which resulted from the training sessions rather than the transfer of the specific task learning.

At the present time, although Michael's development is still spotty, he continues to show much progress in many areas. He is able to establish eye contact and to pay attention to simple commands. He can attend to a task as long as it takes to complete the task. He has good form and color discrimination although the names of forms and colors have as yet no meaning. He has number concepts up to five. Michael is still learning many of the self-help skills. His accomplishments include feeding himself, using the proper utensils, dressing himself in simple clothing, and independent toileting. His parents find it easier to work with Michael at home since he no longer whines and fumes. He continues to be free of temper tantrums.

## Discussion of Results

The illustrative case history of Michael takes on more importance when his achievements are regarded as a measure of the effectiveness of training given him. The relation between operant techniques and the effect upon behavior have been adequately established. Concurrent changes in behavior following use of operant techniques can reasonably be attributed to the individual using the operant techniques.

The above analysis when used to evaluate the effectiveness of Michael's teacher gives strong support for her effectiveness. Prior to the training program given to the mothers, Michael's teacher gave no evidence of ever having systematically applied operant techniques. She was given the techniques in the training program; thus, one can conclude that the results gave positive evidence for the training program.

The additional significance of the success of the training program comes from the fact that the direct cost to the community was nominal. The time required for training both mothers and children was volunteered. All training provided to the mothers was given after the regular University clinic hours.

The program execution further emphasizes the availability of community manpower resources that have not been fully utilized. There seems little doubt that full mobilization of community resources to combat such problems as mental retardation will require the involvement of parents. Furthermore, the involvement of the parents probably will eventually be shown to have personal-social value in its own right.

Finally, the program described in the report demonstrated that there are physical facilities in the community that for one reason or another are not fully utilized. Many of the community facilities, notably the churches, would probably be willing to provide without charge space for programs similar to the one described in this paper.

## REFERENCES

Baer, D. M., Peterson, R. F., and Sherman, J. A. 1967. The development of imitation by reinforcing behavioral similarity to a model. *J. Exp. Anal. Behav.* 10(5):405.

Bensberg, G. J., ed. 1965. *Teaching the mentally retarded: A handbook for ward personnel.* Atlanta: Southern Regional Educational Board.

Chisholm, M., Haar, D., and McCarty, K. December 1966. *Symposium on Mental*

*Retardation*, p. 703. The Nursing Clinics of North America. Philadelphia and London: W. B. Saunders Co.

Ellis, N. R. 1963. Toilet training the severely defective patient: An S.R. reinforcement analysis. *Am. J. Ment. Def.* 68:98.

Girardeau, F. L., and Spradlin, J. E. 1964. Token rewards on a cottage program. *Ment. Retard.* 2:345.

Headley, L., and Leler, H. 1964. A nursery school for cerebral palsied children. Mental Retardation during the decade 1954–1964. Children's Bureau, U.S. Department of Health, Education and Welfare Administration, 276.

Hundziak, M., Maurer, R. A., and Watson, L. S., Jr. 1963. Operant conditioning in toilet training of severely mentally retarded boys: A controlled study. Unpublished manuscript, Columbus, Ohio, State School.

Spradlin, J. E. 1964. The premark hypothesis and self-feeding by profoundly retarded children—a case report. Parsons Research Center, Working Paper 79.

# Experimental Approach to the Role of Monoamine Deficiency as a Cause of Mental Retardation

MAUNO M. AIRAKSINEN, M.D.

*Division of Biological Research, Texas Research Institute of Mental Sciences, Houston, Texas*

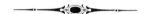

A long-lasting decrease in the transmitter substances—a chemical denervation of the brain—may well be the point at which several metabolic disorders can cause mental retardation. This conclusion is logical if we suppose that the normal transmission is necessary for normal development of the nervous system. Although it is almost certain that acetylcholine is one of the transmitters in the brain (Votava 1967), the biological amines seem to be closer to several amino acid disorders. Hypotheses about the role of these amines have been made in some specific diseases because the concentration of these amines and their metabolites are changed in blood, urine, and cerebrospinal fluid. The changes of catecholamines in Down's syndrome and the concepts about 5-hydroxytryptamine (5-HT) deficiency in phenylketonuria are well-known (Pare *et al.* 1958; Woolley 1962; Pare 1967). Although γ-amino butyric acid is also suggested as a neurotransmitter and may be decreased in some amino acid disorders (Tashien 1961), I will discuss only 5-HT and catecholamines.

In this institute we have tried to reduce the transmitter amines in rats, starting from birth (in some animals even earlier), and have evaluated

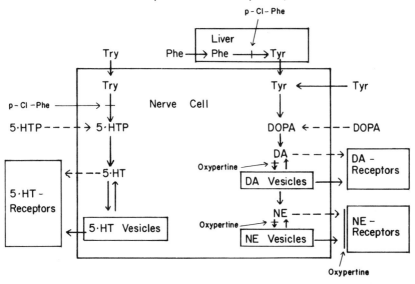

FIGURE 78. Scheme of the synthesis of 5-hydroxytryptamine (5-HT), dopamine (DA), and norepinephrine (NE) in the nerve cell and the sites of action of p-chlorophenylalanine (p-Cl-Phe) and oxypertine.

the effects on learning. The idea is not new, and our results are still scanty. Better possibilities for these kinds of studies now exist because of the availability of more specific compounds that block the synthesis or metabolism or release of one specific amine (instead of all). We still have great difficulties in producing only a transmitter amine decrease without producing other effects (impairment of the availability of amino acids for protein synthesis, for instance).

We have used p-chlorophenylalanine as an inhibitor of 5-HT synthesis. It blocks brain tryptophan hydroxylase effectively *in vivo* (Fig. 78), but unfortunately it also blocks liver phenylalanine hydroxylase (Koe and Weissman 1966; DeGraw *et al.* 1967) and causes the chemical manifestations of a "true phenylketonuria" (Lipton *et al.* 1967); therefore, this alone can hardly be used for the evaluation of the role of 5-HT in the growing brain. However, in this way we may have a good "experimental phenylketonuria" and the decreased 5-HT level can be corrected by continuous administration of 5-hydroxytryptophan (5-HTP). I do not think the syndromes that are made by feeding high amounts of 1-phenylalanine or phenylalanine and tyrosine are good models of phenylketonuria. They correspond rather to tyrosinemia or tyrosinosis, and permanent impairment of learning tests has not usually been found (Polidora 1967).

In phenylketonuria, and probably in other disorders where a neutral amino acid and the corresponding keto- and hydroxy-acids are increased (in maple syrup urine disease, hyperhistidinemia, and hyperglycinemia), there is some evidence that the main cause of 5-HT decrease is the inhibition of tryptophan absorption and uptake to the brain (Pare 1967; Smyth 1967) rather than the inhibition of tryptophan-5-hydroxylase (Freeland *et al.* 1961; Perry *et al.* 1964), 5-HTP decarboxylase (Pare *et al.* 1958; Davidson and Sandler 1958), or 5-HT storage mechanisms. The inhibition of hydroxylation may, however, be a contributing factor. Because the same seems to be true of the uptake of tyrosine (Guroff, King, and Udenfriend 1961), there is a corresponding shortage in the substrate for catecholamine synthesis as well as for 5-HT synthesis in brain cells. Only slightly decreased blood levels of tyrosine (Smyth 1967; Linneweh and Ehrlich 1962) do not refute this hypothesis. It is not known whether the carriers of phenylalanine, tryptophan, and tyrosine into nerve cells are the same; in the intestinal absorption at least two carriers of neutral amino acids seem to be present (Smyth 1967). Some authors (Yuwiler, Geller, and Slater 1965; Geller and Yuwiler 1967) have suggested that the inhibition of 5-HTP and DOPA uptake is the cause of 5-HT and dopamine decrease in their experimental hyperleucinemic and hyperphenylalaninemic rats and in patients with corresponding clinical diseases. It seems questionable if significant amounts of 5-HTP and DOPA normally go from other tissues to the brain because they are present in the plasma only in very low concentrations, if at all (Garattini and Valzelli 1965; Erspamer 1966), when compared to the real amounts of tryptophan and tyrosine. Recent studies (those with intracerebral tryptophan administration) show that the amount of substrate can be critical for brain tryptophan hydroxylase activity (Jequier *et al.* 1967; Consolo *et al.* 1965; Airaksinen *et al.* 1968). The same may be true for tyrosine hydroxylation, the limiting point of catecholamine synthesis (Levitt *et al.* 1965; Udenfriend 1966; Sarri *et al.* 1967).

Tyrosine hydroxylase inhibitors (Udenfriend 1966; Sarri *et al.* 1967) can be used to block catecholamine synthesis, and high doses of DOPA can be used to increase it. The action of these compounds is reflected by dopamine, and to a lesser extent by noradrenaline, formation (Carlsson 1964; Corrodi and Fuxe 1967). For specific decrease of NE synthesis, we

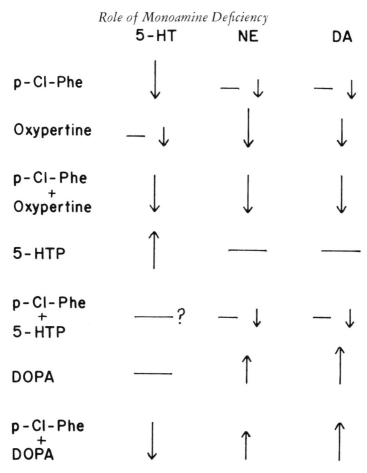

FIGURE 79. Direction of the changes of brain amines after the administration of p-chlorophenylalanine, oxypertine, 5-hydroxytryptophan, and dihydroxyphenylalanine and some of their combinations.

would need a specific inhibitor of dopamine-$\beta$-hydroxylase (Goldstein 1965; Van der Schoot and Crevelling 1965), but *in vivo* effective inhibitors of this enzyme (disulfiram) have other disturbing effects. We can try to increase brain NE specifically with dihydroxyphenylserine, a partial precursor of NE (Carlsson 1964), but H. Corrodi and K. Fuxe (1967) received only a small and temporary NE increase with this compound.

We have used oxypertine (Win 18,501) to block central NE mecha-

nisms in our infant rats. This compound was first reported to decrease
'brain NE specifically without any effect on dopamine or 5-HT (Spector
*et al*. 1962; Matsuoka *et al*. 1965). Unfortunately, it was not so specific;
it has also been shown to decrease brain dopamine levels, and high doses
decrease brain 5-HT (Fuxe *et al*. 1967). It seems to release NE from the
store vesicles (Fuxe *et al*. 1967; Hassler and Bak 1966). The effects of
chronic amine release generally are difficult to interpret because different
opinions exist as to whether there is increased or decreased flow of the
free amine to the receptor site. The central effects of reserpine are usually
explained as resulting from the decrease of free NE (Holzbauer and
Vogt 1956; Karki and Paasonen 1959) or dopamine (Bertler 1964;
Sourkes 1964) or all monoamines (Carlsson 1964; Pletscher 1965) or
increase of free 5-HT (Brodie and Shore 1957; Brodie 1968) in the
brain. In the heart of developing rats, chronic administration of reserpine
has been shown to make a permanent impairment of NE uptake like im-
munosympathectomy (Iverson *et al*. 1967). Because oxypertine also is
a peripheral and central adrenolytic compound (Wylie and Archer
1962), it, unlike reserpine, simultaneously blocks NE receptors when it
decreases the amount of NE (Fig. 78).

Figure 79 gives an approximate picture of the changes of brain amine
levels in the rat with our drug combinations. The actual results depend
largely on the dose and methods of administration. We do not yet have
clear results about all combinations because the ideal dosage has not always been found, and we cannot conclude much about learning if the
animals are in poor physical condition. The preliminary results suggest
that 5-HT deficiency plays a role in rats made "phenylketonuric" with
p-chlorophenylalanine; 5-HTP addition makes them do better both physically and in learning tests. On the other hand, in a series where all the
rats had d,l-phenylalanine in drinking water and the controls already
showed a deficiency in learning, the additional decrease of brain 5-HT
with p-chlorophenylalanine did not show much effect. This time, however, a rather low dose of p-chlorophenylalanine (0.5 mg. per ml. in
drinking water) was used.

Oxypertine did not seem to have much effect in doses that decrease
brain NE more than in p-Cl-Phe-induced phenylketonuria. We do not
yet have data about the possible role of dopamine deficiency in our
retarded rats.

Several compounds, mainly $\beta$-carbolines, are synthesized in this institute (McIsaac *et al*. 1967), and their effects on brain monoamines as

well as on some pharmacological properties are being studied. Some of these compounds seem to increase or decrease one amine only. Little is known at present about their mechanisms of action, but some of these neatly synthesized compounds may be useful tools in this type of study in the future.

## REFERENCES

Airaksinen, M. M., Giacalone, E., and Valzelli, L. 1968. Hyroxylation of tryptophan in the brain *in vivo*. *J. Neurochem.* 15(1).

Bertler, A. 1964. Dopamine in the central nervous system. In *Proceedings of the Second International Pharmacological Meeting*, ed. E. Trabucci, R. Paoletti, and N. Canal. 2:5. Oxford: Pergamon Press; Prague: Czechoslovak Medical Press.

Brodie, B. B. May 1967. Considerations on the role of brain serotonin. Symposium on the biological role of indolealkylamines. *Adv. Pharmacol.* 6B.

Brodie, B. B., and Shore, P. A. 1957. A concept for a role of serotonin and norepinephrine as chemical mediators in the brain. *Ann. N.Y. Acad. Sci.* 66:631.

Carlsson, A. 1964. Functional significance of drug-induced changes in brain monoamine levels. *Prog. Brain Res.* 8:9.

Consolo, S., Garattini, S., Ghielmetti, R., Morselli, P., and Valzelli, L. 1965. The hydroxylation of tryptophan *in vivo* by brain. *Life Sci.* 4:625.

Corrodi, H., and Fuxe, K. 1967. The effect of catecholamine precursors and monoamine oxidase inhibition on the amine levels at central catecholamine neurones after reserpine treatment or tyrosine hydroxylase inhibition. *Life Sci.* 6:1345.

Costa, E., Gessa, G. L., Hirsch, G., Kunzman, R., and Brodie, B. B. 1962. On current status of serotonin as brain neurohormone and in action of reserpine like drugs. *Ann. N.Y. Acad. Sci.* 96:118.

Davidson, A. N., and Sandler, M. 1958. Inhibition of 5-hydroxytryptophan decarboxylase by phenylalanine metabolites. *Nature* (London) 181:186.

DeGraw, J. L., Cory, M., Skinner, W. A., Theisen, M. D., and Mitoma, C. 1967. Experimentally induced phenylketonuria I. Inhibitors of phenylalanine hydroxylase. *J. Med. Chem.* 10:64.

Erspamer, V. 1966. Occurrence of indolealkylamines in nature. In *Handbook of experimental pharmacology*, ed. V. Erspamer, pp. 132–166. New York-Berlin-Heidelberg: Springer Verlag.

Freedland, R. A., Wadzinski, J. M., and Weissman, H. A. 1961. The enzymatic hydroxylation of tryptophan. *Biochem. Biophys. Res. Comm.* 5:94.

Fuxe, K., Grobecker, H., Hökfelt, T., Jonsson, J., and Malmfors, T. 1967. Some observations on the site of action of oxypertin. *Naunyn-Schmiedebergs Arch. Pharmakol. Exp. Path.* 256:460.

Garattini, S., and Valzelli, L. 1965. *Serotonin.* Amsterdam-London-New York: Elsevier.

Geller, E., and Yuwiler, A. 1967. Brain amine decrease in leucine-fed rats. *J. Neurochem.* 14:725.

Goldstein, M. 1965. Inhibition of norepinephrine biosynthesis at the dopamine-$\beta$-hydroxylation step. *Pharmacol. Rev.* 18:77.

Guroff, G., King, W., and Udenfriend, S. 1961. The uptake of tyrosine by rat brain in vitro. *J. Biol. Chem.* 236:1773.

Hassler, R., and Bak, I. J. 1966. Submikroskopische Catecholaminspeicher als Angriffspunkte der Psychopharmaka Reserpin und Mono-Amino-Oxydase-Hemmer. *Nervenarzt* 37:93.

Holzbauer, M., and Vogt, M. 1956. Depression by reserpine of the noradrenaline concentration in the hypothalamus of the dog. *J. Neurochem.* 1:8.

Iversen, L. L., deChamplain, J., Glowinski, J., and Axelrod, J. 1967. Uptake, storage, and metabolism of norepinephrine in tissues of the developing rat. *J. Pharm. Exp. Ther.* 157:509.

Jequier, E., Lovenberg, W., and Sjoerdsma, A. 1967. Tryptophan hydroxylase inhibition: The mechanism by which p-chlorophenylalanine depletes rat brain serotonin. *Molecul. Pharmacol.* 3:274.

Karki, N. T., and Paasonen, M. K. 1959. Selective depletion of noradrenaline and 5-hydroxytryptamine from rat brain and intestine by rauwolfia alkaloids. *J. Neurochem.* 3:352.

Koe, B. K., and Weissman, A. 1966. p-Chlorophenylalanine: A specific depletor of brain serotonin. *J. Pharmacol. Exp. Ther.* 154:499.

Levitt, M., Spector, S., Sjoerdsma, A., and Udenfriend, S. 1965. Elucidation of the rate-limiting step in norepinephrine biosynthesis in the perfused guinea pig heart. *J. Pharmacol. Exp. Ther.* 148:1.

Linneweh, F., and Ehrlich, M. 1962. Fur Pathogenese des Schwachsinns bei Phenylketonurie. *Klin. Wchnschr.* 40:225.

Lipton, M. A., Gordon, R., Guroff, G., and Udenfriend, S. 1967. p-Chlorophenylalanine-induced chemical manifestations of phenylketonuria in rats. *Science* 156:248.

McIsaac, W. M., Ho, B. T., Estevez, V., and Powers, D. 1967. Chromatography of $\beta$-carbolines. *J. Chromatography* 31:446.

Matsuoka, M., Ishii, S., Shimizu, N., and Imaizumi, R. 1965. Effect of Win 18,501-2 on the content of catecholamines and the number of catecholamine-containing granules in the rabbit hypothalamus. *Experientia* 21:121.

Pare, C. M. B. May 1967. 5-Hydroxyindoles in phenylketonuria and non-phenyl-ketonuric mental defectives. Symposium on the biological role of indolealkyla-mines. *Adv. Pharmacol.* 6B:159–165.

Pare, C. M. B., Sandler, M., and Stacey, R. S. 1958. Decreased 5-hydroxytrypto-phan decarboxylase activity in phenylketonuria. *Lancet* 2:1099.

Perry, J. L., Hansen, S., Tischler, B., and Hestrin, M. 1964. Defective 5-hydroxy-lation of tryptophan in phenylketonuria. *Proc. Soc. Exp. Biol. Med.* 113:817.

Pletscher, A. 1965. Biogenic amines. In *Neuropsychopharmacology*, eds. D. Bente and P. B. Bradley, pp. 16, 52. Amsterdam-London-New York: Elsevier.

Polidora, V. J. 1967. Behavioral effects of phenylketonuria in rats. *Proc. Natl. Acad. Sci.* (U.S.A.) 57:102.

Sarri, W., Williams, J., Britcher, S. F., Wolf, E. E., and Kuehl, F. A., Jr. 1967. Tyrosine hydroxylase inhibitors. Synthesis and activity of substituted aromatic amino acids. *J. Med. Chem.* 10:1008.

Smyth, D. H. 1967. Amino acid absorption through intestinal epithelium. *Protoplasma* 63:26.

Sourkes, T. L. 1964. Action of DOPA and dopamine in relation to function of the central nervous system. In *Proceedings of the Second International Pharmacological Meeting*, ed. E. Trabucci, R. Paoletti, and N. Canal. 2:35. Oxford: Pergamon Press; Prague: Czechoslovak Medical Press.

Spector, S., Melmon, K., and Sjoerdsma, A. 1962. Evidence for rapid turnover of norepinephrine in rat heart and brain. *Proc. Soc. Exp. Biol. Med.* 111:69.

Tashien, R. E. 1961. Inhibition of brain glutamic acid decarboxylase by phenyl-alanine, valine, and leucine derivatives: A suggestion concerning the etiology of the neurological defect in phenylketonuria and branched chain ketonuria. *Metabolism* 10:393.

Udenfriend, S. 1966. Tyrosine hydroxylase. *Pharmacol. Rev.* 18:43.

Van der Schoot, I. B., and Crevelling, C. R. 1965. Substrates and inhibitors of dopamine-$\beta$-hydroxylase (DBH). *Adv. Drug Res.* 2:47.

Votava, Z. 1967. Pharmacology of the central cholinergic synapses. *Ann. Rev. Pharmacol.* 7:223.

Woolley, D. W. 1962. *The biochemical basis of psychoses or the serotonin hypothesis about mental diseases.* New York: John Wiley & Sons.

Wylie, D. W., and Archer, S., 1962. Structure-activity relationship of 1-[(3-indolyl)alkyl]-4-arylpiperazines, a new series of tranquilizers. *J. Med. Pharm. Chem.* 5:932.

Yuwiler, A., Geller, E., and Slater, G. G. 1965. On the mechanisms of the brain serotonin depletion in experimental phenylketonuria. *J. Biol. Chem.* 240:1170.

# Catecholamine Metabolism in Mongolism

DOMAN K. KEELE, M.D., CONSTANCE RICHARDS, B.S.,
JAMES BROWN, M.S., and JANE MARSHALL, R.N.

*Denton State School, Denton, Texas*

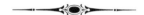

While we were at the Denton State School we studied some aspects of catecholamine metabolism in mongolism. Figure 80 shows the two well-known major pathways in the formation and metabolism of norepinephrine and epinephrine. We have performed the following determinations: dopamine, norepinephrine, epinephrine, dihydroxymandelic acid, metanephrine, normetanephrine, and vanillylmandelic acid.

The subjects with mongolism were paired with nonmongoloid mentally retarded patients as control subjects according to weight, sex, and height. The I.Q. of the subjects with mongolism ranged from zero to 39 with a mean of 28. The I.Q. of the control subjects ranged from zero to 73 with a mean of 38. There was a difference of ten points between the two groups, $p = .001$, so the data indicates that the subjects with mongolism had a lower I.Q. than the control subjects. All the subjects were residents of the Denton State School, an institution of mentally retarded individuals. All were well during collections and were under no known stressful situations. Subjects were admitted to the institutional hospital for urine collections. Subjects were placed on a vanillin-free diet four days prior to and during the urine collections. Consecutive twenty-four–hour urine collections were made until two consecutive twenty-four–hour total creatinine determinations were similar. These two specimens were

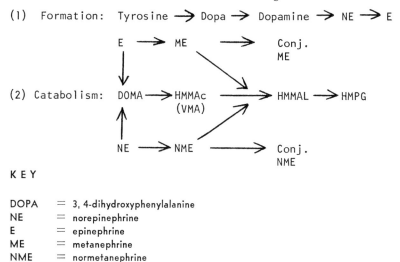

## Catecholamine Metabolism in Mongolism

(1)  Formation:   Tyrosine → Dopa → Dopamine → NE → E

E → ME → Conj. ME

(2) Catabolism:   DOMA → HMMAc (VMA) → HMMAL → HMPG

NE → NME → Conj. NME

**KEY**

| | | |
|---|---|---|
| DOPA | = | 3, 4-dihydroxyphenylalanine |
| NE | = | norepinephrine |
| E | = | epinephrine |
| ME | = | metanephrine |
| NME | = | normetanephrine |
| DOMA | = | 3, 4-dihydroxymandelic acid |
| HMMAC | = (VMA) = | 3-methoxy-4-hydroxymandelic acid |
| HMMAL | = | 3-methoxy-4-hydroxymandelic aldehyde |
| HMPG | = | 3-methoxy-4-hydroxyphenylglycol |

FIGURE 80.   Steps in the formation and catabolism of norepinephrine and epinephrine.

pooled for catecholamine determinations and results reported as amounts per twenty-four hours. Urine was collected in a brown glass bottle that contained 50 ml. of 6 normal hydrochloric acid. The urine was stored in the refrigerator. All determinations were done in duplicate with per cent recovery done on each.

Urine epinephrine and norepinephrine determinations were done according to the method of J. R. Crout (1961). Recovery experiments showed a mean of 84.2 per cent for the controls and 86.5 per cent for the subjects with mongolism. Mean urinary dopamine recovery experiments were 88 per cent and were done according to the method of A. Carlsson (1959). Urinary 3,4-dihydroxymandelic acid determinations were done according to the method of V. DeQuattro and his associates (1964). Recovery experiments showed a mean of 90 per cent.

Urinary metanephrine and normetanephrine determinations were done according to the methods of S. Brunjes, D. Wyberger, and V. J. Johns

Table 39

Mean Urinary Creatinine Excretions
mg/kg/day (25 pairs)

|  | Control Subjects | Subjects with Mongolism |
|---|---|---|
|  | 22.50 (3.90) | 22.07 (5.34) |
| r(wt/cr) = | 0.90 (p=<.01) | 0.92 (p=<.01) |

r = Pearson's Moment Correlation Coefficient

(1964). Mean recovery was 88 per cent. Urinary VMA determinations were done according to the methods of W. Sunderman, P. D. Cleveland, and N. C. Low (1960). Mean recovery was 87 per cent. Plasma epinephrine and norepinephrine were done according to the method of H. L. Price and M. Price (1957). Mean recovery on these were our lowest, 84 per cent.

All statistical analyses were made on an Olivetti Underwood Programma 101 High-Speed Electronic Calculator and Automatic Computer.

Table 39 shows that the mean urinary excretion values for creatinine on twenty-five pairs were practically the same, 22.50 and 22.07. Correlation between creatinine excretion and body weight was very high, being 0.90 and 0.92. Both of these were, of course, significant. In view of the high correlation, it was decided to present all subsequent determinations in terms of body weight. The weights ranged from 10 kg. to 88 kg. with a mean of 48.20 kg. for the mongoloid subjects and 48.46 kg. for the control subjects.

In these and all subsequent tables, the number of pairs will be given in the title. Values in parentheses will give the standard deviation. Pearson's Moment Correlation Coefficients between the determination and the body weight is r and the level of significance, p, for the correlation coefficients will be given in parentheses by the value for r.

Urinary excretion of dopamine was not significantly different between controls and experimental subjects (Table 40). Correlation between urinary dopamine and body weight was highly significant, r being 0.606 for controls and 0.707 for the mongoloid subjects.

Excretion of conjugated and free norepinephrine between the two groups was not significantly different (Table 41). Correlation of norepinephrine excretion with body weight was significantly positive at the 0.05 level. Norepinephrine, then, in the two groups was not significantly

## Catecholamine Metabolism in Mongolism

### Table 40

Mean Urinary Dopamine
μg/kg/day (22 pairs)

|      | Controls | Mongoloids |
|------|----------|------------|
|      | 3.700 (2.29) | 3.050 (1.14) (p=0.20+) |
| r=   | 0.606 (p=.01+) | 0.707 (p=0.01+) |

### Table 41

Mean Norepinephrine (NE) and Epinephrine (E) Excretions
μg/kg/day (25 pairs)

|           | Controls | Mongoloids |
|-----------|----------|------------|
| Free NE   | 0.640 (.38) | 0.690 (.43) |
| p=        |          | <0.7 |
| r=        | 0.595 | 0.482 |
| Conj. NE  | 1.400 (.95) | 1.250 (.66) |
| p=        |          | >0.3+ |
| r=        | 0.406 (p=.05) | 0.512 (p=.05) |
| Free E    | 0.150 (.10) | 0.080 (.121) |
| p=        |          | <0.05 |
| r=        | 0.373 (p=.10) | 0.160 (p=.10+) |
| Conj. E   | 0.200 (.12) | 0.120 (.08) |
| p=        |          | <0.01 |
| r=        | 0.440 (p=<.05) | 0.040 (p=<.05) |

### Table 42

Mean Plasma Catecholamines
μg/L (21 pairs)

|                | Controls | Mongoloids |
|----------------|----------|------------|
| Epinephrine    | 0.07 (0.04) | 0.06 (0.04) (p=0.3) |
| Norepinephrine | 0.37 (0.14) | 0.38 (0.18) (p=0.3) |

different; however, epinephrine was lower in the experimental subjects, 0.15 and 0.08 μg. per 24 hours, p=.05. The same thing was observed with conjugated epinephrine, 0.2 and 0.12 μg. per 24 hours, p=.01.

Plasma catecholamines were not significantly different between the two groups (Table 42).

Table 43

Mean Urinary 3,4-Dihydroxymandelic Acid
$\mu$g/kg/day (22 pairs)

|  | Controls | Mongoloids |
|---|---|---|
| Conj. | 10.770 (6.65) | 9.890 (6.23) |
| p= |  | <0.4 |
| r= | 0.519 (p=<.02) | 0.489 (p=.01+) |
| Free | 9.890 (6.86) | 9.230 (5.48) |
| p= |  | 0.5+ |
| r= | 0.467 (p=.01+) | 0.430 (p=.01+) |

Table 44

Urinary Normetanephrine (NMN) and Metanephrine (MN)
$\mu$g/kg/day (25 pairs)

|  | Controls | Mongoloids |
|---|---|---|
| NMN | 7.470 (3.46) | 6.450 (4.38) |
| p= |  | 0.1+ |
| r= | 0.343 (p=<.05) | 0.307 (p=.10+) |
| MN | 3.450 (2.32) | 2.890 (1.70) |
| p= |  | <0.2 |
| r= | 0.378 (p=<.05) | 0.458 (p=.01+) |

Table 45

Mean Urinary Vanillylmandelic Acid
mg/kg/day (22 pairs)

|  | Controls | Mongoloids |
|---|---|---|
|  | 0.090 (.08) | 0.080 (.07) |
| p= |  |  |
| r= | 0.365 (p=<.05) | 0.275 (p=.1+) |

Urinary excretion of 3,4-dihydroxymandelic acid likewise was not significantly different from the controls (Table 43).

Urinary normetanephrine and metanephrine excretion was also not significantly different from the controls (Table 44). Urinary VMA values were also the same for the two groups as shown in Table 45.

Table 46

Summary of Findings

| Determination | Variation |
|---|---|
| Urinary Dopamine | Same as controls |
| Urinary VMA | Same as controls |
| Urinary DOMA (Conj. and Free) | Same as controls |
| Urinary ME | Same as controls |
| Urinary NME | Same as controls |
| Urinary NE (Conj. and Free) | Same as controls |
| Urinary E (Conj. and Free) | Low |
| Plasma NE and E | Same as controls |

In summary then, these results indicate that in all determinations the mongoloid subjects were the same as the controls except for the conjugated and free urinary epinephrine levels, which were low (Table 46).

One criticism that can be made of this data is that the I.Q. is slightly higher, 10 points, in the control subjects than in the subjects with mongolism. We have subjected these data in each group of subjects to statistical analysis, and there is no correlation between I.Q. and any of the determinations that were made. We had from twenty-five to twenty-two subjects in each group for each determination. The I.Q.'s ranged from 0 to 73, and there was no correlation between I.Q. and any of the data studied.

Does the low epinephrine excretion in mongolism have any significance? The answer is not apparent from our data.

Injections of radioactive epinephrine have shown that less than 7 per cent is excreted in urine as the unaltered amine (Axelrod 1963). If the excreted unaltered amine in these experiments reflects what is happening endogenously, it is apparent that excreted epinephrine may not represent a reliable indicator of production, and I think the same thing could be said of plasma levels. In this experiment, the plasma levels were too low to detect a significant difference if it existed. In addition, the plasma level is taken at a single moment in time and does not reflect what is going on all the time. Epinephrine excretion or plasma levels may not, therefore, represent reliable production indicators. The quantity of unaltered epinephrine excreted in urine may, however, correlate with epinephrine release. V. S. von Euler (1964), F. Elmadjian, J. M. Hope, and E. T. Lampson (1957) and S. Levi (1964, 1965) measured the excretion of epinephrine and norepinephrine under normal circumstances and demonstrated significant changes in excretion values in a variety of stresses including change of gravitation, muscular work, insulin, and various mental states. It may be reasonable to postulate, then, that low values for urinary epinephrine in mongolism represent a decreased release of epinephrine from the adrenal glands. This hypothesis is capable of being tested. Epinephrine excretion response to insulin hypoglycemia in mongolism is feasible. Indeed, A. Bergsman (1959) has reported such experiments in two mongoloid subjects with a low epinephrine excretion response to insulin hypoglycemia.

Would the diminished release of epinephrine have any physiological significance in mongolism? A diminished release of epinephrine appears to have significance in two other conditions. C. J. Light and his associates (1967) have shown that severe hypoglycemia seen in some infants of diabetic mothers is accompanied by a diminished excretion of epinephrine, and they postulated a failure of epinephrine release. A. A. Smith and J. Dancis (1967) have shown that higher levels of epinephrine and norepinephrine exist in the adrenal glands of children dying of familial dysautonomia than in controls. Life in this state is accompanied by low excretion of VMA and postural hypotension. These investigators assumed a deficit in the reflexive release of catecholamines in dysautonomia preventing not only the normal response during life but also the exhaustion of the adrenal glands at death.

At the Denton State School we had over 150 mongoloid patients under our medical care, and we were impressed with the fact that these children seemed to be sicker with an ordinary infection (of course it is well known that they are subject to more infections than are controls). Unlike non-mongoloid patients, an ordinary infection seemed to put these children in the hospital. We wondered if perhaps part of the difficulty might be due to some sort of deficiency in an ability to respond to stress with increased epinephrine production; in part we undertook these experiments to discover if this hypothesis were true.

We do not really know whether or not our data have any physiologic meaning. We are still worried about the fact that epinephrine as excreted in the urine, the unaltered amine, only represents 7 per cent of the radioactive amine injected intravenously in *in vivo* experiments.

# REFERENCES

Axelrod, J. 1963. The formation, metabolism, uptake and release of noradrenaline and adrenaline. In *The clinical chemistry of monoamines*, ed. H. Vasley and A. H. Gowenslock, pp. 1–18. New York: Elsevier.

Bergsman, A. 1959. The urinary excretion of adrenaline and noradrenaline in some mental disease. *Acta Psychiatrica et Neurologica Scandinavica.* 34(suppl. 133):1–107.

Brunjes, S., Wyberger, D., and Johns, V. J., Jr. 1964. Fluorometric determination of urinary metanephrine and normetanephrine. *Clin. Chem.* 10:1–12.

Carlsson, A. 1959. *Detection and assay of dopamine*, p. 300. Symposium on Catecholamines Held at National Institute of Health, Bethesda, Maryland, October 16–18, 1958. Baltimore: Williams and Wilkins Co.

Crout, J. R. 1961. *Catecholamines in urine: Standards of clinical chemistry*, ed. David Seligson. 3:62–80. New York: Academic Press.

DeQuattro, V., Wyberger, D., Studnitz, W. von, and Brunjes, S. 1964. Determination of urinary 3,4-dihydroxymandelic acid. *J. Lab. Clin. Med.* 63:864–878.

Elmadjian, F., Hope, J. M., and Lampson, E. T. 1957. Excretion of epinephrine and norepinephrine in various emotional states. *J. Clin. Endocr. & Metab.* 17: 608–620.

Euler, V. S. von. 1964. Quantitation of stress by catecholamine analysis. *Clin. Pharm. Ther.* 5:398–404.

Levi, S.
1964. The stress of everyday work as reflected in productiveness, subjective feeling, and urinary output of adrenalin and noradrenalin under salaried and piece work conditions. *J. Psychosom. Res.* 8:199–202.

1965. The urinary output of adrenalin and noradrenalin during pleasant and unpleasant emotional states: A preliminary report. *Psychosom. Med.* 27:80–85.

Light, C. J., Sutherland, J. M., Loggie, J. M., and Goffney, T. E. 1967. Impaired epinephrine release in hypoglycemic infants of diabetic mothers. *New Eng. J. Med.* 277:394–398.

Price, H. L., and Price, M. 1957. The clinical estimation of epinephrine and norepinephrine in human and canine plasma. *J. Lab. Clin. Med.* 50:769.

Smith, A. A., and Dancis, J. 1967. Catecholamine release in familial dysautonomia. *New Eng. J. Med.* 277:61–64.

Sunderman, W., Jr., Cleveland, P. D., and Low, N. C. 1960. A method for the determination of 3-methoxy–4-hydroxymandelic acid (vanillylmandelic acid) for the diagnosis of pheochromocytoma. *Am. J. Clin. Path.* 34:293–312.

# A Classical Conditioning Model for the Assessment of Intellectual Deficits in Young Animals

M. MARLYNE KILBEY, Ph.D.

*Texas Research Institute of Mental Sciences, Houston, Texas*

Although observations of the effects of drugs upon behavior are centuries old, psychopharmacology as an active, formal discipline is a contemporary development. The initial impetus to the development of psychopharmacology came from reports of clinical use of psychoactive chemical agents in the treatment of mental illness. This, in turn, gave rise to basic questions of the mechanisms of drug action within the organism and concomitant changes in various properties of living organisms—questions that require the correlation of drug administration with anatomical, behavioral, biochemical, and electrophysiological data. A significant portion of the ongoing experimental program of the Behavioral Pharmacological Research Laboratory of the Texas Research Institute has had as its goal the assessment of drug effects on animal behavior using traditional behavioral pharmacological research strategy. This traditional research method incorporates two basic features: operant conditioning techniques and drug administration.

A brief description of operant conditioning illustrates its appropriateness to the kinds of questions generally asked in behavioral pharmacological investigations. Formulated by B. F. Skinner (1938) operant conditioning theory is based upon observation of animal performance in an experimental situation devised by Skinner: the bar pressing of a rat in an operant chamber. Since the consequence of reinforcing a response emitted by an animal is to increase the rate of that response, the experimenter can establish stable, reliable behavior by scheduling the manner in which reinforcement is made available to the animal. C. B. Ferster and Skinner (1957) have outlined sixteen major classes of reinforcement schedules which allow elaboration of a wide range of behavioral patterns in the rat. The major advantage of Skinner's system is the stability and reliability of responding achieved by the animal. Once the animal is trained to any of these reinforcement schedules his behavior is characterized by a unique slope and pattern on the cumulative record of responses over time.

Drug effects on this behavior are indexed by disruptions of this characteristic slope and pattern. Generally the drug dosage level necessary to disrupt behavior is first determined. Next, dosage levels that modify the behavioral pattern are explored. The effects of time elapsed since drug administration upon the behavioral patterns are evaluated. Using this strategy the Behavioral Pharmacological Research Laboratory has established dosage-response and time-response relations for a series of $\beta$-carbolines, a class of monoamine oxidase inhibitor which alters serotonin and norepinephrine levels. In summary, traditional psychopharmacological research strategy utilizes normal, mature animals conditioned under normal experimental, drive level, and reinforcement conditions. In these animals conditioned performance is temporarily disrupted by administration of drugs, and the relations of dosage and time since administration to the disruption and/or modification of performance are ascertained. Behavioral indices are then correlated with biochemical indices of drug effects obtained from control animals. Correlations between dosage and time response relations for behavioral and biochemical indices, of course, lend support to the hypotheses that the drug is affecting underlying processes related to the animal's behavior.

Recently the laboratory staff has become interested in a kind of question not amenable to traditional pharmacological research strategy and technique. In working with mature rats (from the laboratory of Dr. William Schindler of Baylor University) which had been given radioactive iodine, [131]I, during the first day of life and were as a result functionally cretin, it became apparent that the conditioned performance of these animals was being affected by nonspecific factors relating to motivational and performance variables. We concluded that when long-lasting effects are produced by chemical intervention during critical periods of behavioral development traditional methods of assessment, which assume a normal behavioral pattern elaborated in a biologically normal animal, become inappropriate and ineffectual.

The kinds of questions we raised at that time relate to the area of developmental psychopharmacology, a subject so new that the literature consists of only one review by R. D. Young (1967) and some 150 related studies. In general, developmental psychopharmacology seeks to answer basic questions concerning biochemical intervention during the developmental process. Our specific research interests lie in the development of appropriate animal analogs to human conditions of mental retardation for which physiological and/or biochemical correlates can be demonstrated. Of these, two that may be simulated in animals are endemic cretinism and phenylketonuria.

In humans, endemic cretinism is defined as a deficiency of thyroid hormone due to lack of dietary iodine during infancy which leads to marked and chronic mental retardation. Phenylketonuria is the result of an inborn error of metabolism characterized by inadequate conversion of an essential amino acid, phenylalanine, to tyrosine. The disease is generally accompanied by mental subnormality, although the literature documents cases in which biochemical symptomatology is present in the absence of behavioral correlates.

In dealing with animal analogs of these conditions, cretinism is clearly the most easily established and has the longest experimental history. The cretinoid rat is produced by injecting 150 microcuries of radioactive iodine, $^{131}I$, on the day of birth. The iodine is almost exclusively concentrated in the thyroid gland, which is completely destroyed by its radiations. The effect is rapid. Our initial study carried out with two groups of normal-cretin littermates was concerned with the establishment of a developmental behavioral protocol that can be used to record such information as daily weights, food intake, activity as measured in a stabilimetric chamber, opening of the eyes, the external auditory meatus and the vagina, development of the grasp, righting, and startle reflex, the appearance of spontaneous play behavior, onset of estrus, and development of sexual functions.

While much of this information has been previously reported for normal and cretinoid animals, it is not available for simulated PKU animals. Our initial data support previous reports that the opening of the external auditory meatus and vagina are retarded in cretinoid rats and that the righting and grasping reflexes are significantly delayed. However, on several points our previous findings differ from those reported by J. T. Eayrs and S. H. Taylor (1951) and J. T. Eayrs and W. A. Lishman (1955). For example, in our second group of cretin-normal littermates the age of eye opening was not significantly different. We found no differences in the preweaning activity levels between groups. In addition, contrary to Eayrs and Taylor (1951), who report that growth determined by body weight is little affected until twelve to fifteen days of age, we found stable differences between groups from day six.

The observations of smaller size in cretinoid rats, an observation also reported for simulated PKU rats (Karrar and Cahilly 1965), of decreased appetite in both groups, and of retarded motor development have lead us to question the appropriateness of experimental designs employing appetitional rewards as reinforcers in learning situations designed to assess intellectual deficits in cretinoid and simulated PKU groups. By the same token speed measures or those requiring the expenditure of a great amount of energy appear inappropriate. We suggest that studies of habituation and classical conditioning which de-emphasize performance variables related to motivational and reward factors would offer a better assessment of intellectual deficit in these animal analogs of mental retardation. In addition these paradigms can be used with animals from the neonatal stage onward.

In human cases of cretinism and PKU, the reports of J. H. Means (1948) on the endemic cretin infant and W. E. Knox (1966) on the PKU infant maintain that the diseased infant, if untreated, shows normal development during the first few months of life and then demonstrates a rapid, progressive decline in intellectual functioning. These observations imply an initially normal intellect that is later debilitated by continued central nervous system development in an abnormal hormonal and biogenic milieu. In this light the logic of the habituation paradigm becomes compelling. Habituation may be characterized as the fundamental intellectual process. In the habituation paradigm the animal learns to stop attending to a stimulus over time if that stimulus is not noxious and if it signifies nothing. Learning in the form of habituation has been demonstrated in the human neonate (Engen and Lipsitt 1965). The neonatal period in rats is the first ten days of life. We propose to assess habituation during this period by repeatedly presenting tactile stimuli and by measuring the general activity evoked by the stimulus. If clinical observations of normal intellectual processes during the neonatal period in cretin and PKU humans are correct and if experimental cretinism and PKU parallel this state we would not expect differences in the habituation process between normal, cretinoid, and simulated PKU groups.

In a further attempt to control motivational and performance factors, we are investigating classical conditioning in the neonatal and infant rat groups. L. P. Lipsitt (1963) has reviewed classical conditioning experiments involving human neonates. Classical conditioning requires the use of an unconditioned stimulus that elicits a specific innate response pattern. In one of the experiments reported by Lipsitt (1963) the unconditioned stimulus was shock, which elicited a leg withdrawal response. The to-be-conditioned stimulus is one that initially elicits some general response that can be shown to habituate. In these experiments the conditioned stimulus was a tone. With repeated paired presentations of first, the tone, and second, the shock, a conditioned response was obtained; when the tone was presented without the shock the neonate was observed to make a leg withdrawal response to it. D. F. Caldwell and J. Werboff (1962) have similarly demonstrated that the unconditioned response of leg flexion to shock stimuli can be conditioned to vibrotactile stimuli in the day-old rat. It should be noted that the levels of conditioning obtained in these two investigations do not approximate those obtained by investigators using mature animals. Both neonatal investigations showed about 30 per cent conditioning; that is, the conditioned response appeared about 30 per cent of the time when the conditioned stimulus was presented. In mature organisms a 70 to 80 per cent level of conditioning is generally established. Our pilot studies using Werboff's paradigm have shown that 70 per cent conditioning can be established in thirty-day-old rats. This age coincides with the time of maximal cerebral cortical thickness in the albino rat (twenty-five to thirty days of age) and of histologically evidenced cortex maturity (Himwich 1962). We are currently involved in parametrically investigating the classical conditioning phenomena in normal, cretinoid, and PKU-simulated rats ranging in age from birth to thirty days. Since it is known that the human endemic cretin and phenylketonuric demonstrate intellectual deficit by the time cortical development is complete, we hypothesize that differences will be found in conditioning among the different experimental groups.

The advantages of our present research strategy are twofold. First, the habituation and classical conditioning paradigms de-emphasize motivational and effort variables allowing truer assessment of intellectual deficit.

Secondly, the anatomical and electrophysiological correlates of habituation and classical conditioning have been extensively investigated and make the search for behavioral-biochemical relations in these paradigms an intriguing proposition.

# REFERENCES

Caldwell, D. F., and Werboff, J. 1962. Classical conditioning in newborn rats. *Science* 136:1118.

Eayrs, J. T., and Taylor, S. H. 1951. The effect of thyroid deficiency induced by methyl thiouracil on the maturation of the central nervous system. *J. Anat.* 85:350

Eayrs, J. T., and Lishman, W. A. 1955. The maturation of behavior in hypothyroidism and starvation. *Brit. J. Anim. Behav.* 3:17.

Engen, T., and Lipsitt, L. P. 1965. Decrement and recovery of responses to olfactory stimuli in the human neonate. *J. Comp. Physiol. Psych.* 59:312.

Ferster, C. B., and Skinner, B. F. 1957. *Schedules of reinforcement.* New York: Appleton-Century-Crofts, Inc.

Himwich, W. A. 1962. Biochemical and neurophysiological development of the brain in the neonatal period. *Internatl. Rev. Neurobiol.* 4:117.

Karrer, R., and Cahilly, G. 1965. Experimental attempts to produce phenylketonuria in animals: A critical review. *Psych. Bull.* 46:52.

Knox, W. E. 1966. Phenylketonuria. In *The Metabolic Basis of Inherited Disease*, eds. J. B. Stanbury, J. B. Wyngaarden, and D. S. Fredrickson, p. 258. New York: McGraw-Hill.

Lipsitt, L. P. 1963. Learning in the first year of life. In *Advances in Development and Behavior*, eds. L. P. Lipsitt and C. C. Spiker, p. 147. New York: Academic Press.

Means, J. H. 1948. *The thyroid and its diseases.* Philadelphia: Lippincott.

Skinner, B. F. 1938. *The behavior of organisms.* New York: Appleton-Century-Crofts, Inc.

# Basic Research in Mental
# Retardation: An Overview

WILLIAM M. MC ISAAC, M.D., Ph.D.

*Texas Research Institute of Mental Sciences, Houston, Texas*

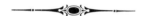

In 1930 K. S. Lashley (see Lashley 1960) wrote, "The facts of both psychology and neurology show a degree of plasticity, of organization and of adaptation and behavior which is far beyond any present possibility of explanation." During the intervening forty years, however, great advances have been made in unraveling the genetic code for inherited physical characteristics. The relatively recently discovered biochemical basis of a number of syndromes associated with mental retardation, so well covered in other articles of this symposium, and the tremendous technological advances of the last decade give us some hope at last that we may yet arrive at an understanding of what may well be the most complex problem of all, namely, the neurochemical basis of learning and memory.

Basic research in the field of mental retardation can, of course, help in the search for new metabolic errors and new causes associated with retardation. In addition, basic research must be responsible for providing the laboratory models for the evaluation of hypotheses and therapeutic possibilities. Emphasis must, therefore, be placed on inducing specific neurochemical changes in animals which may stimulate the clinical condition and on evolving adequate experimental psychological tests for the associated behavioral changes.

Considering the number of metabolic errors associated with mental retardation that have been discovered in the last few years, it would be surprising if there were not others waiting to be found. It is possible that these may not be obvious primary errors of the metabolism of carbohydrate, lipid, or protein but may affect other fundamental processes. The existence of such abnormalities is indicated by a number of reports such as that of indolylacroyl glycine excretion by children in a family where varying degrees of mental retardation were associated with a familial chromosomal abnormality, thus indicating an abnormality of tryptophan metabolism (Mellman *et al.* 1963).

Hitherto unknown pathways for the metabolism of purines and methionine have been suggested by the discovery of 5-amino-4-imidazole-carboxamide-5'-S-homocysteinylriboside in the urine of homocystinuric patients (Perry *et al.* 1966). Absence of specific enzyme systems such as glucuronyl transferase have also been linked to mental retardation by J. F. Crigler and V. A. Najjar (1952) and by others. These types of metabolic errors will not necessarily be detected by current routine screening procedures but are more likely to be revealed by in-depth individual case studies.

Although emphasis has been placed on genetically inherited errors of metabolism, we should not overlook possibly increasing incidence of induced errors caused by viral infections, radiation, drugs, and other chemical agents. Thalidomide certainly focused attention on the teratogenic hazards of drugs, but the less obvious sequel of decreased learning ability which may follow the use or abuse of other agents may not be so easy to document. The fact that compounds like LSD can induce chromosomal aberrations should alert us to this possibility.

The role of the nucleic acids in learning and memory has attracted much attention in the last few years. The transfer of memory in planaria was reported by J. B. McConnell in 1962. Later, H. Hyden and E. Egyhazi (1963) reported data relating to RNA base composition in selected regions of the brains of trained versus naive rats; these data indicated a relationship between RNA in brain cells, learning, and memory; many other studies including inhibition of RNA synthesis with actinomycin have been utilized for corroberation.

A compound called Pemoline, 2-imino-5-phenyl-4-oxazolidinone, has been reported to enhance brain RNA polymerase and to facilitate the acquisition and retention of conditioned avoidance behavior in rats (Plotnikoff 1966). This effect on RNA polymerase, however, could not be confirmed by N. Morris and his associates (1967), and many other investigators, in attempts to transfer learned behavior by injection of RNA-containing fractions from trained donors to naive recipients, have consistently obtained negative findings (Byrne *et al.* 1966).

Although the possibility that memory may be consolidated in the form of base sequences in fashion analogous to the genetic code is most attractive, the evidence available at this time is insufficient to warrant any conclusions and instead should act as a stimulant to further work in this area. No matter what the primary metabolic error may be or how the basic memory patterns are encoded, we are dealing here with a common symptomatology, namely, mental retardation. Perhaps then we should concentrate more attention on the possible secondary effects such as the integrity of the synapse and, in particular, the biosynthesis, release, effectiveness, and metabolism of the neurotransmitters which may prove to be the focal point where the subnormal mentational effect is caused.

Although the mental defect and impaired myelination found in phenylketonuria may be the result of the primary metabolic error on total cerebral metabolism, it is possible that the crucial obstacle to normal cerebral activity is a deficiency of the essential neurotransmitter, serotonin (Hilliard and Kirman 1965). A markedly reduced level of serotonin has been reported to be associated with phenylketonuria (Pare, Sandler, and Stacey 1957 and 1968); it has been found that the level can be elevated to normal either by administration of the precursor 5-hydroxytryptophan or by a low phenylalanine diet (Kirman and Pare 1961).

In animals in which a chronic serotonin deficiency has been produced, either by overloading with phenylalanine and tyrosine to cause a model PKU or with reserpine, a reduced ability to learn has been noted. This subnormal maze-learning ability was found to be largely prevented if 5-hydroxytryptophan was administered continuously from birth to maturity. These results have been interpreted by D. W. Woolley and T. van der Hoeven (1964) to mean that the learning deficit in this experimental PKU is directly attributable to the 5-hydroxytryptophan deficiency in infancy.

There are indications that tryptophan and serotonin metabolism also are abnormal in mongolism. Tryptophan metabolism in Down's syndrome has been extensively studied by a number of investigators who report anomolies at various steps of the metabolic pathway (Tu Jun-Bi and Zellweger 1965).

Children with trisomy-21 have been reported to have depressed levels of serotonin (Tu Jun-Bi and Zellweger 1965; Rosner *et al.* 1965.

M. Bazalon and his co-workers (1967) reported that the administration of 5-hydroxytrytophan reverses the hypotonicity in infants with mongolism, but it is yet too early to judge whether any improvement in cerebral function may also result from attempts to restore serotonin levels to normal. Since much of the data relating learning deficiencies to changed brain amine levels are based upon the use of reserpine or iproniazid, which have nonspecific effects on several amines, it is not easy to disentangle the exact role played by any particular amine. Fortunately, more specific agents have recently become available. Oxypertine has been shown to reduce specifically brain norephinephrine levels without affecting serotonin (Wylie and Archer 1962), and p-chlorophenylalanine reduces brain serotonin while the norepinephrine levels remain normal (Koe and Weissman 1966). These compounds then provide us with the tools to explore the behavioral and learning correlates of a specific amine deficiency.

To fill in the other end of the spectrum, we at the Texas Research Institute of Mental Sciences have been devoting much time and effort to the design, synthesis, and testing of compounds that will specifically elevate either brain serotonin or norepinephrine. Not only should such agents help in the basic understanding of the relationship between brain amines, learning, and retention, but also such compounds would appear theoretically to have a great potential therapeutic value.

# REFERENCES

Bazelon, M., Paine, R. S., Cowie, V. A., Hunt, P., and Houck, J. C. May 1967. Reversal of hypotonia in infants with Down's syndrome. *Lancet* 1:1130–1133.
Byrne, W. L., Samuel, D., Bennett, E. L., Rozenzweig, S., Wasserman, E., Wagner, A. R., Gardner, F., Galambos, R., Berger, B. D., Margules, D. L., Fenichel, R. L., Stein, L., Corson, J. A., Enesco, H. E., Chorover, S. L., Holt, C. E., Schiller, P. H., Chiappetta, L., Jarvik, M. E., Leaf, R. C., Dutcher, J. D., Horovitz, Z. P., and Carlson, P. L. 1966. Memory transfer. *Science* 153:658–659.

Crigler, J. F., and Najjar, V. A. 1952. Congenital familial nonhemolytic jaundice with kernicterus. *Pediatrics* 10:169–179.

Hilliard, L. T., and Kirman, B. H. 1965. *Mental deficiency.* Boston: Little Brown and Co.

Hyden, H., and Egyhazi, E. 1963. Glial RNA changes during a learning experiment in rats. *Proc. Natl. Acad. Sci.* 49:620.

Kirman, B. M., and Pare, C. M. B. 1961. Amine-oxidase inhibitors as possible treatment for phenylketonuria. *Lancet* 1:117.

Koe, B. K., and Weissman, A. J. 1966. Antiamphetamine effects following inhibition of tyrosine hydroxylase. *Pharm. Exp. Therap.* 154:499.

Lashley, K. S. 1960. *The neuropsychology of Lashley,* eds. F. A. Beach, D. O. Hebb, C. T., Morgan, H. W. Nissen. New York: McGraw-Hill.

McConnell, J. B. 1962. Memory transfer through cannibalism in planarians. *J. Neuropsych.* 3:S 42.

Mellman, *et al.* 1963. Indolylacroyl glycine excretion in a family with mental retardation. *Clin. Chim. Acta* 8:843.

Morris, N., Ronald, A., George, K., and Bloom, F. E. 1967. Magnesium pemoline: Failure to affect *in vivo* synthesis of brain RNA. *Science* 155:1125–1126.

Pare, C. M. B., Sandler, M., and Stacey, R. S.

1957. 5-hydroxytryptamine deficiency in phenylketonuria. *Lancet* 1:551.

1968. *Lancet* 2:1022.

Perry, T. L., Hansen, S., Bar, H.-P., MacDougall, L. 1966. Homocystinuria: Excretion of a new sulfur-containing amino acid in urine. *Science* 152:776.

Plotnikoff, N. 1966. Magnesium pemoline: Enhancement of brain RNA polymerases. *Science* 151(3711):702–703.

Rosner, F., Ong, B. H., Paine, R. S., and Mahanand, D. 1965. Blood serotonin activity in trisomie and translocation Down's syndrome. *Lancet* 1:1101.

Tu Jun-Bi, and Zellweger, H. 1965. Blood serotonin deficiency in Down's syndrome. *Lancet* 2:715.

Woolley, D. W., and Hoeven, T. van der. 1964. Serotonin deficiency in infancy as one cause of a mental defect in phenylketonuria. *Science* 144:833–834.

Wylie, D. W., and Archer, S. J. 1962. *J. Med. Pharm. Chem.* 5:932.

# INDEX

aberrations of human chromosomes. SEE chromosomal anomalies
abortions
and LSD, 232
acentric fragments, 123
acetate buffer. SEE chromatography
acidosis, 76, 77, 84
acrocentrics, 126
actinomycin, 333
activity level
in drug research, 231
adaptive development. SEE malnutrition; development
adenine, 120
adrenaline. SEE epinephrine
affective reaction. SEE maternal deprivation
age
and drug use, 299
effect of, on offspring, 130
of mother in mongolism, 128, 137
vulnerability of, to malnutrition, 266
aggressiveness
and chromosomal anomalies, 124
in hyperuricemia, 106, 113
agitation (postnatal), 238, 239
Airaksinen, Eila, 33, 102, 162, 203, 204; paper by, 191–208
Airaksinen, Mauno M., 242; paper by, 310–317
alanine
α–alanine in histidinemia, 65
β–alanine in histidinemia, 62
position of, in chromatogram, 196
alcohol, 229, 232, 237, 239
aldehyde, 243
allopurinol, 107, 108, 110, 112, 116
Alt, Jean, 25, 31
amidopyrine, 228

amines
biological, 310
and chromatograms, 194
amino acids
analysis of
in plasma, 191–206
in whole blood, 153
analyzer and diagnosis, 191, 201
chromatogram, 193, 194, 195, 196, 202
detection of errors in, 195
disorders of metabolism of, 72, 191, 196, 197
in histidinemia, 68
in homocystinuria, 50
in hyperglycinemia, 84
multiple toxicity of, 77
in phenylketonuria, 6, 13
testing for, 168
SEE ALSO plasma amino acids
aminoaciduria, 75
α–aminobutyric acid, 196
γ–aminobutyric acid, 196, 310
β–aminoisobutyric acid, 196
α–amino nitrogen, 173
aminopterin
and embryogenesis, 235
amitriptyline (Elavil), 239, 293
ammonia intoxication, 155
amniotic fluid
testing of, in mongolism, 139, 149
amphetamine, 293
An, Rong, 205
analysis technique
of plasma amino acids, 191–206
SEE ALSO plasma amino acids
anaphase, 132
Ando, Toshiyuki, paper by, 72–86
anemia
and hemoglobin, 276

337

# Index

oxalic acid, 72
oxypertine, 313, 335
oxypurines
  in hyperuricemia, 112

pachytene, 134, 137
palate
  arched, 40, 126, 212, 213
  cleft, 187
pallor, 94, 276
paper chromatography. SEE chromatography
paper electrophoresis, 191
parenteral fluids
  in hyperglycinemia, 76
parents
  age of, and anomalies, 222
  as carriers, 127, 218
  consanguinity of, 218
  and homocystinuria, 51
  and hyperuricemia, 116
  and intelligence, 247
  and malnutrition, 264, 265, 284
  metabolic disorders of, 159
  and phenylketonuria, 9, 10, 26, 28
  in training of retardates, 302, 303
Parkland Memorial Hospital, Dallas, 108
Parnate, 293
Pauly reagent, 181
pediatrician, 162, 267
Pemoline
  and brain RNA polymerase, 333
penetrance
  of anomalies, 214
pentobarbital
  and maze learning, 230
pentose sugar (ribose), 120
pentoses, 182
peptides, 168, 194
performance
  conditioned, 327
  control of factors of, 330
peripheral blood culture technique, 147
perphenazine (Trilafon), 299
personality
  in hyperuricemia, 113
  patterns and drug treatment, 291
personnel. SEE training programs
*pes cavus*
  in homocystinuria, 41
pesticides
  effect of, on amino acids, 204

phasic myotatic reflexes
  in malnutrition, 277
phenacetin
  and metabolism of drugs, 228
phenelzine (Nardil), 293
Phenistix test, 171
  in histidinemia, 58, 65, 66
  in phenylketonuria, 25, 33
phenobarbital
  distribution of in central nervous system, 228, 230, 231
phenolic acids, 168
phenothiazine
  effect of, on offspring, 237, 239
  hazards of, 299
  during pregnancy, 237
  as treatment, 291, 299
phenotypic alterations, 122
phenotypic spectrum, 216
phenylalanine
  densitometer pattern of, 201
  in histidinemia, 58, 68
  levels
    determination of, 152, 181, 196, 201
    in mothers, 187, 188
  in phenylketonuria, 3, 4, 9, 12, 13
  and serotonin, 334
  serum, 9
  tolerance for, 152
phenylalaninemia
  and malnutrition, 206
*p*-phenylenediamine hydrochloride, 177
phenylketonuria (PKU)
  atypical, 58
  biochemical characteristics of, 4
  and cerebral metabolism, 334
  control of, during illness, 16, 17
  and death, 13
  diagnosis of, 3–8, 152, 162, 168, 200, 206
  experimental, 311
  and family, 6, 10, 20, 26
  genetics, 27
  heterozygotes, 6, 32
  incidence of, 3
  infections in, 31
  Lofenalac and diet, 6, 9, 12, 13, 14, 15, 18, 24, 26, 27, 34
  long-term management of, 18–22
  maternal, 157
  and mental development, 4, 18, 21
  in older patients, 18, 20, 32, 33

## Index